THIRST FOR FREEDOM

THIRST FOR FREEDOM

DAVID A. STEWART

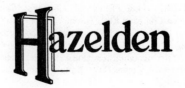

ACKNOWLEDGEMENT

Professor John Macmurray's concepts, *person*, *event*, and *action*, found in many of his publications, have been in part adapted to the empathic theme of this book. He gave liberally of his time in discussions with me during 1951-52 in the University of Edinburgh. It was he who suggested the value of Dr. Ian Suttie's *Origins of Love and Hate* (Kegan Paul, Trench, Trubner & Co. Ltd., London, 1948). Dr. Suttie's concept, the *tenderness taboo*, is basic to my theory of pre-addictive behaviour.

Dr. E. M. Jellinek's remarkable insight into every aspect of the alcoholic's behaviour was of great value in the making of this book. He has given me important technical advice and moral support. The section on the woman alcoholic refers to views of Dr. G. Lolli who has been encouraging in personal talks and exchange of letters. Dr. John Bingham and Dr. David Pratt have kindly assisted on technical points of psychiatry and medicine. Dr. Marie Nyswander generously consented to the use of material quoted from her book, *The Drug Addict as a Patient* (by permission of Grune and Stratton, New York). Dr. Harris Isbell and Dr. A. Wikler, whose clinical work in the addictions is well known, are cited and quoted. The book, *Opiate Addiction*, Principia Press, 1947, by Professor A. R. Lindesmith, is confirmed and cited with reference to the genesis of the drug addict. I have combined Dr. Harry Tiebout's concept, *surrender* with similar insights of Wm. James in my description of the alcoholic's readiness for sobriety. The sections quoted from Stephen Crane's *George's Mother* are drawn from *Stephen Crane: Stories and Tales*, edited by Robert Wooster Stallman, a Vintage book originally published by Alfred A. Knopf, New York, 1952.

Wise counsel and practical assistance have come from Dr. John Griffin, Professor Wm. Line, Dr. R. G. Bell, Dr. Milton Gregg and Mr. R. H. Cook.

More has been learned from members of A.A. than it is possible for me fully to express.

VI   ACKNOWLEDGEMENT

Among the settings, other than private practice and personal talks, in which material for the book was gathered were these: The Yale School of Alcohol Studies; the Crichton Royal Hospital, Scotland; the Provincial Hospital, Campbellton, N.B.; the Bell Clinic, Brookside Clinic, Harbour Lights Clinic, Mercer Clinic, Mimico Clinic, Toronto; Atascadero State Hospital, California.

David A. Stewart

PREFACE

THE effort to quench personal thirst—the longing to be yourself—can take two forms.

(1) You can indulge in drink (or drugs). For some, the bottle is a flight from life; for some, it is a defiance of life. For others, it is a symbol of "kicks". Book I is a study of the meaning of addiction, and of the way to freedom.

(2) You can indulge in empathy—the art of putting yourself in the other fellow's place—and know what it means to accept yourself and be yourself. This it is to quench personal thirst—to be free, productive, and happy in abundant living. Creative sobriety through empathy is the theme of Book II.

Each chapter of Book I is balanced by each chapter of Book II. The story of Drink is matched by the story of Sobriety. Few people realize that sobriety is an action of insights and skills far beyond mere abstinence. Sobriety is a creative discipline in the art of freedom of growth, and of love. To be yourself is to become yourself.

CONTENTS

BOOK I

Acknowledgement   v

Introduction   1

1. Why Do People Drink?   60
2. The Drinking Pattern of the Alcoholic   67
3. The Alcoholic—What Sort of Person Is He?   80
4. Allen's Story   94
5. The Alcoholic's Insight   100
6. Surrender and the Follow-Up   109
7. Alcoholics Anonymous   121
8. Personal Growth—the Basic Issue   143

BOOK II

1. Why Be Sober?   151
2. The Search for a Creative Clue   169
3. The Goals and Ideals of the Sober Person   197
4. Allen's Story—Twelve Years Later   226
5. From Insight to Action   240
6. The Practice of Freedom   283
7. Alcoholics Anonymous—A Clinical View   316
8. The Gifts of Adventure   340
Index   361

INTRODUCTION

MAN is a curious creature. He is a thinking animal, he is a human being, and he has within him the capacity to be a person. He is conscious, self-conscious and visionary. Sometimes he is urged to throw off the demands of conscious life and revert to an earlier stage of his growth where the instincts and impulses operate without benefit of form and direction. Sometimes he suffers under the burden of those reflections which make him human in organized social life. His capacity to reflect enables him to change the environment and to control his living conditions, but it also makes him fearful. Fear always accompanies control—fear lest the controls are reversed and turned upon him. With the fear there is guilt, shame, anxiety, depression and a sense of inadequacy. So he often wishes to discard the burden and return to a simpler life. Or he may wish, too, to go beyond himself, to become more than he is now, to delve into uncharted areas where he can be free, creative, and adventurous.

Plato spoke of an ideal experience called *sophrosyne*. By this is meant an easy and graceful harmony among the three basic urges of man's inner nature, and a delightful rapport with the world around him. Essentially, it means a clear sense of personal identity within, and an amiable at-one-ness with the world in which he lives. Such an ideal state is a far sounder basis for the meaning of sobriety than the stiff, abstinent and gloomy aspects that the word has taken on in recent history.

Sophrosyne can be related to the current use of the word "cool" that has grown so popular as an admirable state of feeling among younger people. "Cool, man, cool" is a phrase of the highest praise among those who aspire to be neither stodgy nor excited, but serenely at peace with oneself and the world. It was natural that many of the "cool" set should turn to Zen Buddhism with its doctrine of apathy, after despairing of pleasure as known in the "square" world.

(This pose would appear more sincere if they really sought a goal higher than the pleasure they disdained.) And it is fitting that the tranquillizing drugs should have become famous for their ataraxic qualities. *Ataraxia* is a state of feeling described by the Stoics and Epicureans and can be traced to the doctrine of Zen Buddhism. It means repose of mind, tranquillity. It seeks, not pleasure, but something more akin to apathy—the avoidance of feeling.

The "cool" set have not been alone in the search to break the limits of the "square" world, and to know peace, adventure and happiness in a golden Arcady. Millions of people all over the world, throughout history, have striven to find some magic way to disown their burdens and to reach for "something more" than they know in the grey routine of their daily lives. They look for short cuts. Their longing is natural and justified in their capacity as persons. But their mistake is to suppose that so great an adventure can be reached without effort. *Sophrosyne* or sobriety is indeed a goal and an adventure of priceless value, when you blend it with the experience of fellowship. But there is only one way to know it—through religion. By religion here is meant the search for the meaning of one's life, one's relations to his fellowman and the world, and one's relations to a power greater than oneself. Religion, thought about, is philosophy. Philosophy lived is religion. Ways and means to understand our feelings and attitudes and actions make up one's personal psychology. These three, then, religion, philosophy and psychology are the sources of wisdom in achieving *sophrosyne*.

Man cannot deny his need for happiness, so he cannot live on apathy, on a diet of *ataraxia*. But he cannot, either, stand the excitement of overstimulation. Man cannot survive as a slave, so he cannot depend on the ersatz "coolness" of the sedating drugs, which in the end, have no semblance of serenity but bring, instead, a chronic condition of the fear he sought to escape in his search for something more.

Failing to learn and to believe deeply in the three proper avenues of his adventure in freedom—religion, philosophy and psychology—man turns to ersatz means of finding himself. Among these are alcohol and the addicting drugs.

When you work, for years, among alcoholics and other addicts you are certain to confront the problem of addiction to many forms of many drugs. Some alcoholics unwisely turn to stimulants, barbiturates and tranquillizers, after they stop drinking. Some even become addicted to morphine or heroin. But besides alcoholics, there are thousands of respectable citizens all over North America and elsewhere who develop a "pill" problem quite innocently, without a conscious desire for kicks or thrills. There is a special group of addicts who do indeed seek thrills and "out-of-orbit" adventures in the deliberate pursuit of pleasure, only at last to be hounded by the law, and to grow miserable in the awful grip of the powerfully addicting drugs.

Addiction prevails, then, among three classes of people (1) thrill seekers (2) a large class of seemingly well-adjusted people under stress of various kinds (3) alcoholics.

The addicting drugs can be classified as *stimulants* and *depressants*.

The Stimulants

The stimulants include cocaine, benzedrine, mescaline and their variants. Users of stimulants are temporarily elated, bright, relieved of tiredness, and made to believe that they are exceptionally capable and superior. Cocaine is taken in the vein, or snuffed. Benzedrine (and dexedrine) are usually taken orally. Mescaline, in natural form, the buttons of the peyote cactus, is taken orally; LSD, a synthetic drug similar to mescaline, can be taken orally or in the vein.

The signs of intoxication with all the stimulants are similar, with differences in onset and duration of symptoms and in the type of hallucination.

Cocaine, a white crystalline powder, is prepared from a coca plant found in Brazil and Java. Its users become paranoid, believing that they are being watched and threatened. They develop a persecution complex which they fear and dislike, because it often leads to violence. Thus, many of them resort to "speedballs"—a combination of cocaine and one of the opiates which reduces the unpleasant effects of pure cocaine.

The effects of benzedrine and dexedrine intoxication are similar to those of cocaine intoxication. The difference is that a benzedrine user may go for months or years before he is aware that he has a real problem. This he discovers in depressed states when he stops taking his usual daily doses.

Mescaline, and the clinically similar substance, LSD, produce vivid colourful hallucinations. Mescaline, used by the Indians in South Western United States and Mexico, is part of their religious ritual. LSD is described by Aldous Huxley in his book "Doors of Perception". In higher doses, mescaline, LSD and benzedrine produce hallucinations similar to the disturbed behaviour of schizophrenics. The merits of mescaline and LSD are questionable in the light of facts which reveal their adverse unpleasant effect on certain emotionally disturbed people. And if people are not emotionally disturbed, these drugs can do nothing that empathic therapy cannot do better, among alcoholics and other addicts. There is always a risk involved in substituting one drug for another, even if used only for treatment purposes. It may well be that a mild, reputedly non-addictive drug appears to be helpful in easing the patient's tension, and gaining rapport with him. But the tendency to move on to stronger drugs, often increased doses of the one in use, fails to bring the desired results. LSD is said by some researchers to be valuable in controlled use by both therapist and patient in the treatment situation. I believe the same danger exists here as in the use of tranquillizers which were first hailed as a cure-all, and now are known to be addicting and disturbing to thousands who took them neither for thrills, nor for serious illness, but simply to ease the strain of a fast-paced life.

All the stimulants tend to lead their users to the stronger

more dangerous depressants. They cannot, then, be regarded as harmless or as non-addicting when crucial psychological conditions are considered as well as the physical factors of addiction.

Habitual use of the stimulants brings the kind of hang-over one would expect of the human body after it has been artificially over-stimulated for a period of time. Withdrawal of the drug leaves the user depressed as darkly and miserably as he was elated in his intoxication. As with any drug, the user discovers to his dismay that the desired effects decrease as the habit grows. Terrifying experiences play an increasingly larger role in the images and hallucinations of the user.

The Depressants

Marihuana, leaves of the female hemp plant, is smoked in the form of cigarettes made of the dried shredded leaves known as "reefers". It is popular among some jazz musicians and young enthusiasts who believe that it improves musical skill and appreciation. Friends of mine in show business tell me that such a belief is entirely false. Smokers giggle and laugh over pointless jokes, are easily amused, and enjoy listening to "hot" music. The need of a drug to appreciate music casts some doubt on the sincere capacity to enjoy it. The great danger of marihuana is that it leads to the stronger drugs. The smoking usually begins among a set of young people who consider it smart to cultivate the language and ritual of the beatnik outlook on life.

In a spirit of denial, rather than revolt, they turn away from the "square" world to the escape routes of the full-fledged addict. The beatnik attitude is not so much wrong as it is tragically incomplete. Many youngsters have good reason to question the values of modern society, but to resort to drugs is simply to follow the logical trend of the very society they wish to reject. It is intelligent to doubt the worth of many current social values, but to become an addict is simply to confirm the psychological truth that pleasure as a basic value leads directly to pain and misery and to the loss of that precious freedom the young enthusiast sought when he felt that the "square" world cramped his style. Actually, the world is not square at all, but only some of the people who are in it. The beatnik attitude is healthy when its devotees go a step beyond their dissatisfaction to make changes in themselves. The logical trend of modern society in the sixties in North America and elsewhere has been to make pleasure and the acquisition of goods the sole aim of life. The natural outcome of this trend is an addiction-prone society. Youngsters who turn to alcohol and drugs, by no matter what route, are simply aping a widespread social trend which places the highest value on creature comfort and the authority of money. This is not the way to freedom of any kind. It is the way to the addiction, the obsessions and personal slavery.

The depressants of traditional interest in the problem of addiction are alcohol, opium and its derivatives, morphine, codeine, heroin, dilaudid, metapon, diorin, pantopon and the synthetic opium equivalents, demerol and methadone. (Alcohol is discussed at length throughout the book.)

Opium smoking and snuffing are now relatively rare in North America, though still a common habit in the Far East. The most common addiction outside of alcoholism among the thrill seekers of America is the "main line" (intravenous) use of morphine and heroin. Of these two, heroin has, in recent years, become the more popular. In the treatment of more than 200 addicts in an Ontario clinic, and in private practice, I found that addiction to heroin was most common among them. There were also some who were addicted to morphine, demerol, codeine, and paregoric. The accounts which follow were furnished by the patients themselves. Most of them concern heroin. These accounts were written at my request in an effort to gain understanding of the problem from the patients' point of view. Not all, but most of these men, were in search of kicks. A few reported that they came to the habit through an effort to overcome pain. Others graduated to heroin addiction from alcoholism, and still others ran a wide range of addicting substances from 222's to heroin. The last type reveals that an addict can never satisfactorily substitute a milder drug for one to which he has grown habituated. It also shows that it is dangerous to treat an addict with a drug stronger than the one to which he is habituated.

The accounts describe initial addiction, switches from one drug to another, and the experiences of withdrawal and relapse.

Initial Addiction

"I first started using drugs when I was twenty years old. It was more or less out of curiosity that I started to use them. I had heard quite a bit about it and the feeling it gave you. I had often thought of trying it as it was very easy for me to obtain, seeing that I knew others who were using it themselves. I went around with two guys who happened to be wired, and I always seemed to be in the same room when they were fixing. One day they had just finished fixing, and they looked so relaxed and carefree that I thought it wouldn't hurt me to try a little bit. Well, I had a fix, and I don't think I have ever experienced anything that felt so wonderful in my life. I enjoyed that first fix so much that I made it a point to be back there the next day. I fixed again then, and started to use it more often. I must admit I started bringing up whenever I had finished fixing. I stopped doing this after I had gotten used to it. Finally I discovered I was wired."

. . . . .

"I listened to addicts talking in a reformatory. 'If there is anything better, God kept it to himself.' They said they were happy when using it. It seemed pretty rough to me that they were serving four years for their fun. Still, believe it or not,

I thought I'd try it when I got out. I was nineteen years old.

"I met one of them when released. He was sick and needed a fix. I bought it for him, I knew him on a "kibitz" basis. We both went to a hotel room and I had my first fix. I couldn't see myself putting out five bucks and not getting something out of it. He had his and thanked me. Then his girl tied up my arm, and he injected it into the main line. There was no effect for ten or fifteen minutes. Then I felt a burning sensation under the skin, I was lightheaded, inflated like hot air in a balloon, it felt like falling onto a big comfortable bed while standing up. I was quite happy and content. I agreed with the guy that it was wonderful stuff. Then I ran to the bathroom and was violently ill at the stomach. I went into a coma 'on the nod', I was conscious of everything going on, with my eyes closed. I was ill several times in the next five hours, I tried to eat but couldn't keep anything down. I didn't mind being sick until I started bringing up blood and retching. I sneaked home and crawled into bed. It felt more or less like an alcohol hang-over next morning—hollow, completely cleaned out and pooped out.

"I went on using it, off and on, for six weeks after the first fix. Then one day at work, my whole body ached. My legs were the worst. And my back was sore like I'd walked for miles. My eyes watered, nose ran and I brought up a few times. I had done without a fix for a whole day before, and didn't feel that rough. I talked to a guy who used a lot and he said I was "wired". I had a fix shortly after that and I felt much better. I never thought of myself as an addict before. It never occurred to me that I'd get wired. Now I just went on using it, figured I had to have it, and I wasn't worried about it. I was off four days since then, in hospital, but I fixed again the day after I got out. I used up until I got arrested."

⋅ ⋅ ⋅ ⋅ ⋅

"I came to narcotics through pain. It started over a migraine headache I had endured for about sixty-one hours that I tried to find some relief for but could not. I had taken quite a few bromo's, 217's and 222's but no relief. I wandered up to a friend's room and there encountered four addicts that I had known for some time. I explained my problem to them of my headache and they offered me some drugs. At first I refused as I had a dozen or more times previously. But their talk was so convincing and my pain so severe that I figured I had nothing to lose at the time, so I gave in and sniffed some heroin in one nostril and cocaine in the other. Within ten minutes my head was as clear as a whistle. I did not touch it again for some time. I did not want any part of the needle as I was more or less needle shy. After a little over four months of steady sniffing I was told by a woman addict that I was addicted, and even then I did not know what she meant until I got more sick by the hour. All she had was heroin solution to give me, but I wanted not even one hypo. She felt sorry for me suffering so much and finally persuaded me to take a hypo. I never felt a thrill so comparable in all my life, not even from a woman."

A Variety of Addicting Substances

"Following a long period of total abstinence from narcotics, I started using alcoholic beverage moderately. I gradually became a periodical social drinker and continued to live a normal life, working and taking an active part in social and recreational activities. This did not last very long as I began to enjoy the stimulation of alcohol. Then I started drinking heavily on weekends and holiday periods. Immediately following these drinking bouts I became very restless and craved for liquor. Since it was not possible to drink on the job, I began taking barbiturates such as nembutal, tuinal, seconal and sodium amytal for a few days after I stopped drinking. When I stopped taking barbiturates I again became nervous, anxious, irritable and depressed. The latter I knew to be sure signs of addiction but I kept on drinking to get stimulation. The hang-overs were longer and instead of taking barbiturates for only a few days I stretched it for a week or more. Finally I stopped drinking and instead took two grains of sodium amytal four times daily for a period of about three months. I tried to withdraw suddenly from sodium amytal but addiction had set in and I experienced withdrawal symptoms similar to those of narcotics; although not as severe. By then I was losing all interest in social activities, and although I was working steadily my efficiency was impaired and I could not face responsibility or difficult situations. My condition was aggravated by constant setbacks financially and socially. Sodium amytal was no longer effective, I also noticed this drug affected my memory the same as nembutal did. I then decided to take an injection of morphine. In a matter of a few weeks I was readdicted."

. . . . .

"Prior to addiction I had periodical feelings of nervousness, anxiety and insecurity. My addiction began through acquaintances who sniffed cocaine and smoked opium for stimulation.

"I sniffed cocaine periodically. This was followed by a feeling of exhilaration. Excessive use created extreme nervousness and hysteria. I began taking morphine hypodermically to alleviate this condition.

"My first injection of morphine made me sick for about two hours. I had nausea, excessive sweating, vomiting and drowsiness. This was followed by a feeling of well-being, confidence and optimism. This lasted for about twelve hours. Then came a feeling of depression and craving for more. When I repeated the dosage, it produced further stimulation but no nausea or vomiting. There was the same feeling of well-being. Thus addiction began at the age of eighteen years. Over a period of several months injections were more frequent (from four to six a day) and the dosage was increased. Drugs were very cheap those days and easy to obtain, but as they came in powder or cube form I was not able to determine the quantity used. I believe I used about six grains a day.

"I had the first withdrawal in prison. I was arrested for

theft—a first offence. The sentence was two months. It was a sudden withdrawal with the exception of two daily doses of chloral hydrate and paraldehyde. I was suffering from intense nausea, vomiting, cramps, diarrhoea, insomnia and general restlessness for about fifteen days. During the balance of the two months I was in a continuous state of depression, with aches and pains, in the arms, back and legs. I was physically weak, and constantly craving for morphine. My condition prior to addiction was aggravated by the withdrawal of drugs. On completion of my sentence I immediately resumed addiction and continued on morphine for about three years.

"Then I took my first injection of heroin. This produced a stronger stimulation and better feeling, but I had to take it more frequently than morphine. The latter lasted longer for me although this may not be so with other addicts. The same applies to withdrawal, as I found it easier to withdraw from heroin. All the injections of morphine and heroin were in the skin and not in the vein.

"The total length of addiction was eleven years with the exception of a total of four years spent in prison and sanitariums periodically.

"When morphine or heroin were not immediately available, I used gum opium, tincture of opium, paregoric or any other product which contained opium derivatives. They all had the same effect if taken in sufficient quantity. Cocaine never at any time could be used as a replacement for morphine or heroin, but it could be used simultaneously for added stimulation.

"I finished my first addiction at twenty-nine years of age, and remained abstinent for twenty-one years.

"I became readdicted when I started taking sodium amytal for nervousness and stress caused from pressure. Then I began to use nembutal and other potent barbiturates heavily.

"My first injection of morphine after readdiction was a skin injection which produced the same feeling as in the very first shot. As before, continued use resulted in addiction. I had the same symptoms on withdrawal but this time for a longer period due to my advanced age. As addiction advanced, I noticed I wanted to sleep most of the time and had a tired feeling although I was taking morphine in tablet form in quantities of one half to one grain. I changed to injections of heroin in the vein; this was again stronger stimulation as I had experienced in the past, but was accompanied by the same feeling of drowsiness. In other words, I could never get the same feeling of well-being as I did at the beginning of my first addiction."

First Symptoms in Stages of Withdrawal

"The first signs of an addict being addicted to narcotics either in the stages of withdrawal or having to wait for an extra long period of time until they obtain a new supply of drugs, are as follows: as the last injection slowly leaves the body, the first signs of needing another hypo are when the addict starts to yawn quite often although not being in need of any sleep. Then the addict's eyes will water and his nose will ooze fluid as though having a cold. He will also sneeze repeatedly. He will also become very restless, having to endure stomach cramps, usually followed by diarrhoea. Although his stomach may be empty of food or water, he will vomit something awful, bringing up a green substance from his stomach. He cannot sit still or lie down or keep still as every nerve in his body is demanding just a small shot and that is when the monkey really is on the addict's back. He is clawing, scratching or biting for all he is worth."

Acute and Chronic Withdrawal

"In the acute phase I am yawning, sneezing, my eyes and nose are watering, I have periodical vomiting, nausea, cramps, diarrhoea, an inability to eat or sleep and a general restlessness, an aching of the body and a constant craving for drugs. This phase lasts for about one to ten days according to the amount of drugs I have used or the length of addiction.

"In the chronic phase I have aching in the arms, legs and back with a general weakness with it. I am tired most of the time with a feeling of lassitude. I have a desire to lie down most of the time. Eventually my appetite comes back and I eat everything I can get and more. There are often certain cravings for some particular food, such as sweets, ice-cream, milk shakes, etc. even dry bread tastes like cake. About this time my sleep comes back gradually. The first nights are very restless, with dreams mostly about drugs, such as getting ready to take it, and then awakening in cold sweats and chills. Gradually, however, my sleep returns to normal after a period of about two months from the beginning of my withdrawal. It is usually three months before the craving for drugs stops, with the exception of periodical desires.

"The chronic phase is very difficult for the addict because the shock of sudden withdrawal and forced abstinence affects the nervous system to such an extent that you become irritable, suspicious, making unimportant things or situations seems important. At least this is so in my case.

"After three months I am on the mend, my confidence comes back with physical and mental strength and while there may be the odd bad day or night the chronic stage is over.

"If I work after that period at something useful, I feel much better. Good books, recreation of some kind such as good music, a good TV show, act as a sort of self-administered psychotherapy.

"If I am given methadone in doses of ten to fifteen milligrams two or three times a day for the first three days, and ten milligrams twice daily for the next three days, then the acute phase is almost entirely eliminated in my case. I do not know of anything that can eliminate the chronic phase after complete withdrawal from any drug."

Withdrawal Symptoms after Addiction is Established

"The following is a personal experience of withdrawal after addiction was established for about two months. I had a regular dosage (one capsule of heroin) at 11 p.m. I had disturbed and restless sleep most of the night.

"The following morning I awakened at about 7 o'clock. I had a feeling of depression immediately on awakening with a sense of urgency to establish contact to obtain drugs. Then I experienced the first real symptoms of withdrawal—I was sensitive to odours, my eyes and nose were running, I was yawning, extremely nervous and had a general feeling of despondency. This lasted until about 9 o'clock. Then followed sneezing, nausea, vomiting, cramps periodically until noon; then I had weakness in the arms and legs with restlessness increasing. I had a morbid fear of not being able to stay on my feet until I could make a contact. Diarrhoea started around 2 or 3 o'clock with nausea and cramps getting worse. All this was experienced while on my feet or sitting in various places waiting for the contact. In spite of the intense suffering, I never lost my sense of direction and I knew what I was doing at all times. I was close to physical exhaustion when the contact was made at 3:30 p.m. The time of continuous sickness was eight hours, and the time from the last shot sixteen hours."

Relapse

"In ten years there have been many reasons for a relapse but the one I remember more than any other happened in 1951. I was released from a West Coast prison and made my way to Ontario for the sole purpose of visiting my wife, who at the time was serving in Kingston Penitentiary. I had not used narcotics since my release as I was afraid of not being able to carry out my plans regarding a visit to the Penitentiary.

"After my visit I started drinking and eventually started to use drugs again. Fortunately, however, the drugs I was purchasing were very poor and there were days of waiting between fixes so I kicked what small habit I had on the street. Being fed up and with several months to wait for my wife, I started to worry about my broken condition and what I had for her upon release. I thought of various ways to increase my financial affairs but was afraid of being arrested before my wife was released, so I left Toronto and went to London, Ontario. Here the problem of drinking got out of hand, and I went to the bottom in the first month. But once again I got a break as some people I met gave me the boost I needed and with one month left before my wife's discharge I started to work. Work to me was a foreign matter as I had never worked outside of some that I had done while in the Army or in prison. At first I found it very hard to take, but I had to make good for my wife was expecting that much of me. I felt this was the least I could do.

"I was able to meet my wife at Kingston on the morning of her release and we settled down in London with both of us going to work. We soon had a new car and furniture and other things it takes to enjoy life. We had borrowed money from a Finance Company and at first had no trouble making payments, but with other bills to pay it got increasingly difficult to make payments and we started worrying. That led to arguing, and then drinking. Up until that time, we never thought about narcotics too much. That is, it never became an obsession.

"In one of my drinking bouts I met a wine hound that had been a junker and he told me about a doctor he had been able to secure some morphine from. I thought of giving it a try, but put it off for a while. Then one night I suggested to my wife that we see if it was possible, not that it mattered, but just to see if we could get some drugs from this doctor. Up to this time I had been off narcotics for one year, and felt good except for the messes I got into with drinking. For an ending I'll simply say that we were successful with the doctor and from that day to this present situation there has been no end of problems, including the same Finance Company, that I blamed it all on."

. . . . .

"I was released from jail after serving six months and returned to live with my wife and family. I got a job driving a truck and was quite happy with the job and with the way my home life was going. It was after three months of this that I got the occasional moods of despondency. I shrugged them off and thought that they had nothing to do with drugs so I had nothing to worry about. But one night at home I got in an awful state of despondency, and asked my wife what could possibly be the matter. I couldn't sit down and my mind was in a whirl. She thought I was working too hard, but I knew it wasn't that. After she had retired and I thought she was asleep I started pacing the floor. The more I paced the floor the more I knew that I was going down to score. Knowing that I shouldn't go, but for every reason why I shouldn't go there remained that stronger feeling that I must, and would go. My thoughts were interrupted when I heard my wife say: 'If you go where you're thinking of going, then don't bother coming back.' I flew into a rage and accused her of bringing up a subject that wasn't even on my mind. She tried to apologize, but I wouldn't let it die. I had found my excuse to get out and I wasn't going to let it slip by. Needless to say, I dressed and went very promptly to score. Why shouldn't I, I thought. She hounded me into it, didn't she? That's what I tried to tell myself, anyway. Knowing even then, that it was a feeble excuse at the best. Anyway, that was the end of the job, and everything else. It was only a matter of time until I was back in jail."

. . . . .

"I was discharged from prison after a short period of incarceration. My desire was to stay off drugs. Immediately upon release the craving came back and my thoughts were all centred on a fix and how to go about getting one as soon as possible. I was in the company of an ex-addict who strongly advised me not to take it or go looking for it. As we talked, the old symptoms came back in the form of extreme restlessness, sweating of the hands, palpitation and a feeling of despondency. I continued to crave for drugs, knew where to go to get them, and yet I was fighting a fierce mental battle to try and overcome the craving. I fully realized my position, and the more I argued against taking it, the more I wanted a fix. Suddenly I realized the consequences of that first fix, then I decided not to take it. Instead, immediately proceeded to a friend's home, where I stayed in the house for four days. The first day was quite a battle but this I attributed to change in environment and reaction after being released from prison. The second day was better and by the end of the fourth day I was feeling much better; the craving and discomfort were gone. It was then I realized the importance of being careful on being discharged from any institution. The ex-addict, although not the reformer type, and my friends in that house were most helpful. I was most thankful for their help, as I am sure had those facilities not been available, I would have gone straight for a fix.

"I stayed off for six and a half months. During that time never once did I take a sedative or narcotic. There was an odd day when I did not feel too well, but on those days I was most careful avoiding certain districts, or kept myself occupied by work or recreation.

"Relapse came when I least expected it. I got a very bad cold, then the grippe. Instead of staying in bed, I went out, knowing it was dangerous for me; it was; I called on an acquaintance and took a quarter grain of morphine hypodermically with the excuse it would relieve my sickness and at the same time I wanted that kick. It turned out to be a 'tragedy pop'. In a week or two, I was back in the horror chamber again, addicted."

· · · · ·

The accounts given by the patients, discussions with them,

and observations of them in all stages of addiction enable us to see the pattern that traps them, in the following table:

The "Experimental" Stage (1)

Association with drug addicts.
Curiosity (hearing about it from others).
Imitation.
Illness, injury or pain.
To relieve hang-overs from drink.
Experimenting while drinking.
Mental strain (nervousness, anxiety).
Initial doses followed by sweating, nausea, vomiting, drowsiness (1-2 hours).
Then a sense of well-being (8 hours).
"Floating" everything fine, life acceptable.
"On the nod" unaware of clock time elapsing.
"Relaxed" free of worry.
"Coasting" imaginative, free—puts oneself into any desired situation, in fantasy.
Chippying, joy popping (experimental).
First fixes are the best in most cases.
These fixes produce "bangs" "drives" "jolts" "kicks".
(Various terms for the drugged sensation.)
"The greatest feeling" (They hesitate to compare it with other human pleasures such as sex, wealth, recognition, etc.).
First reaction (next day) hollow, empty, cleaned out, beat.
When nausea and vomiting cease after a fix, you know you are "wired" (addicted) or if vomiting continues, it ceases to be unpleasant.

Withdrawal—Acute Stage (2)

Yawning, sneezing.
Eyes and nose watering.
Periodical vomiting.
Nausea, cramps.
Diarrhoea.
Inabilty to sleep or eat.
General restlessness.
General aching of body.
Constant craving for drugs.
Very cold chills up and down the spine.

Possible contraction of pneumonia or severe cold.
Hot and cold sweats (very sour odour).
Depressed (suicidal thoughts and attempts).
Phase lasts from 3 to 10 days, varying with age, amount of
drugs used, and length of addiction.

Withdrawal—Chronic Stage (3)

Aching arms, legs and back.
General weakness, tired.
Desire to lie down most of the time.
Sleepless, restless for a period of 4 to 6 weeks.
Appetite returns. "Chuck horrors"—dreams of food, espe-
cially personal favourites in the sweet line, such as ice
cream, milk shakes, desserts. Even bread tastes like cake.
Dream often about delicious steaks and sweets. Raven-
ous for food.
Sleep comes back gradually.
First nights are restless. (During sleep, erections and org-
asms occur.)
"Dream horrors"—dreams very realistic, about getting a
fix. Awaken in a cold sweat.
Heavy sleep follows early restless period.
Sleep returns nearly to normal after 2 months' withdrawal,
or more.
Craving for drugs does not cease, in less than 3 months.
Even then periodical desires persist past the 3 months of
withdrawal.
Chronic anxiety.
General bodily debility—no ambition, no drive.
In the fourth month, confidence returns gradually, and one
gains physical and mental strength.
One feels much better after fourth month, if interests are
aroused in something useful.
Good books, recreation, music, T.V. shows, are helpful.
Group therapy is of the greatest value.

The Pill People

Far more extensive than addiction to the opiates is the widespread problem of addiction to that class of
depressants known as the hypnotics and sedatives—chloral,
paraldehyde, bromides, the barbiturates and tranquillizers.

An alcoholic, whom I once treated, succeeded in gaining abstinence from alcohol. He was evasive and soon dropped therapy. After several months, a mutual acquaintance informed me that Bill had been acting very strangely at A.A. meetings recently. Shiny, glassy eyes, very slow in his speech, very quiet. Then one night, he collapsed while speaking to his group. I discovered he had taken to chloral. He came to realize that his therapy had to include abstinence from all addicting substances. This was several years ago. Experienced A.A. members now inform recruits of the danger of substitute drugs, and urge upon them abstinence from injections and pills whose substances are known or suspected to have addictive properties.

A patient I found to be addicted to paraldehyde confessed to me at last that he went on drinking sprees expressly to wind up in a nursing home where they gave liberal portions of what he most wanted, in their treatment of alcoholism— "The feeling I want," he said, "is that numbness starting in the toes, and going all the way up."

One of the worst withdrawals I ever saw was that of a patient addicted to one of the popular bromide variants. He had become psychotic, believed he was back in the Air Force about to go on a dangerous mission. He irritated the nurses with violent criticism of his "quarters". Whenever he could, he scrubbed the floors and walls, complaining that the NCOs in this unit were terribly negligent. His withdrawal lasted six weeks before he could be said to be normal again. There was no history of psychosis in his record.

Another bromide variant was the drug of choice of a woman alcoholic. She died several months ago without having broken her addiction. She had never wanted to undergo long-term treatment.

While such cases appear from time to time, the really prevalent addictions, excepting only alcoholism, are found among the heavy habitual users of the barbiturates and tranquillizers. Withdrawal from these can be more painful and more serious than withdrawal from morphine and heroin, if the addiction is deeply ingrained. Usually the barbiturates and tranquillizers are taken in pill form. Hence such addicts are called the pill people, to distinguish them from the addicts who take drugs intravenously.

The barbiturates and tranquillizers, like morphine, have justified uses under the control of medical doctors in the treatment of a great variety of human ailments. But the alarming use of these drugs, outside the control of medicine, has made of them a serious problem in North America.

The morphine and heroin addicts are singled out for special notice in any popular account of drug addiction, along with the marihuana smokers. These stories dwell on sensational underworld activities, and are much over-dramatized when related realistically to the hundreds of thousands of pill people who have made major industries out of the barbiturates and tranquillizers. A million pounds of barbiturates were manufactured in the United States in 1951. If this figure levelled off since 1954, it can largely be explained by the phenomenal rise in the use of tranquillizers, which have more than matched the popularity of barbiturates. The Kefauver Report (1960) reveals that Americans spend at least 400,000,000 dollars a year on tranquillizers. When this figure is compared with the 500,000,000 dollars spent yearly on morphine and heroin in illicit trade, we see how much greater is the use of the tranquillizers. The Kefauver Committee reveals that the new drugs are costing the public far too much, but even so, their cost is small compared to the "retail" price of a heroin addict's "fix". A fix ranges from six to ten dollars. The average addict spends at least $30 and more likely $50 a day to support his habit. It is conservative to conclude that the number of tranquillizer users is far greater than the number of opiate addicts—a number extending into every class of American culture.

The barbiturates of choice among addicts are nembutal and seconal. The tranquillizers appear under so many trade names that it is impossible to keep up with them. Meprobramate, Promazine, Chlorpromazine and Reserpine are among the main ingredients of the popular tranquillizers. I have classified the tranquillizers as depressants because they relieve tension and are conducive to sleep, when properly prescribed under competent medical supervision. Some preparations contain stimulants, as well as the depressant barbiturates, or tranquillizers, in the effort to counteract the loggy and stuporous effect of the depressant drug.

One young woman addicted to a "pep" pill—depressant and stimulant combined—was under my care and abstinent from these drugs for more than two months before she was thinking and feeling normally. It required six more months of psychotherapy before she could say honestly that she was comfortably free from drugs, resolved never to use them again. She came to me emaciated, with an ugly rash of carbuncles, and very disturbed emotionally. She told me that her pill was "like champagne". She grew so dependent on it that every occasion of the slightest challenge induced her to take it. A worry about her child, a visit to a friend, the prospect of a dutiful phone call, a shopping trip, even a party among congenial people—any occasion at all was a fearful experience prompting her to take that pill. Then she described the awful panic she suffered when her supply ran out. Finally, like the opiate addicts, she came to fear the terrible suffering of withdrawal more than she valued the intoxication of the pill. The drug eventually did no more than enable her to feel nearly normal, even in increased dosages. When this happened, the pill ceased to do the job it originally had done. Desperately she sought help, physically and mentally exhausted. This young woman, after the concerted efforts of medical dotors and psychologists, slowly regained her health, but it was a tremendous task. If she had not been able to take advantage of concentrated care, the story might well have been different.

Barbiturate addicts reveal signs of intoxication similar to those of alcoholics—mentally sluggish, unstable, confused, irritable, slurred speech. In addiction, they often show gross disturbances in coordination of speech, space and time, more serious than the similar disturbances of alcoholics. A prominent banker, who shifted from alcohol to barbiturates, would walk towards one door meaning to go through another. He lost all track of time, and he was as incoherent in his speech as an infant. His intoxication by pills was far worse than his drinking sprees, and his withdrawal from barbiturates required three times as long as his withdrawal from alcohol.

Convulsive seizures, resembling grand mal epilepsy, often occur among barbiturate and meprobramate addicts, after they appear to be improving. Delirium, usually at night, with vivid hallucinations, is sometimes experienced, in a variety of striking colours.

In August, 1959, the Federal Government of Canada placed thirty-two types of tranquillizers on the prescription list. This action revealed the alarm of the Canadian authorities over the dangerous widespread use of these drugs. Officials reported that the pills have critical cumulative effects. As a means of reducing tension or anxieties, these drugs had become a menace, with many serious harmful effects. They induce severe depression and then suicidal tendencies when taken indiscriminately. Also reported by the drug advisory board were cases of damage done to the kidneys, liver and stomach by the tranquillizers.

These findings can be supported by anyone who specializes in the treatment of addiction. At the time the Canadian ruling went into effect, I had six patients in therapy, all of whom were tranquillizer addicts. Three of them took my advice and went to a private sanatorium for treatment. They required six weeks to be withdrawn. While there I kept in touch with them, and resumed psychotherapy with them when they were released. One was much under-weight, another had suffered liver damage, and a third had developed serious stomach trouble. The others did not undergo supervised withdrawal: from these I have heard nothing. In my experience it is very difficult to withdraw a drug addict, no matter what the drug, at home, or by "cold turkey" (complete abrupt withdrawal). Any plan for a competent drug clinic should include barbiturate and tranquillizer victims as well as opiate and stimulant addicts.

Many innocent persons grow dependent on tranquillizers without realizing what is happening to them, until they suffer from addiction just as severe in its reactions as those from the barbiturates, and worse than the hang-overs of alcoholism. They often say one thing and mean something else, and become utterly unintelligible in severe intoxication. In withdrawal or in decreased dosages, they suffer muscle pains, hot and cold sweats, extreme agitation and convulsive seizures. When deeply intoxicated, they walk unsteadily, and often fall unless closely watched.

Intoxicated or withdrawing, I have never seen addicts more disturbed than those addicted to the barbiturates or tranquillizers.

The pill people of America are drawn from all ranks of society. Here we are not dealing with sinister underworld characters, but with the respectable rank and file of men and women in business, industry and the professions. Alcoholics and drug addicts come similarly from all walks of life. Only lurid sensational stories represent the addict as a psychopathic type and a renegade from respectable living. It is true that some addicts have had a bad time from childhood throughout their lives. But this is not to identify them as criminals or outcasts.

What, then, underlies the addiction of thousands of people of every class all over the world today?

The Addict—What Does He Want?

Dr. Marie Nyswander, in her book, "The Drug Addict As A Patient", makes it clear that treating the drug addict requires more than withdrawing him from his drug. She agrees with Dr. Harris Isbell who has said "Withdrawal of drugs is merely the first phase of treatment and is the only easy one.

Unfortunately it is frequently regarded as being synonymous with complete treatment. It is no more rational to consider withdrawal as being a complete treatment for addiction than it is to consider mere 'drying out' as being completely adequate treatment for alcoholism".[1]

Dr. Nyswander believes that "the most crucial stage in the treatment of a drug addict begins at the moment he is released from the hospital where he has been withdrawn from drugs and has spent from six weeks to four months in a drug-free environment. His return to social and work life depends to a great extent on beginning this part of the treatment at once".[2]

Every experienced clinician in addictions will readily agree with Drs. Nyswander and Isbell. This is not to minimize the essential task of acute withdrawal, and it is not to ignore the personal discomfort of the addict, which can be extremely distressing. Every clue is being searched to make acute withdrawal less distressing, but such efforts lose their greatest value if one fails to take into full account the complex task of long-term withdrawal and enduring sobriety.

Both Dr. Nyswander and Dr. Isbell refer to the theory of Dr. A. Wikler regarding opiate addiction. Deeper than personality classification, and more basic than the theories which attempt to explain the addict's traits, is the urge to alleviate pain, to avoid sexual troubles, and to tone down aggression.[3]

There is no doubt about the pain killing properties of the opiates, and the power of these drugs to soothe and reduce aggressive feelings. As to sex, Dr. Nyswander observes "Studies of the subjective reactions of addicts to a single dose of morphine reveal that many of them experience a feeling of exhilaration, akin to an orgasm discharged in the abdominal region. It is entirely possible that the intensity of this pleasure exceeds any pleasure known to non-addicts".[4] I can say, on the basis of reports to me by addicts that a "fix" does indeed exceed in quality any known sexual pleasure.

The problems of money, power and sex with their attendant pain and aggression create problems for addicts of all kinds (including alcoholics); in addition to these reasons for indulgence, there is also the strong drive of wanting something more than they seem able to get through the usual channels of society at large. It is this positive reason that I stress in all my work with addicts, whether it be alcoholism or addiction to other drugs.

Dr. Nyswander observes that addicts in the younger group are sensitive to material wealth, commenting often on Cadillacs, clothes and money. Again I can confirm this from my experiences with the younger group. Several of my patients commented kindly on the shabby car I drove. They felt I should be doing better than that. They were noticeably neat, and well turned out, though the wardrobe of a reformatory is restricted. When I first began treating addicts I was astonished to see that as a group they were clean cut, intelligent and personable. Like other people, I had formed a sinister image of the skulking dope fiend. I couldn't have been more surprised and relieved when I knew the facts. Moreover, that group was made up of the so-called "criminal type". Not one of them was what you could really call a criminal. Though they had been thieves, they stole to support their habit, not to make it a profession by choice.

Deeper than their concern for money, or their interest in power, prestige or sex; deeper, too, than their avoidance of the problems presented by pain, physical or psychological, was their search for *something more* in a positive experience, beyond the alleviation of their troubles. In discussing the alcoholic I call this urge or search, *personal thirst*. Among addicts of other kinds, I call it *personal craving*. It is in the meaning of this personal craving that we find what the addict really wants.

It is well here to note what Professor A. R. Lindesmith has said in his book "Opiate Addiction"[5] about the genesis of any drug addict. It includes (a) exposure to the drug; (b) recognition of withdrawal distress and (c) the use of the drug to alleviate such distress. This simple and practical guide serves many useful purposes. It takes us beyond the area of any one drug, and beyond any one class of people. It is common to all addicts to alleviate their distress, in the only way they know, with the drugs of their choice. In addiction, the whole trouble lies in this fact—the need to reduce distress finally overcomes the urgency to seek that "something more", the original core of personal craving.

Thus addiction at last belies its original promise, earning the label "monkey on the back", when all the increasing hazards of access and fear of withdrawal yield little more, at best, than the feeling of normalcy. Even this feeling of normalcy is threatened, for all the addict's energy and cunning have to be devoted to securing his next fix; chronic fear of the pain of withdrawal becomes the key note of his daily life.

It is essential to think of the addict's main problem in terms of purpose rather than cause. This is the upshot of all the work I've done in therapy. By this I do not mean that researchers should neglect the study of cause. It is just that a practical scrutiny of purpose yields a working basis for treatment of all classes of addicts.

Let me illustrate in the experience of exposure. A drug addict once said that the most upright clergyman, or the most reliable citizen one can produce, can become an addict if exposed to morphine or heroin often enough. I agree with him. (Exposure includes not only availability of drugs, but also ignorance of their dangers.) What, then, happens to theories which represent the addict as a special kind of emotionally disturbed person? Of course it is true that many emotionally disturbed people become addicts, but what of those who become addicted in whom no serious sick traits were originally present? Many doctors, nurses and others who have easy access to drugs have become addicts. And many youngsters exposed to persons who are addicts are moved by curiosity to try drugs. A socially permissive scene, or a situation where drugs are easily available, where some of them enjoy immunity from criticism, or when a drug is represented as harmless and health-producing—all these situations lay the ground for potential users in any walk of life.

The tell-tale experience occurs after the candidate has indulged. Exposed often enough he may soon get "hooked". (I'm told that eight fixes of heroin are enough to addict a person to that drug.) Now the intoxication brings a feeling that no one can experience, in just that way, by any other means. Let me go back to the youngsters who were so devoted, soberly, to money, clothes, and beautiful women. From chatting with them, week after week, fascinating views emerge. They grow more serious as you gain their confidence. They tell you, when they are sure you are with them, about the mysterious lure of the feelings they have when they are well "fixed". You begin to realize that what they grope to express are the ideals of every sensitive and imaginative human being in his depths. Then you sense that these ideals go beyond the urges of money, power and sex with their attendant pain and struggle, to the hope for freedom and adventure and love. This is the core of personal craving —a universal dream. Who is there who would not like to by-pass his inadequacies, fears and tensions and become at peace with himself and the world?

One youngster told me, and there was a chorus of agreement among the others, that the most desirable woman, the fattest wallet, the best clothes, and the most illustrious prestige are as nothing compared to the clarity, peace and adventure of the right "fix". I tried to get a description of this "pleasure". They cooperated and studied the problem for me. At last they said: "It is no good comparing it with any pleasure you can think of—women, dough, status, a yacht, power. There is just no comparing it, Doc, that's all." So I gave up trying to conduct therapy on the basis that sobriety primarily was a source of more pleasure than addiction. It is easily demonstrated that sobriety can indeed yield more pleasure, in the long run, than addiction, but this fails, of itself, to impress them. It was only when I spoke of "being yourself, free and easy, to seek what you really want—harmony within, and at peace with the world", that they began to respond with interest. This approach works equally well among all addicts, not just those who are found in a reformatory. It works, I believe, because it appeals to the hope of every sensitive person in the world, and every such person might well become an addict if exposed enough in a permissible climate, not knowing the danger of drugs.

My clients are drawn from every class of society. Many of them are wealthy people of status, with no sexual problem other than that of most non-addicts. They are people who have no sound reason to be upset by problems of pain, sex, or aggression. They dimly sense the deceptions of money, power and sex, but know not where to turn for "something more". One patient tell me he wants more "bubbles". When he tried to explain this, he is perplexed. He admits that his money and prestige have lost their glamour and he confesses that sex is less urgent than it used to be. He is impotent when intoxicated, but he has no problem satisfying his sexual urges when he feels them. What does this man want? The return of young sexual virility? No. The making of more money and the gaining of more status? No. Something attractive and real, in sobriety, besides the reduction of pain, of aggression, and of sexual conflicts, is what he must find.

The most reliable citizen, who copes well with his human problems and pains, could become an addict if exposed. Of course it is true that likely candidates for addiction are those with obvious problems of pain, of sex and of aggression. But both the normal and disturbed groups would crave the illusion of "something more", beyond the problems of pain and struggle, that, once the physical dependence was established, would lure them back to drugs again and again. Addiction is an experience running much deeper than conscious control. It strikes deep into the strongest feelings. And these, then, are what have to be aroused for long-term recovery. I have outlined this procedure in detail in the treatment of alcoholics. The same approach works with all other addicts.

They really want *to be* themselves, as they think they'd like to be. In this feeling, they confuse *having* with *being*. This is why the penniless addict supposes that he wants wealth when he is sober. This desire is belied when he describes the state of *being* of intoxication, and reveals that what he really wants is not what he supposes he wants. This evidence is further supported in the treatment of addicts who are wealthy. They value their money as highly as penniless addicts do, chiefly because, by over-compensation, they know—both the wealthy and the penniless—that society at large treats them better, and accepts them more graciously, if they can pay their way. It is notoriously true that all addicts, including alcoholics, are very conscious of what money and clothes they have, as you may observe in a clinic when they are sober. They go into a fussy mood, the reverse of the care-free abandonment they display when intoxicated. The great respect of the addict for wealth, whether he has it or not, is an over-compensation for his neglect of the demands of society at large—to be up and at it, to be aggressive, and to get there. Naturally, with the pressure of society upon him, and his respect for it, albeit grudging and even hostile, he supposes, as also many non-addicts do, that *to be* himself is *to have* as much as he can. To a limited extent, he is right. It takes money to support addiction, lots of it.

The enjoyment of intoxication reveals his true needs. At its best, apart from the misery and cost of addiction, intoxication gives him a feeling of being himself, oblivious to the struggle of getting and having things, as he most wants to be. The addict then, has to see, in his own way, that addiction eventually is not the route to *being*, but to having and being had. To be an addict, in the full scope of its meaning, is *to be had*. But the meaningful core of personal craving, the justifiable purpose of it all, was to be himself, certainly not to be had. So a therapist works into the heart of the matter when he helps patients to understand the whole play of having and being in their proper relations to each other. It requires, not only intelligence, but an awareness of feelings at their depth, to overcome the years of addiction with a strong dynamic urge to be and to become oneself in sobriety.

This plan, as with alcoholics, involves insight and action through the technique of empathy. The withdrawal period of drug addicts is much longer than that of alcoholics. It requires usually about four months, in an ideal treatment plan. During this time, lectures and psycho-therapy dwell ideally on practical clues to lifetime sobriety. The *purpose* of personal craving, and the way in which this purpose can be realized, constitute the bulk of my efforts in clinical work. The personal problems engendered by the use of drugs cannot be cleared by another drug or any other physical substance, in long-term sobriety. The self-intoxication that has taken place—confusion of feelings—needs to be treated before real freedom from drugs can be known. Drug addiction is a slavish devotion to the need for the habituating drug more powerful and more compelling than the dictates of all the rest of one's known highest values and principles. It is essential then, to explore with patients their deepest feelings to locate, if possible, a feeling that can be made stronger than the urge to indulge their habit, and to study with them the *purpose* of this feeling. I believe that this feeling in every addict, no matter what his background, and no matter what his type of personality, is the core of his personal craving—the urge to be himself. In the actions required by the purpose of this craving he first learns that he must, at all costs, avoid being had. Nothing has taken him so completely as his addiction. So he sets up a personal discipline enabling him to abstain completely. Second, he learns that such abstinence has its main value as an instrument for what he really wants. Third, the goal he works towards is his self-realization, the only authentic source of that freedom and adventure and peace that he formerly believed could only be found in "fixes". This self-realization is what he really wants. The way to it, as I've stressed throughout this book, is through acts of empathy.

The techniques of empathy require insight into identification, resistance, imitation, and growing out of these the creative act of putting yourself in the other fellow's place. This is empathy, and it invites empathy in return.

Let us glance back to the experimental or initial stage of addiction. It is here that we get our best clues to recovery. We notice that the pattern begins with three tell-tale experiences—association with others, curiosity or desire to know something new or adventurous, and imitation.

Identification, the first phase of the process that eventually can grow into empathy, takes place in association with others. As association with addicts deepens, identification with them grows stronger, and resistance against the "square" world also grows deeper. (The addict cannot see that this resistance is really a self-resistance. This is not seen until he strives for recovery.)

After the potential addict imitates his addicted exemplars often enough, he becomes a victim of *imposed imitation*. By this is meant that he no longer has to imitate anybody in order to behave as he does, because now the compulsive nature of his physical dependence has imposed itself upon his behaviour such that he is powerless to direct it by conscious control. You may wonder why I say than imitation is a phase of the creative and worthwhile act of empathy. Well, there are two main types of imitation in human behaviour—imposed and free. Imposed imitation, as in addiction, is the control of one's life by forces which do not operate in healthy behaviour. Free imitation, on the other hand, is the choiceful modelling of our behaviour on that of others whom we respect and admire. All good learning, all good art, is based on free imitation. It is free imitation which we stress as one of the techniques of empathy. In the recovery programme then, the addict is encouraged to replace the imposed imitations of his addiction with healthy deliberate acts of free imitation.

The difference between imposed imitation and free imitation is the difference between "Do as I say, or else" and "Do as I do, if you like". It takes a lot of patience and understanding to convince a man that it is in his own best interests to switch from imposed imitation to free imitation. And it requires a lot of practice to imitate freely rather than compulsively.

Even after he has practised free imitation, for example, the following in the footsteps of recovered associates, he has still to reach the heights of his recovery by moving from free imitation to empathy. By developing the act of putting himself in the other fellow's place he develops his own personal style. He has passed from imitation to the great goal of all sensitive human beings—he learns to be himself, unafraid and curious about the adventure of life which lies ahead. The most curious lesson he learns is that he can only really be himself in concert with others in fellowship.

Now let us sum up the techniques of empathy, as developed throughout this book.

The recovering addict identifies deliberately with others like him in their common defect, addiction, and common goal, sobriety. The ground of this identification is good will.

Then he learns that resistance is chiefly self-resistance. He has been fighting himself vainly for years. So he learns to accept himself, addiction and all. The only genuine resistance worthy of his study and effort is respect for others. Genuine resistance, that which is left after self-resistances are accepted, is respect for the other.

Next he imitates his exemplars consciously and freely; the examplars who are now recovered and recovering. This is free imitation. And finally he becomes a helper, as well as a person helped, when he practises empathy in his efforts to understand the plight of others.

The fact that empathy works equally well with alcoholics and drug addicts does not mean that clear differences between the various addictions are ignored. Drug addiction is deeper, more treacherous, much more difficult to treat than alcoholism. If it is true that nothing short of a new way of life is required by alcoholics, then it is even more clear that a new way of life is required by drug addicts. If you probe deeply into the values of an alcoholic, you run to the depths of the addict's values. Alcoholics who are well recovered know that life-time follow-up is essential to their freedom. Drug addicts, whose problems are often worse, because of their greater physical dependence, can hardly be expected to have enduring freedom more easily than alcoholics.

The exploration of empathy, with all its bypaths, is the best approach to all the addictions that I have discovered in assisting patients to realize the purpose of their craving. There is no discipline I know of which better enables a human being to be and to become himself.

Drug addicts who develop real insight will follow up their freedom in Narcotics Anonymous. This therapy is similar to A.A. and can bring the same effective results when it secures the support it richly deserves. Within these therapies, empathy flourishes when the groups cooperate with the programme. Recovery rates for drug addiction have not been startling. They are low compared to known recoveries from alcoholism. But the fact is that the drug addict can recover if he really wants sobriety, if he gives himself over to the real purpose of his personal craving—the desire to be himself.

Guilt, shame, fear and stigma envelop any drug addict in North America today. These are what a therapist must try to remove in his acceptance of his patient as a sick human being.

It is most difficult to operate well among drug addicts, to create a free and easy climate, when social forces militate against both patient and therapist. Our laws concerning the use of drugs and our attitude towards addicts could well be patterned on the British approach to this problem. This approach is grossly misunderstood here. Many believe it to be a legalized way to indulge addiction. This is entirely false. It is simply an intelligent way to handle addicts in the process of helping them to recover. It reduces the illicit drug traffic to a minor problem. An addict who rejects treatment will go to illicit sources. And if he is caught, he is charged with illegal possession, but he may be put on probation provided he is willing to undergo medical treatment. Drug addiction is no real problem in Great Britain, compared to the situation in North America. There are social and personal forces in North America of a sort different in many ways from those of Great Britain, but there is no doubt that a different attitude towards distribution would go far to reduce the problem here. As long as the illicit traffic flourishes, we can expect youngsters to seek forbidden adventures, and to engage in criminal activities to support their habit. But let us not suppose that the addicts who began as thrill seekers are the main problem. We must create a new social attitude towards *all* addicts, including the larger class of pill people, if we are to encourage every candidate for treatment to seek his freedom.

More Government-operated clinics, a new drug law, and the encouragement of Narcotics Anonymous are the three essential public projects, from a therapist's point of view, in coping with the drug problem in North Amercia today. Like the alcoholic, the drug addict deserves to be accepted as a sick person, not a criminal.

Throughout this book, I have been concerned chiefly to describe the inner personal experience of addiction to alcohol and drugs, and to chart the way to freedom from these addictions in the growing adventure of sobriety. The prevention of addiction is somehow to be found in deeper understanding of empathy, just as recovery from addiction is found in the practice of empathic acts.

I have said no more about the scientific approach to alcohol and drugs than appeared relevant to the problems of empathic treatment and prevention, and no more than I feel qualified to report. Besides the works cited, there are competent sources of scientific, medical and legal material as well as good descriptive accounts in Maurer and Vogel,[6] De Ropp,[7] Murtagh and Harris,[8] The Quarterly Journal of Studies on Alcohol,[9] and the British Journal of Addiction.[10] There are numerous other excellent references, and new studies continue to appear. In the ten references supplied at the end of this introduction, the serious student can be sure of thorough guidance and of exhaustive bibliographies, in his effort to understand all aspects of the alcohol and drug problem, especially if the stress falls on the objective aspects of addiction.

THE MYSTERY OF ADDICTION

FROM the start of a person's addiction, no matter what the addicting substance may be, there are evasive forces at work concerning his desires, needs and values. These are made complex and resistant to study as addiction deepens, and as physical dependence is fused with the pattern of his life's problems. Some of these forces yield to scientific order, some do not. In his recovery, also, some needs yield to organized effort, such as diet and rest, but others do not.

The response to this act, in an age like ours, may well be that we just have not gone far enough. More effort in the scientific area will, it is thought, clear all problems and all uncertainty.

At the outset of this book, I wish to make clear that there are aspects of addiction, from start to finish, and on into the programme of freedom from drugs, which make of it a mystery. This mystery prevails, not because we do not know enough about the problem, but because there is inherent in the nature of the addict's purpose and of his recovery an experience which has always been, and always will be, a personal meaning beyond scientific knowledge. This need not deter scientific effort. We need to know as much as science can tell us. It certainly will have more to tell us as the years go by, and we shall make the best use of every insight that science can provide.

I wish to illustrate in several ways the presence of the mystery of addiction. It can be understood, it can be worked with, and real meaning can emerge from it. A mystery is not confusion and darkness; it is a meaningful experience if we can be bold enough to believe that there are areas of knowing other than those cultivated by twentieth century science.

Follow-Up and the Problem of "Results"

The recovering addict makes real progress when you observe him shifting his main interest from disease, disorder, and other related problems, to growth, learning, the rewards of sobriety, and creative interpersonal activities. Only well along in follow-up can you adequately assess freedom from any of the addictions. The reason is this: statistics are too often made on abstinence only, with little regard for the sounder, more elusive state of the patient's personal health. When such statistics refer to a period short of two years, they fail to measure the critical shift from after-care to rehabilitation. It is conceivable, for example, that a patient may relapse several times within a year, and yet be better recovered than the abstinent one whose mental health resembles a man sitting on an active volcano. I do not wish to be misunderstood. I am not implying that the tense abstinent patient has not improved. His abstinence alone is noteworthy. I want, rather, to point out that improvements can be observed in patients who, though relapsing, are proceeding towards sobriety in the best way they can. I try to remember my own instructions to patients about personal differences and difficulties, my effort to secure an open-minded attitude on *degrees* of sickness.

Perhaps the best criterion of recovery and sound rehabilitation is *loss of the desire to indulge*. For evidence of this, the clinician must depend on personal testimony, in addition to the fact of abstinence. (Even evidence of the fact of abstinence will require the honesty of the patient and the trust of the clinician.) Loss of the desire to indulge, though it appears negative in form, is far from negative in fact, for it means that the patient no longer needs to indulge, no longer depends on his drug, and has found a creative way to solve the problems which were formerly dissolved in intoxication. Loss of desire to indulge means, therefore, that the person has now a liking for sobriety, a creative act.

But there is a difficulty. Clinicians stress, from time to time, the dynamic nature of human behaviour. A creative desire today will not remain strong and clear without effort, for tomorrow is another day with new challenges and new adventures. There is no neat solution enduringly to guarantee consistent behaviour or consistent statistics about behaviour.

Yet, we have to be practical, though we cannot be rigidly certain about human behaviour or about our statistics on it. Clinicians, like other persons engaged in practical work, have to have some guide and faith in what they do, if their efforts are to be productive and worthwhile.

My guide and faith in what I have done, and will continue to do, is based on three important beliefs.

(1) The recovery and follow-up of the addict is a life-time adventure, grounded on an irreversible permanent sensitivity to drugs such that the addict may never safely indulge again. Fused strangely with all the trouble a patient has had, is an experience of relief or pleasure, long lost, but triggered into recall in moments of stress or of nostalgic longing. Under stress, or in a period of great ease and relaxation, this urge may take hold—any time, anywhere, in the first year of sobriety, or the tenth, the addict never knows. The response to this urge can be a slip, or the daily personal effort that goes into his sobriety. Well into recovery, there must be effective sources other than the clinic to which a patient can choose to turn. He may live at a distance from the clinic, or he may be away from the clinic location for the weekend when such an urge strikes him. As the years pass, the contacts a patient makes, the persons he turns to, the activities he develops, will be more and more his own decisions, and less and less the suggestions of his clinic.

(2) Clinicians only *participate* in a patient's recovery and follow-up. We could not produce statistics to prove that we have been solely responsible for recovery. We fail to practise our own principles if we fail to convince patients that their personal and interpersonal efforts are essential to their rehabilitation. What the patients put into their sobriety, they will get out of it. This is a paraphrase of an A.A. belief. I believe it is sound, and if it is, who exclusively, other than the patients themselves, can say he has effected their rehabilitation?

When a patient fails to improve, given an adequate testing period for our efforts, we must re-examine our procedures and techniques, and try to improve them, or change them, or experiment with new techniques. We must assume that we have been at fault, provided the patient has been sincere in his desire for help. Any assessment of results, therefore, must be qualified by the fact that, in a dynamic approach to recovery, what we do in this situation with this patient, may not be the same as what we do in a similar situation with another patient. What there is in a set of lectures or group therapy or interviews this week may be modified the next week. And also, clinicians, human beings, may be more effective today than they are tomorrow, even when techniques and procedures remain the same. Clinicians must undergo growth as patients do. A great problem in a busy private clinic is lack of time and facilities to do much needed research.

(3) I am utterly convinced of the importance of "timing" in the therapy of alcoholism and other addictions. A patient with many relapses on his record may be indefinitely blocked from recovery by a brusque though well-meaning refusal to treat him again. Dynamically, he may be more ready for real insight than he appears to be. It is often hard to know. And his slips may even be interpreted as stages through which he had to pass in order to experience a genuine softening of resistance. Such a process, even when soundly understood, cannot be included in a statistical statement.

On the other hand, a patient abstinent for two years or more, *does* look impressive as a recorded recovery, though we may have many misgivings about the quality of his sobriety, from reports we get on his tensions, fears, and resentments.

Within any clinical programme itself—the in-patient programme—there are also important timing factors to watch. We have known patients so resistant the first few days, that special personal attention was required to convince them to stay. Without exception, these patients have done splendidly. But it was more a practical sense than a scientific technique that gave us the clue for those special interviews. Then, too, there are those who respond too well right from the start. They assure you there was never an experience in all their life to compare with the value of the instruction they are getting at the clinic. You feel wonderfully encouraged. They appear to have over-identified, which may well mean they never effectively identified at all! These patients are not actually discharged until some time after the routine course is finished. The reason is that they may "slip" in a matter of days or weeks after they complete the normal three-week period of the course. They have still to show the resistance that appears to be required before any real improvement can be marked, and then to work their way through this resistance.

Then there are those who are neither resistant nor teachable, while in clinical residence. They are genial, amiable, rather cavalier, and always obliging. They are likely to miss lectures, or group sessions, or slip quietly away just after lunch to avoid the afternoon programme. The human tendency of the clinician here may be to resent such patients if they happen to be missing his part of the programme. A neglect of timing among these hazards may well threaten the clinician's mental health. To remind yourself that this patient is sick, that it is silly to be annoyed, that to be annoyed is to contradict your belief in the clinic's diagnosis, is timely and a necessary "timing". This kind of patient is on our hands for a long time, but we cannot abandon hope in his ultimate recovery if we see any signs, at all, of improvement. These signs show in his quiet manner during the second admission when more attention is directed to those aspects of treatment he formerly ignored.

Timing also relates to the degree of severity in a disorder of a nutritional or organic kind, the fear of which, breeding other fears, may induce the patient to slip frequently. Only when the fear factor is eliminated can we hope to see any genuine improvement. We have had several patients, for example, whose heart disorders were such that our consultants could truly say "Stop drinking, or you'll die". Now they continued to drink, not because they wanted to die, but because their fear of abstinence was greater than the fear of death. Any way you take it, fear of any kind leads to drinking—never away from it. They were afraid indeed about their heart condition, but they were more afraid of sobriety. Such patients require a "timing" stretching all the resources of a clinician.

Finally, there are those who need to suffer more before they can make any step towards recovery. Of this type, most are patients who have no real desire for sobriety, and to whom, at this stage, it is difficult to communicate the worth of the desire for sobriety. They have come to us under pressure of family, associates, or the courts, may even appear to be cooperative at times. They stay throughout the course, neglect most features of the follow-up, and return, again under pressure. Time is required to keep faith with them until they themselves come up with the desire for freedom.

Any assessment of therapy should be qualified by the above three basic beliefs in order to provide as true a picture, as possible, of results. Those three beliefs, as outlined above in some detail, are (a) Sobriety is a lifetime job; (b) Clinicians are participants in recovery and follow-up, not controllers of these acts; (c) The importance of "timing".

Because I lack the techniques to record clear dependable

differences between patients, dynamically improved, but suffering relapses, and patients, abstinent but unhappily sober, I can only offer a clinical opinion with regard to the three main criteria of good sobriety; abstinence, a change of attitude, and an enjoyable sobriety.

This clinical opinion, though it is impossible to base it on precise statistics, is drawn from the observation of the behaviour of about one thousand patients over a period of ten years. Patients who have followed up in A.A. or Narcotics Anonymous after the completion of a clinical course, and concurrently with the clinical programme of after-care, are those who have the best record of abstinence, creative change of attitude, and most enjoyable type of sobriety. The next best group are those who cooperate with the entire clinical programme excepting the suggestion to join A.A. These people do quite well, but fail to equal the quality of recovery and rehabilitation observed in the first group. The third group include those who cooperate with the requirements of the in-patient course, but do little or nothing about follow-up, either in the clinic or in A.A. The fourth group are those who come to a clinic for a short "drying-out" period and leave, though properly advised that much more is required of them where lasting recovery is concerned.

Patients in group one have a better than fifty percent prospect of indefinite, life-long sobriety in accordance with the three criteria. Those in group two do not exceed thirty percent expectancy of sobriety, comparable in quality to that of group one. Those in group three do not exceed ten percent of lasting sobriety of any kind. All patients of group four continue to have trouble until they decide to give serious attention to long term recovery.

Being Oneself

In rehabilitation efforts I encourage the patient "to become and know himself through others". This means that he will more and more take the initiative in seeking the help and support he will need, as long as he lives. The action initiated in self identity is in accord with the three basic therapeutic beliefs set forth in the previous section.

Just as the therapist, in treating addiction, finds it effective to experience, by imaginative discipline, the feelings of his patient, so, too, the patient, in rehabilitation, will find it helpful to participate in the problems of the fellow addict, recovered, recovering, or groping for assistance. There is a distinctly creative effort here involved, a personal form distinct and different from the scientific instructions given to the patient during the period of after-care. It is not opposed to scientific techniques. It rather supplements them. The nature of the act is such that you cannot prescribe it, as you do vitamins or protein-intake. You can suggest it, talk about it, point ostensibly to those patients who engage in this creative act, and thus encourage others to try it, if they are interested in long-term, life-long sobriety. The following is one of the ways in which the worth of this creative act is explained.

Within addiction, there has been, and still is, an experience of value to the addict. The addict's anxiety is reduced if you can assure him he is not "crazy", eccentric or simpleminded in the prizing of intoxication. You do not have this "prizing" in the experience of pain when, for example, you suffer from "flu". If one has flu, he knows well that others have it, and that everyone finds it consistently unpleasant. The doctor does not have to feel as you do in order to prescribe effectively for your physical distress. The main issue in physical distress is the control or alleviation of pain. The competent doctor diagnoses the trouble, and treats the effect from a knowledge of cause and symptom. Between cause and effect in the patient there is no intermediary experience of value, of pleasure, of release, of satisfaction.

The medical doctor, treating a simple physical disorder for which there is a clear diagnosis, and a clear physical aid to recovery, does not have to make much of the feeling of his patient except to exercise the usual finesse of a good bedside manner. He does not have to cultivate deliberately the skill of imagination required to identify his feelings with those of the patient, as therapists do who are primarily concerned with *personal* disorders.

Now in personal disorders, and addiction in a personal disorder, the experience of the patient in between scientific cause and effect is not just an experience of discomfort. Far from it! Here, the doctor must reckon with those important experiences that have grown, both from the scientific causes and the total personal needs of the patient, healthy as well as unhealthy. Thus, not only "causes" but also the purposes and needs and experiences following causes will throw much light on the nature of recovery.

The experiences following causes of addiction are sometimes pleasant and rewarding as, for example, in intoxication, in early addiction, at its best, when the addict feels comfortably high, companionable, at one with the world. Such experiences resist classification in our usual ideas of space, time and cause. The addict, usually an intelligent person, has no trouble seeing the logic of the causes which led him into trouble. But this scientific picture, no matter how clear and logical, is unimpressive compared to the value of intoxication *as an adventure outside of the usual framework of space, time and cause;* the pursuit of pleasure or the avoidance of pain or both may be only the route to the joys of its mystery. The old theory of escape does not fit the facts. Escape indeed there may be, but there is something more here in the urge to create—if only in an illusory way—a clearer sense of personal identity, to *form* one's life in a fashion that the "scientific" world cannot allow.

Added to the original causes of addiction, there is something more important in such experiences than in causes in the past. Moreover, the active addict keeps *looking forward* to richer experiences, though increasing addiction always reveals the evidence of more misery and less pleasure, quantitatively measured. Surely, then, it is important both for professional therapist and recovering patient to understand this process, and to realize that a patient cannot easily be persuaded to recover on the grounds alone of scientific fact.

To the question "How does the addict react to scientific lectures?" you may well be able to answer, "He is intellectually cooperative, nods logical agreement to the causes of his trouble, and yet *feels* blithely indifferent both to cause and effect."

When this is the case, as it often is, in slip after slip, you know that such an addict is concerned chiefly with the feeling itself of intoxication (not to mention the lure of the entire ritual of addiction). He is absorbed with an experience, indifferent to "time" as measured by a clock, and to space as respected by practical people. (Here helpful allusions can be made to St. Augustine, Bergson and George Mead in examples easily understood. "One crowded hour of joyous life is worth an age without a name." The three abovementioned writers have been credited with reputable theories of personal time from which clinical psychologists have still much to learn.) This experience is so important that a therapist or recovered patient does well to cultivate every means possible to identify, in a deliberate discipline, with the feelings of an active addict in need of help, and in pursuit of recovery.

The nature of addiction, therefore, is such that the practice of empathy is essential in recovery and to life-long sobriety, not just in order to be kind and to help the other fellow, but also to fulfil oneself by a method other than intoxication. Thus, full recognition is given the urge to be oneself and to form, creatively, the sort of life that the cause-effect world of scientific measures fails to provide. (I refer to "science" as understood from Newton to present time. It is possible that science, some day, may enlarge its scope to include what Plato called "the principle of action" and Aristotle called "the formal cause"; I refer to this as the personal creative form of the rehabilitated patient, in this context.)

(With regard to fulfilling oneself, it is a mistake to suppose that the obviously extroverted addict is necessarily a good mixer. Such an extrovert may often be a person who uses others, or who superficially *mixes*. He does not really mix. His avoidance of his own meaning as a person keeps him from knowing others because he is unconsciously afraid that knowing others will tell him more about himself than he cares to know. The so-called extrovert is in as much need to empathize with fellow addicts as the introvert.)

When scientific efforts are made to assess the effectiveness of recovery one must, in the interest of good science as well as a good recovery, observe the difficulties and obstacles that limit these efforts. If it is true that the recovered patient must know and cope with his feelings in a way similar to the therapist's exercise of empathy, an elusive variable presents itself to the rigorous statistician. In every case, if dependable quantification, based alone on scientific method, is sought, the figures would have to take into account the therapist's attitude, during the clinical course, to each one of his patients—and, indeed, the attitudes also of all the clinical staff—together with the nature of the patient's progress in self knowledge through others. To what extent has the patient cultivated his personal form of therapy in helping others through the practice of empathy?

I do not say that such a survey cannot be made. On the contrary, clinicians have to make qualified appraisals and practical assessments all the time, and seek to improve their methods on these bases. But these, strictly speaking, have to be called opinions or evaluations. It would be unscientific to present them as undeviating statistics. Until we are able to construct a frame of reference including the elusive effort in which the patient creates a personal form of recovery, we can offer qualified opinions but not scientifically sound statistics.

But even if such a new frame of reference were ready at hand, or even if with present methods, ingenious researchers conceived a complex structure to provide us with better statistics, a great difficulty would remain. The difficulty is therapeutic, and it is this: The therapist or rehabilitated patient who grows too concerned with *his* success or failure in helping others, or with the success or failure of the team in which he works, will find, in time, that his empathic skills suffer from over-concern with neat models, and predictable results.

The reason for this inverse ratio of scientific control to empathic skill lies in the elusive creative form of personal life. The personal form is not essentially an ego development as is concern with success and failure. The skills of empathy are *created* not in concern for the ego, but in concern for personal growth. Personal growth consists of experiences relating oneself to others, not in a relation of control by one over others, but in a relation between oneself and others. Neither ego, super-ego, nor id, nor any combination of them in subtler scientific models, can describe the personal form created by human beings in the practice of empathy. (Ego can, however, aptly describe our activities as scientists.) Empathic acts cannot be located neatly in single units of human beings, such that one is subject, the other, object. Empathic acts are interpersonal. The feelings of the other are required for the feelings of the one who performs the empathic act. The great paradox is that this intermingling through deliberate identification is what gives each of us his personal identity, inclusive of ego, super-ego, and id, and that "something more" essential to being a person, in which a human being strives to be free to be himself, to communicate with others, to respect them as he hopes he will be respected. This act includes techniques of science and of art, but goes beyond them in the religious nature of fellowship. This it is which obliges us to give clinical opinions and personal evaluation, and to refrain from any pretension to furnish statistics, known as "scientific", as that word is understood in the twentieth century.

But the problems posed to the conscientous scientist need not stand in the way of the clinician or the recovering patient. There are always *practical*, as distinct from theoretically perfect, clues to follow, in pursuit of recovery and in ways to improve this pursuit into lasting rehabilitation. Thus, we will not stay in the dark regarding our honest appraisals of what is helpful, what fails to work, and what changes to make when some technique fails to register its alleged worth. The best guide here is always the personal testimony of the patient (or therapist) in his appraisal of what helped *him*. Concern with failure is in order regarding awareness of his own private defect. But failure in ego activities is not important enough to warrant our primary attention in a context where personal problems are more pressing.

What is Addiction?

No one can say scientifically what addiction is, whether to alcohol, narcotics, tranquillizers or anything else. There is, however, no doubt about the seriousness of the problem, and there is no doubt about the effectiveness of treatment, when the addict has the desire to "recover".

I mean "recover" in a special sense, because freedom from addiction means much more than just recovery of a former state of health; it means also the experience of growth. In the whole person, growth is an action involving change of feeling and attitude towards oneself and others, an action amounting to a way of life, a practical philosophy applied to one's behaviour from day to day.

A philosophy or way of life is developed when a person makes intelligent plans about his behaviour based on conscious principles, techniques and goals. This is illustrated in the group therapy of Alcoholics Anonymous, where recovery and personal growth are well evidenced among those who sincerely follow their sobriety programme. A way of life, lived and practised, is what we usually understand by religion. Religion, thought about, is philosophy; philosophy lived is religion.

What are we to say about the prevalent belief that addiction is a sickness? There are three facts to face in the light of present knowledge, if our thinking about this problem is to be productive and sound:

Addiction is not, exclusively, a medical problem;
Addiction is not, exclusively, a psychological problem;
Addiction is not, exclusively, a social problem.

Any addict will tell you that medicine alone will not cure his illness. He may regain good physical health only to relapse. Many addicts report that they got in good shape the better to enjoy their next binge. Psychological insight, if it were the only required remedy, would enable addicts to resume their habit. The records show it is impossible for an addict to indulge with control, no matter how enlightened he may be about his emotional trouble, and no matter how well he may control his feelings. Social adjustment similarly fails to bring recovery, if it is thought that a suitable job, and harmonious social relations alone are the answer to alcoholism or the drug habit. Many socially satisfied patients I have known to deepen and worsen their problem. They report they "never had it so good." Then they relapse.

What do these facts tell us? First of all, the facts are no criticism of the valuable services provided by the three great disciplines. We need medicine, we need psychological counsel, we need social perception, where these services are relevant to the study, research and treatment of addiction. And we need them, too, in the great task of education for prevention.

But it is a great mistake to suppose that medicine, psychology and social work will by themselves solve the problem. You do not necessarily come up with a way of life when you add medicine, psychology and social work.

Something more is required than the insights of these three disciplines, valuable though they are in the treatment of addiction. That "something more" is a cohesive set of values melding and directing the facts revealed by the scientific disciplines. There are addicts, clever ones, who can use the facts to support and foster their addiction! One "wet" intellectual once told me that every time he came away from his therapist he had another reason to drink.

Though we cannot say precisely what addiction is, we can say what it is not. Addiction is not a way of life, although it may appear to be. No way of life, philosophy or religion, can be soundly built on a disorder revealing loss of control, impairment of brain activity, memory lapses and behaviour generally at odds with what the addict would otherwise desire. Still, the intensity of addiction and its invasion of the whole person in every aspect of his life resembles so much the intensity and pervasiveness of a genuine religion that we may, for practical purposes, call addiction a pseudo-religion. To be even more practical, we can call addiction a religious disorder.

In the addict there is deep and thorough devotion to the experiences of his drug, as in the genuine religionist there is deep devotion to a faith which yields the working values of a free sober life. The difference, however, is important. In the addict, the devotion is compulsive; in the religionist, when he is healthy, the devotion is free and deliberate. The condition necessary to the practice of religion is freedom. Freedom is what the alcoholic or drug addict conspicuously lacks. He is a slave to addictive behaviour. So addiction is a religious disorder if it is true that the impairment of personal freedom is its chief symptom.

What the addict who wants to recover must strive for, more than anything else, after he realizes he cannot be free alone, is a richer experience of personal freedom. This is far more important, in my experience as therapist, than anything he may learn from medicine, psychology or sociology. It is, of course, true that scientific facts can help him in his pursuit of sobriety, provided he has already developed some desire for the freedom which sobriety will give him.

How does the addict acquire his freedom? He begins to acquire freedom from addiction when he desires to be sober, and he will usually desire to be sober only when he realizes that in active addiction he has lost his freedom, lost his capacity to make choices and decisions because of slavery to his habituating drug. Without the desire to be sober, no amount of skilful instruction will bring him recovery. The most important act in the treatment of addiction is fostering the desire to be sober.

Negative teaching on the evils of addiction, the ruining of health, and the disgrace awaiting him induces fear and is worse than useless. Though addiction cannot be precisely defined, it is clearly a pattern of fear. So, more fear only worsens the addict's problem. Perhaps the most rewarding experience in therapy is the change you see registered in the addict when he comes to see sobriety as more attractive to him than his addictive pattern. To do this, I have used a common sense idea I call *personal thirst*.

By personal thirst I mean the desire to feel better, to be oneself, to be capable of mixing easily with others and to sense adventure and mystery not commonly known in the daily rounds. The essence of all this is the desire to feel free and easy. It is utterly natural in any vital person and there is nothing necessarily sick or abnormal about it. Up to the time he loses control and realizes that he is now sick, hung over and remorseful, the addict, in resorting to alcohol or drugs, innocently supposed he had found a way to satisfy his personal thirst.

In treatment he is encouraged to see that sobriety is a more attractive and rewarding response to personal thirst than drinking or taking drugs. The appeal must not be made on the grounds that sobriety gives more pleasure than addiction, because pleasure is the yard-stick he uses in pursuit of his addictive ends. The standards used in alcoholic drinking and bouts with drugs cannot be used in seeking sobriety, for the practical reason that pleasure, deliberately sought as a primary goal, usually leads to pain and misery.

What works best in fostering a desire to be sober is the promise the addict is going to be free! This makes personal freedom the main goal of recovery that endures and fosters personal growth. To become free and easy—the original healthy drive behind personal thirst—one needs others in fellowship, and fellowship is a human and practical aspect of religion. "I cannot be free alone" the addict discovers in his isolated and lonely bouts. Personal thirst is best satisfied through the good will and help of others. Good will is the condition of free will, and only in the capacity to exercise free choice, can man find real happiness.

The answer to the religious disorder of addiction, then, is genuine religion, as experienced in fellowship and in the recognition of a power transcending any of the individuals in the fellowship. This therapeutic truth is used most effectively by Alcoholics Anonymous. It is to be hoped that a similar group, Narcotics Anonymous, will flourish, in time, among drug adicts.

Another strong force in the effective recovery of addicts is the active capacity to put yourself in the other's place and thereby better understand both him and yourself. This is the technique of *empathy* and is at work constantly in Alcoholics Anonymous where is goes hand in hand with fostering fellowship.

I believe the modern clinic in the treatment of addictions is doing its best work when it recognizes the priority of personal freedom, fellowship and empathy over scientific controls and takes its direction accordingly. This does not imply criticism of the valuable work done by medicine, psychology and social work. It is a suggestion for a frank reappraisal of what constitutes the chief interest of those of us dedicated to solving the problems of addiction: the freeing of addicts in productive recovery, and the greater task ahead of prevention through education.

Addiction is a sickness, as the clinics and A.A. well know, but it is a sickness with a difference. This difference vitally involves impairment of the act of choice. Treatment must bring into play the practical role of religion, for religion in human practice is an adventure in freedom, only to be found and fostered in fellowship. Because addiction impairs the human capacity for making choices and brings about loss of control in many areas, I call it a religious disorder.

Addiction is a mystery for the same reason religion is a mystery. As there is always something unknown in religion, there must also be something unknown in a disorder marked by religious defect. I believe that no matter how far we go in science, and it is important that we go as far as we can, we will never rout the mystery that marks both addiction and the recovery that puts it right.

It is unfortunate that many people feel threatened by the term "mystery". It does not mean confusion but simply the recognition of a power greater than ourselves, although at work in and through ourselves. Mystery means recognition of human limits, and of the futility of human controls where those controls do not work. The human controls of medicine, social insight and psychology are necessary and useful, but something more needs to be understood in the experience of addiction and in freedom from it. This understanding requires (a) recognition of a power greater than oneself (b) a benevolent attitude toward one's fellowman and (c) self-realization.

Postulates of the Personal Treatment of Addicts

Though a man may grow to the stature of a person, he cannot forget the needs of his animal and human nature. The regulative—as distinct from the creative—task of personal life is indeed, to discipline one's animal and human tendencies, to make the best use of them as means to personal growth.

Therefore the necessary (as distinct from sufficient) condition of enduring health and of proportionate personal growth is optimum physical form. Other necessary, but alterable, conditions of personal growth, serving human needs, are the values of the community in which one lives—traditions, customs, morals, norms of power, of prestige, of sexual taboos and practices.

But physical and human needs serve the higher experiences of personal life. It is in the creative choiceful actions of a person that recovery from addiction is best assured, because addiction is a personal disorder.

This view of the nature of man as animal, human and personal, and the belief that addiction is a personal disorder involving physical, mental, social and religious problems, together constitute the basic ground of the personal treatment of addicts. This ground was gradually discovered in the course of studying and treating addicts over a period of ten years. It yields the following postulates.

1. *It is important to recognize addiction as a disorder in its own right*, in any personal treatment of it.

Emotional or social problems either precede addiction, or arise within it, and have therefore to be properly treated, but the addicting substance will always be the centre of reference. Similarly, physical defects are often associated with addiction, and must also be treated, but also with stress on the addicting substance which the disorder involves. ("By-passing" addiction does not mean underestimating its power. On the contrary, to "by-pass" means avoiding trouble out of an insightful respect for prospective dangers. The discussion on by-passing or forgetting addiction, in the group therapy, had, as its main purpose, insight into the futility of fighting addiction.) Problem drinking or "joy-popping" may be regarded as symptomatic with therapeutic advantage in the pre-disease stage, preceding loss of freedom, but when addiction is definite, the problem has developed into a disorder in its own right, in which the patient has lost his freedom to use alcohol or drugs with attendant disturbances in physical, mental and social behaviour.

2. First attention is given to the incapacity of the addict to drink, or use drugs, a sensitivity permanent and irreversible. The addict is physically incapable of indulging with control,

and often has to be treated for impairment to his health, as a result of indulging, whether or not he really wants lasting recovery. *Proper medical attention can help to make a patient receptive to instructions and psychotherapy in the pursuit of sobriety.* It is not categorically true that an addict "has to be ready" for sobriety. Much can be done to help him want to be ready. With proper timing, neither the therapist nor the patient needs to feel discouraged or frustrated. The addict, acutely or chronically ill, or both, responds readily to all approved techniques for rebuilding his health, restoring his energy, and providing proper rest and nutrition. Physical aids give him strong support at a time when he is not well enough to acquire the insight and to form the intentions which lead to lasting sobriety. It might be impossible or painful for him to resist indulging again were it not for the reliable conditioning of his depleted health by effective medical aids tactfully and kindly administered, at a crucial period in his addictive pattern. If he cooperates with the doctor and nurses, and he begins to improve physically, his mind clears and he can think more effectively about long-term recovery. There are justifiable instances in treatment when a patient's ability to know what is best for him is so confused and impaired that the qualified help of others can do much to restore to him a healthier state of reason and judgement.

3. *Psychotherapy in addictions is primarily concerned to communicate insight into the value of personal freedom, the necessary condition of personal life.* Personal freedom cannot be proved or controlled, but it can be illustrated, lived, imitated and created. A therapist is most effective when he can empathize the plight and problems of the patient.

By freedom is meant what most people understand by the word—the freedom to be oneself, to do as one pleases, and as one wants. Want is need, implies choice, and therefore personal values. The addict's personal freedom, as only he can understand it, is not curtailed by the lack of power to do something he does not want to do. Only the addict who

senses that his freedom is impaired can respond to treatment.
Thus, the best planned programme for recovery from addiction seeks above all, to reach the patient who neither admits
that he is disordered nor desires to recover. The decision of
the patient to remain as he is, to protect his need for alcohol
or drugs, or to recover, is personal. The meaning of his thirst
or craving, what he was and is striving for, has to become
clear in and for himself, in his own way. If sobriety is not
among his strivings, therapy is arrested until it is. Thus the
primary task of the therapist is to make the patient aware
that he is less free than he can be. This procedure cannot be
scientifically controlled because you cannot prescribe freedom. It is achieved through communication by invitation,
good will and testimony, in the growth of interdependent
personal relationships.

It is useful and necessary to communicate facts relevant
to the disorder and to recovery, but there is another value
worth noting about communication. This is *the way* in which
facts or ideals are communicated. In *testimony*, one person
wants to do something for another, over and above the
"cash" value of the experience communicated. A person
assumes the worth of what he says, and expresses himself
through trust in the other person. He relates something of
himself in an action which goes beyond scientific evidence
to a faith in anticipated change and growth. Testimony is
exchanged in an inviting climate. It requires a receiver as
well as a giver. One best offers testimony if, implicitly, he
feels as though he is invited to do so.

4. *Personal freedom, of which freedom from addiction is
but one example, is best illustrated in acts of empathy.* The
therapist, to communicate well and to deepen his own convictions about "the know-how" of sobriety, seeks to know
the plight of the patient, on the patient's own grounds. The
symbol, *personal thirst*, for example, is a term easily understood and felt by the alcoholic, *personal craving*, by the drug
addict. The patient is encouraged to do likewise, with respect to the therapist, in free imitation and in creating his

own pattern of sobriety. This mutual personal relation, grounded in goodwill and creating fellowship, is the act of empathy.

5. *Medicine, psychology and religion are interwoven in every phase of the personal treatment of addicts.* Medicine is concerned with the control of pain, psychology with the control of pleasure and pain, religion with the discipline of pleasure and pain and the expression of freedom in personal life. Medicine is the condition of treatment. The immediate pressing problems of physical impairment have first to be met, then there follows a sound programme of nutritional supplement, of rest, and of relaxation personally suited to the needs of the patient.

Psychology needs to take into account the physical state of the patient in dealing with emotional and social problems, the problem of pleasure as well as that of pain, and anticipates, at every move, the goal of freedom from disorder. Religion—the highest action of persons—requires a wise recognition of one's limits as revealed in physical or psychological disorders, and also in personal disorders, as, for example, in addiction. Creatively, religion is concerned to increase personal growth in pursuit of one's highest values. Whatever these are, they are best achieved through freedom, creative activity and fellowship. "One gains personal growth in and through the act of loving." Religion is the goal of treatment. (In this view, religion has therapeutic meaning. It can, and does, mean other, and more, than its working description in this statement. But religion and also medicine and psychology seem at least to embrace what I describe, though they may well mean more, in other contexts, and in the views of other people.)

Between the condition and goal of the personal treatment of addicts, there is the dynamic concept of a personal psychology intimating, in its role as mediary, that much more effort is required to assess its internal relation both to medicine and to religion. In this view, it is suggested that psychology, at least as therapy, has to incorporate within its discipline the religious core of personal growth as well as the scientific insight provided by medicine.

6. Throughout the above five postulates, it is obvious that freedom from addiction moves towards an active, sober way of life, in every conceivable avenue of behaviour. This is also the goal in the education for *prevention* of addiction. A consciously worked-out psychology of empathy is what will best serve our purposes in training youth for creative sobriety. This plan could begin in the high schools now. It will take years to plan for the use of empathy in primary grades.

Conclusion

The theme of this book, woven in and through the personal plight and sobriety of the alcoholic, can be basically useful in the treatment and programme of freedom of all types of addicts. If life-long sobriety is the goal of the alcoholic, then nothing less is required of all other addicts. I believe, too, that people with no addictive problems who are troubled by recurrent imitative behaviour of other sorts, may well find the book useful and suggestive. The techniques of empathy which release the alcoholic and drug addict can also release people hindered by other problems. These techniques will be amply illustrated throughout the book.

References:

1. Isbell, Harry: Bull. N.Y. Acad. Med. Dec. 1955, Vol. 31, No. 12, p. 897.
2. Nyswander, Marie: The Drug Addict As A Patient, Grune and Stratton, New York and London, 1956, p. 129.
3. Wikler, A.: Amer. J. Psychiat. 105: 329-38. Psychiat. Quart. 26: 270-93, 1952. Opiate Addiction, Charles Thomas, Publisher, Springfield, Ill. 1953.
4. Nyswander, Marie: Op. Cit., p. 44.
5. Lindesmith, A. R.: Opiate Addiction, Bloomington, Principia Press, 1947.
6. Maurer, David W., and Vogel, Victor H.: Narcotics And Narcotic Addiction, Charles C. Thomas, Springfield, Ill. 1954.
7. DeRopp, Robert S.: Drugs And The Mind, St Martins Press, New York, 1957.

8. Murtagh, Judge John M., and Harris, Sara: Who Live In Shadow, McGraw Hill, New York, 1959.
9. The Quarterly Journal of Studies on Alcohol: Yale University, 52 Hillhouse Avenue, New Haven.
10. The British Journal of Addiction: 93 Harley Street, London, W.2., England.
11. McCarthy, R. G. (editor): Drinking And Intoxication, Selected Readings in Social Attitudes and Controls, Yale Center of Alcoholic Studies, New Haven, 1959.

1.

WHY DO PEOPLE DRINK?

MOST people say they drink to feel better. It isn't that simple. We eat, sleep, play, fight, work and love, to feel better.

Why alcohol?

Herodotus, the father of history, records that drinking and drunkenness were going on two thousand years ago. Even then there were those who could take it or leave it alone, and those who became drunkards.

There have been moderate drinkers all through the ages who had no problems and suffered no ill effects. Most drinkers are moderate. You are fortunate if you are one of them.

Yes, it is true. People drink simply "to feel better", alcoholic, occasional drinker or social drinker. But let's be more definite. For every kind of drinker alcohol has certain short-lived attractions. What are these?

(a) Alcohol dulls the pain of disagreeable duties, of personal relations.

(b) It eases tense nerves and tense situations.

(c) It relieves tiredness.

(d) It releases pent-up hostile feelings.

(e) As some people find it difficult to be mature at all times they seek release from grown-up behaviour. Once in a while they want to be childish. Alcohol does the trick.

(f) Some people seek social approval through drinking.

They believe they are more warmly accepted if they drink. "The men and women of distinction" idea is related here to the false belief that "all the best people drink". Alcohol is a quick temporary cover-up of shyness and feelings of inferiority.

All people drink for one or more of the above reasons in wanting to feel better.

For the majority of drinkers a few drinks seem to ease a tense situation, whatever it may be. To loosen up a stiff party, to ease the worry and strain of a hard day's work, to banish shyness, to dull the anxieties of a high-pressure civilization—all these situations are eased by a few drinks. People relax their tense feelings and for a little while forget their troubles.

The drinking habit persists in society because most people seem able to control it. Society puts the stamp of approval on a custom that helps men to ease the strain of civilized living. People value the order and security that society provides, and they pay for this discipline in the control of their natural impulses. But sometimes personal impulses conflict with the prosaic customs of society. This conflict creates a strain. Alcohol, among other means, is an outlet.

In our country, early Indian tribes, like us, found an outlet in alcohol. When drunk they quarrelled, murdered, assaulted their loved ones, and destroyed their property. They repeated the same words over and over again, as they dissipated hours on end. They abused themselves as well as others, inflicting bodily harm on their own persons. All this very rarely happened when they were sober.

Today these actions take other but similar forms when "civilized" men get drunk. There are happy drunks—sometimes—but just as often there are those who criticize abusively, who repeat boringly the same ideas like children learning new words, who indulge in self-pity and go on crying jags. The happy drunk very often is not seen in the other stages of his binge when suddenly he may turn morose, sulk and retire into a shell of loneliness.

The sensible drinker, of course, knows when to stop. He has control over his drinking. He is well disciplined.

All the advantages of civilized living, homes, jobs, entertainment, the getting and using of food and clothes, the orderly business of living in all phases is paid for in discipline.

The tension between natural impulses and social customs urges us to control our impulses in the interests of long range satisfactions. We must not give in to the sexual drive when it starts to assert itself. The customs of marriage and of the family forbid it. All through adolescence and early adulthood, the sex drive must be disciplined until we are able financially and socially to get married.

The impulse to injure those who stand in our way must be curbed in civilized living. So we apologize to a person who steps on our toes, though the impulse, from away back, might be to strike him.

We do not steal the food we need from the grocer. Society has decided in favor of a more orderly method of exchange.

Civilized living is a disciplined living. We want all its comforts. The price we pay for them is the discipline of animal impulses.

A tension develops between selfish desires and social customs. This tension is natural if we look at the problem maturely. It is like a business deal. We examine the merchandise. We want it, so we pay the price. So with living. We examine what society expects of us. We see what we shall get if we pay the price. We shall have its protection and care if we act on its rules.

Some people pay the price willingly. They experience no conflict in living as society wants them to live. They have no need of drugs, of stimulants, or any other form of pain killer. Then there are those who feel a little strain, who enjoy a drink or two to ease their mild pains of adjustment.

These are the people who can drink socially, whose control never permits drunkenness. Very often these people enjoy coffee or tea more than a highball. Liquor does not fascinate them any more than a soft drink or a bowl of soup. They do not *need* alcohol.

Then there is that large class that can be called the problem drinkers. Many of them are not alcoholics—not yet, but they can easily qualify, if they continue to drink. At parties they always drink a little too much. They do not make fools of themselves, they do their jobs well, they are kind to their families and associates. But they are conspicuous around the punch-bowl, they laugh a little too loud. You can't help feeling they are trying to cover something up. They are inclined to be "hangoverish", though they always get to the office in the morning. Somewhere they have heard, "Never take a drink in the morning", so they suffer it out until noon. Others say "I never take a drink until sundown". They say it a little too often and with too much conviction.

This class of drinker includes those who find the price of civilized living too high. They have clashes in sober living that unduly disturb them. They easily grow tense. In their discovery of alcohol they found a quick release of their worries and strains. They turn to it now with a sort of fascination. They are getting to need it in order to make life bearable. Out of this class develops the alcoholic. The drinkers of this class, like all other drinkers, drink in order "to feel better". In the early stages, even the most intelligent alcoholics never suspect what a boomerang their indulgence will later turn out to be. Like the early Indians, they regard their drinking as a great sport while drunk. They know better when they sober up, but they return to alcohol compulsively, as though they could not be reasonable about their problem. And there is the truth of the matter. The alcoholic has no control over his drinking.

Alcoholics form a minority group among drinkers. It is

unfair to irritate the mature citizen who can drink sensibly by moralizing on the "evils" of alcohol. It is also unfair to threaten his right to drink.

But the intelligent moderate drinker will surely agree that alcoholism is a problem, that problem drinking merits the concern of an enlightened community. If you can drink that's your business. But there is a friend of yours who can't. Whose business is that? Anyone who is sick deserves help from some one. Perhaps he does not want help. It's a free country. But if he is seeking help, you can do him a great service in recognizing that alcoholism is a sickness and that it can be treated effectively *if the alcoholic wants to get well.* Your understanding of the problem can do much to encourage him and give him hope.

Problem Drinking

For the alcoholics a few drinks are a joke. They must have the prize in the bottom of the bottle. The fact that they take more than a couple of drinks is proof that they defeat the very purpose of drinking—the easing of tense feelings. They don't ease tension, they make it worse. They are really "tight" whether drunk or not. Their guilt, remorse and worry, their loss of jobs, their waste of money, their damaging of health make the problem of tension more than they can bear. They either stop drinking or drink themselves to death.

Any drinker *may* become an alcoholic if he:—
Drinks to get drunk or "feel high".
Drinks to relieve tiredness, as a habit.
Drinks to escape worry and a job he doesn't want to do.
Drinks because he is shy and simply must have something for the party.
Drinks the price of the bottle that should help to pay bills.
Drinks rather than attend a movie, game or some other pastime he enjoys.

Drinks a morning "eye-opener".

Drinks alone.

Any one or more of these reasons for drinking may create an alcoholic. In healthy use, alcohol is never taken to produce drunkenness. After the drinker takes a 2-oz. drink of standard whiskey or the like, every extra "lift" *within the hour* lets him down twice as hard. This kind of drinking causes the hangover. The hang-over paves the way to alcoholism.

The alcoholic, or the person in danger of becoming one, should totally abstain. There is no half-way solution. For the alcoholic moderation is a joke, but abstinence is within his reach. "Abstinence is as easy to me as temperance would be difficult." In these words, Samuel Johnson recognized that he was an alcoholic. Abstinence for the alcoholic means health; indulgence means sickness of body, of mind, of spirit. Alcoholism is a disorder of the whole person.

The active alcoholic is a person known to drink an amount sufficient to classify him as one "under the influence"; on some occasions he becomes drunk, though he does not always plan to do so. The alcoholic is sometimes able to take a few drinks and stop at that point. But in the evidence of many alcoholics, they do not know, beforehand, whether they can stop after a drink or two, or proceed compulsively to reach a state of intoxication. Briefly, the alcoholic has no control over his drinking.

The chronic alcoholic is one who, from long and excessive use of alcoholic drinks, develops certain mental and physical changes. The physical condition of the chronic alcoholic makes him more susceptible to certain ailments, often nutritional diseases and sometimes pneumonia or heart disorders. He has a shorter average life than the moderate drinker or abstainer.

In this brief chapter *Why People Drink* I have tried to show that there is no issue in sensible drinking. This is no plea for either the wets or drys. The problem to face is alcoholism. The suggestion here is that all intelligent citizens whether "dry" or "wet", for prohibition or against it, will profit by looking at the alcohol problem in the clear light of the facts.

A scrutiny of the alcoholic's problems will reveal many valuable facts about human nature, quite apart from alcohol altogether.

Alcoholism becomes a disorder in its own right. But in early drinking it is also a symptom of many troubles that you may recognize as your own! What helps the alcoholic may, then, help you, though you are a moderate drinker or even a teetotaller.

2.

THE DRINKING PATTERN
OF THE ALCOHOLIC

HERE is Allen, the potential alcoholic at the age of twenty. He likes people but he is sensitive and self-conscious. He wants to be liked and is afraid he won't be. He is at a party, the drinks are passed and after two or three cocktails he feels a warm glow. His tensions and fears fade away, self-confidence rides high. He talks easily, laughs and mixes without strain among the guests. He moves now on enchanted ground.

For about five years this is the kind of party Allen enjoys in the company of his friends, most of whom seem to drink as he does. But gradually he begins to look for drinking occasions.

Allen, at the age of twenty-five, finds himself moving from one party to another, from one companion to another. Without noticing it he is drinking much more than any of his friends or associates.

Now his outlook changes. He is dimly aware that he is not drinking like others. He sneaks many of his drinks. He comes to the party "fortified", carrying a pint in his pocket. He does not admit his drinking pattern has changed.

Why? He vaguely realizes he is no longer a normal drinker. He has something to hide. His guilt deepens, yet he continues to drink like a small boy setting out on a forbidden adventure.

Here appear the signs of his underlying personality disturbance, which centre round six qualities. He is dependent; he is sensitive; he is idealistic. He is impulsive; he is intolerant; he is given to wishful thinking. These six qualities reveal themselves more clearly the more he drinks. He becomes displeased whenever he is opposed; he sneaks his drinks as a boy steals cookies. He feels guilty, growing more sensitive as he becomes more aware of his rebellious behaviour. Allen is no longer a "social drinker".

He makes alibis for his excesses, building a fantastic structure of wishful thinking around his frequent flights from life. He seeks new friends who drink as he does. Confronted by his former friends he feels small, inadequate and resentful. Released from responsibility by alcohol, he reverts to childish ways and dreams. He longs for the affection he had as a child or for the affection he did not have as a child. This reversion to childishness goes on through fantasy or in the unconscious mind till Allen actually reaches an infantile level. He is alarmed to discover, after a drinking bout, that he has wet the bed and lost control over his bowels. His wife spoke truer words than she knew when she remarked that his recent passout reminded her of a helpless baby.

"Yes," Allen may reflect, "I have been having blank spells lately and I forget what I've said and done." But Allen does not yet see the stark fact that drinking for him is dangerous, if not deadly. Conscious of society and its disapprovals, he still values his job and loves his family. In this stage there are the signs of a new process distinct from the former gay social pattern, a process in its own rights, a bond of loyalty between the drinker and alcohol. Alcohol has gripped Allen, mind, soul and body. No other consideration competes with the demands it makes on him; nothing else really matters. But he struggles feebly against this slavery, still conscious of other forces in his life, his friends, his family, his job, the nostalgia of lost interests. So he compromises. He declares a truce in the form of alibis and goes on drinking. As the alibi system grows more elaborate, as he becomes an expert liar, he builds on his sensitive nature a heap of anxiety and fear, only to learn that his wishful thinking and lame excuses save him from precious few difficulties, that his lying is acceptable only because his hearers are either indulgent or indifferent. When he is sober now, he is guilt-ridden and insecure. "I am no good," he says, "I have no friends. I can't trust anyone." In moods like these he indulges heavily, no longer able to stop after a couple of drinks. Will power? It is a joke.

At thirty, he recalls that he handled his liquor quite well about eight years ago. What has happened? Where did his control get out of hand? It is hard for him to realize that his drinking was out of hand from the time he took his first highball.

During one of these tense morbid moods, he becomes very drunk. Suddenly the world is at his feet and he towers above every situation. He is alone, but he feels kindly towards everyone. He feels the urge to expand. He calls a taxi and goes to a nightclub where the patrons and the waiters enjoy his drinks and tolerate his talkative moods. He spends his money and departs, leaving a tip for the waiter in folding change, his last dollar. Back at home, he has another drink and decides to phone his old friend, a thousand miles distant. He does not know how he got to bed. In the morning he is bewildered and resentful. Jack, he hazily recalls, did not seem to appreciate the noble gesture that will run to about fifteen dollars on the phone bill.

In his hang-overs Allen begins to suspect people of trying to persecute and harm him, so guilty has he become in the mixed variety of his alibis, and so sensitive to the slightest sign that he is being ridiculed or criticized. These mounting suspicions make him arrogant and resentful in his misery. He reaches the stage where *he drinks away the symptoms of drinking*[1], and he climbs on the vicious treadmill of the full-fledged alcoholic.

But, now, who can say that it is the personality disturbance made worse in the drinking pattern, or the susceptibility of the body craving the morning drink, or the guilt induced by social disapproval that is behind the compulsive urge of the alcohol in this stage? Surely it is not one factor but all three mixed in one jumbled process. A vague uneasiness of mind, a definite worry, an unexpected joy, a social pressure, may start Allen on that first drink, leading so often to drunkenness. He has now, many mornings, that awful feeling of dryness—the water in the cells of his body is drawn into the spaces between them. The disordered distribution of water, his disturbed nerves, and upset stomach crave the anaesthetic of a soothing "eye-opener". These physical discomforts together create a physical compulsion to drink again. But this physical compulsion does not operate alone. There is also an uneasiness mixed with the physical discomfort, adding to the compulsion and strengthening it. The personality disturbance, with its tensions and conflicts, set him off on his drunk; his dryness, disturbed water balance, frayed nerves and upset stomach complicated by remote personality trouble touch it off again in the morning. But the physical need, though for the moment satisfied, only makes the mind more confused, and now the physical craving joins with the confused "mind", whose control is decreased through depression of the central system, to want more and more to drink. So runs the vicious circle.

Allen drinks away the symptoms of drinking, which induce worse symptoms and longer drunks. He is dismayed and once again appeals to his alibi system. "I'll drink only gin, or rum or whiskey with cream." When this fails, he decides that geography has something to do with it. There is just enough truth in this belief to deceive him into thinking his new scheme will work. He says to himself, "I'll drink only in Ottawa or Montreal, but not in my own home town." The geography alibi works for about six months but fails miserably when he finishes a binge started in Montreal in his own office.

At his wit's end, at the bottom of the alibi barrel, he says, "I will be resolute. I will drink only at certain times of the year. I will go on a keg, behave during the months preceding my vacation, Christmas, and New Year's, and have my bouts without damage to anyone." This last alibi also fails because the dry periods become unendurable. So many kegs are broken that control is finally seen to be hopeless. Life is unbearable when he is dry, he passes out when he is drunk. He is definitely anti-social now, withdrawn into himself when drinking. He begins the furtive lone drinking routine. The pattern started in a gay and friendly social way, back in those rosy days of the first drinks. Now he is unutterably lonely and at peace only when he passes out. The end is death; life is either dull or frighteningly ugly when he is sober. It is oblivion when he is drunk. His last, almost forgotten alibi comes to him, an alibi more honest but less satisfying than all the others. He says, "I am different, I need alcohol; though it brings me nothing but grief, it kills my pain for a while." In his sober periods he has nameless fears and vague feelings of guilt and persecution which he cannot identify with any one person or thing.

He is beginning to suspect that the fault somehow lies within himself. He has lost his scapegoats. Pain, physical and mental, becomes so uncomfortable and the tension so great that to relieve the distress is his main concern, even if to kill the pain means death itself. Formerly he lost only Monday morning after a week-end party. Now it is three or four days at a time, a week or two, even a month if he can arrange it. He no longer pretends that there are pleasant reasons to drink. Drinking is now clearly negative as Allen drinks only to forget and pass out.

He finally comes to choose between life and death, between complete abstinence and hell. He sees himself now as poverty-stricken spiritually, if not materially. It does not matter if he still has money and financial security. He is sick at heart.

"The bum's life," he reflects, "is at least spiritually honest. If I choose it, I become frank and sincere and avoid the pain of hypocrisy, deceit and the hopeless fight with society. As a drunken bum I can commit suicide slowly, without having to use a knife or jump into the river.

"On the other hand, I can try to regain the simple pleasures of the healthy life, face myself, accept myself and do right by other people, by decent folk whose company I once enjoyed so much. The drive to live is so strong I must stop questioning it and stop fighting it. I'm tired. I can fight no longer in this losing battle. No one, not even the scientists, can prove that life is good and sweet. The nearest to such proof is that noble and good people persist in living against the greatest odds. Life is not all a pleasant escapade; actually there must be difficulty and pain to sharpen the meaning of good things. The finest people we know, those who inspire the rest of us, are often those whose lives have been enriched by struggle and tragedy."

So Allen decides in favour of living, with its sorrows as well as its joys. He chooses life and rehabilitation. He remembers the story of all attempted suicides who, having failed in their attempts to die by their own hand, tell us that in the moment when death seemed sure, they suddenly revolted, reversed all their negative decisions, and strove with every fibre of their being to stay alive.

"I'll stop running away," he says, "from job after job, I'll try to mend this wrecked body, and I'll try to regain the normal happiness and peace of mind of sober living. While I am about it, as the struggle seems so worthwhile, I shall look into myself and do something about that person who must have been disordered and confused from the time he took his first drink. I must seek not just a cure for wrecked nerves and a damaged body, not a glib program on how to win friends and mix with people. I must seek a new way of life because only a whole new pattern covering myself, society and the world is big enough to redirect and transform disorders and pains brought on or aggravated by my compulsive drinking."

After learning that no one can fight the battles of life alone, that no doctor can hand him the solution to his problem in a package of pills or bottle of medicine, he resolves, soberly, to examine all the people of his acquaintance who suffer as he does; when he has done that, he will return to himself and see how much the others are like him, how much the others differ from him. "In this way," he reasons, "I'll find out all I can about the problem and so learn how to cope with it."

He finds from his own observations and with the help of a few good books on alcoholism from the library[2], that he can classify his heavy drinking friends into about eight types.

There was Bill. Now there seems to have been some excuse for poor Bill. He suffered from the after effects of infantile paralysis. But for a long time before he died, Bill stopped drinking because, as he said, drink had become more important to him than the relief he got from his pain. So important did it become that he drank even when his paralysis did not disturb him. He saw, in the last stages of his drinking, that the habit had grown from medicinal use to addiction, that all the good things in his life were damaged in alcohol. So Bill resolved to quit drinking, and even suffer at times, in order to regain his peace of mind and to enjoy, when he could, the pleasures of healthy sober living. Bill was what the scientists call the pain-killer type of alcoholic.

Alice and Jim are two very bored people, though they are intelligent and well-bred. Neither seems able to enjoy friends or amusements; neither seems able to feel deeply about anything, pleasant or unpleasant. They are blase. They move from one interest to another, one club to another, one friend to another, restless, dejected, and empty-hearted. The masks they wear for faces are growing blank. There is nothing in their minds and souls but the need to get away from themselves. They knock themselves out in the vain hope that what they can't find here, they will find there until lately it appears that the goal of their weak strivings is always a drink and then more drinks until they become numb and forget why they are living at all.

Harry is a college graduate, intelligent, nervous and idealistic. He cannot reconcile the standards of everyday living with his high hopes and perfectionist ideas. He is disillusioned because the world as it is does not click with his views of what it ought to be. Never has he been able to secure the job he thinks he deserves; lately he has been working with a firm that does not require college graduates. He broods over this as he complains about the injustice of his employers. Women, according to him, fall short of what they should be. He seems to nurse a fantastic ideal about women that he developed in his high school years and appears to forget that women are human beings in many ways sharing the short-comings of men like himself. Harry is a discordant drinker who drowns his worries and forgets his tense ideals when intoxicated. In drinks he forgets his high thoughts, and grows confident of abilities he does not believe in when he is sober. The trouble with Harry is that though he loses fear and grows confident when drinking, his actual performance is cheapened—a performance that you somehow believe would be good if he had the courage to face it when sober. Lately, Harry, in his hangovers, has been looking and probably feeling more inferior than ever. When he drinks now, he tends to talk bigger than he did in the past as though he were trying to make up in grandiose ideas what he lacks in the ability even to think about when he wakes up the next morning.

A friend of Harry's is George, clearly a pampered fellow, a spoilt son. He started drinking to be sociable, but now he drinks on the side and almost always gets drunk at parties. He has a rather good job and has no financial worries. He stopped drinking once for a year because Mary, his wife, a very strong-willed person, threatened to leave him if he ever took another drink. Well, George took that other drink while Mary was visiting her mother, and Mary kept her promise for a time. But she is back with him now in alternate moods of indulgence and anger, and he still drinks. It looks as though he will always drink until he decides to quit for his own sake. As a child and as a husband he has been pampered so much that all his activities seem to hinge on what those closest to him think and on how they will react.

Misbehaviour is impulsive; he makes snap decisions and is intolerant of anyone who criticizes him in the slightest degree. His mother thinks he is the most wonderful boy in the world—"Poor George," she will say, "Mary, you know, has never understood him." Because others have indulged him so long, he cannot stand stress of any kind. The least difficulty serves as a reason to take a drink. The concern of his wife and of his mother he seems in a perverted way to enjoy. It is a sort of parental care such as he had when he was a little boy. Indulgence he must have, though it means getting drunk to have it. George seems to be one of the fellows you can kill with kindness. Personally a likeable chap, he needs to stand on his own feet and make up his own mind about his life and what it means. When he sees this, he may quit drinking.

Perc is an office clerk whose drinking bouts include a group of listeners gullible enough to hear his tales about the big shot—himself. Each time you see him he has a new plan for changing the business. If he had his way the firm would flourish and grow rich in a matter of months. At the office, when he is sober, the office boy laughs at him, and at home he is a tyrant. In drink, Perc can be what he wants to be. He is a self-aggrandizing drinker. His poor cramped life craves attention and prestige. It never occurs to him that alcohol only makes him a laughing stock among everyone except those for whom he buys drinks. His narrow outlook has nothing to do with his job, his family or his friends. He needs outlets other than his work; he needs to get over the obsession that some people are superior, some inferior to him. Perc's pride is too much for him. If Perc would soften and learn to laugh at himself, the office boy would stop poking fun at him, and he'd be able to enjoy his family without dictating to them, and his friends without trying to impress them. But Perc won't learn to laugh at himself until he quits drinking. "I know," thought Allen to himself, "as well as any alcoholic, that the drunk can't take a joke."

About four years ago Ned's wife died. Since then his drinking has grown steadily worse until now he is a sorry spectacle as he mopes despondently in his cups. Ned just can't take his loss. His wife was his whole existence; now that she is gone, there seems to be nothing to live for. He needs to see that life must go on in spite of tragedy and bereavement. And who can give him the encouragement and cheer he needs so much? Perhaps recovered drunks can help him, thought Allen. He has to stop feeling sorry for himself. He should recover because Ned never took a drink before his wife died. Ned is a situational drinker.

Situational drinkers of another sort are the war veterans who became alcoholics under severe stress and strain, boys who never took a drink before they enlisted, but under the unnatural conditions of war drank to forget what they missed most, their homes, sweethearts and peace time values.

Finally there are the periodic drinkers. Don is one of them. Reserved, undemonstrative, kind but pent-up, sensitive, and unable to say what he most truly feels. He is a hard worker and a successful business man but some day he is going to die in one of his frightful prolonged binges. He may be sober for months, even years, and then he breaks forth in what must be truly a sickness because he gets no fun at all out of his drinking. Strangely enough, he seems to go off the deep end in one or other of two extreme moods. At the height of some success, some favorable business deal, he will plunge; in the depths of worry, in a crisis, he will do the same. The periodic drinker is a serious alcoholic and seems to need something to pierce his outward shell, and plumb to the depths of his personality. If Don could only open up, relax, and share his life more intimately with his family and friends, it might help to save him from an early death.

"All these are drinkers I have seen and know. How, now,"

thought Allen, "can I relate all these types of drinkers to myself?"

It shocks him to discover, in his honesty, that all alcoholics share certain tendencies, no matter how much they may differ as persons in their drinking behaviour. He sees that he is like them all in many respects. "All of us," he notes, "are childish, sensitive, grandiose, impulsive, intolerant and given to wishful thinking. Now these qualities appear to be the mark of many non-alcoholics as well as us." So Allen looks more intently at the pattern. He concludes that the alcoholic is anyone who drinks to get drunk, and who often gets drunk whether he wants to or not.

He notes that alcoholics have no control over their drinking. "The non-alcoholics who share the personality defects that we have are able to control them more effectively than we do. They do not run the dangerous risk of expressing them in the letting down of control as we do. The prime disappointment that we alcoholics face is that not one of the things we seek in drink is ever realized. In fact, our needs grow more urgent, more painful. The period of early deception passes." Insight into his sickness comes when Allen realizes that alcohol worsens his pain, it does not ease it. He sees his alcoholic life as a path to suicide—a long drawn out self-inflicted death. This is the result when drinking becomes compulsive.

Some theories assert that alcohol affords release from the burden of some repressed tendency or of some emotional conflict; they add up to the theory of escape and compensation. Briefly, a man drinks to get away from his troubles or to gain in fancy what he is denied in fact. The six qualities of the alcohol personality revolve around this theory of escape and compensation in which alcohol serves to remove the pain of inhibitions, and to fulfill deep needs.

Other theories stress physical causes for drinking in the hope that science can reveal some definite weakness in the body which accounts for the alcoholic's inability to handle alcohol in much the same way that diabetics cannot handle sugar.

A third group of theories stress social customs and morals as the main cause of alcoholism.

These three groups of theories, though different in many respects, are alike in one main belief. *There is nothing for the alcoholic but complete abstinence whether the cause is mental, physical or social or all three.*

For scientific purposes, we seek the theory that suits most cases best. For practical purposes, we seek the personal pattern that best describes the person who is suffering.

We must remember that alcoholics are individuals whose problems are intensely personal. We are wise to be open-minded about science in its search for greater certainty, for "rules" that apply to all alcoholics alike. But we are also wise to note that alcoholics come under the "rules" in different ways, each by the path from his personal background, and lighted by problems uniquely his own.

Personality troubles when not faced head on, realistically, take refuge in various kinds of escapes known as neuroses. All neuroses are unrealistic, negative and destructive unless properly channeled and creatively expressed. At the basis of most neuroses or escapes is the desire for love and self-protection. A lack of affection drives the neurotic to selfish outlets such as drinking. But drinking fails to satisfy the need for love. Actually it makes the need more urgent. A clue for the alcoholic here is that he must learn how to regard love and affection maturely, as giving as well as receiving. Love maturely understood is in harmony with life. When it is not maturely understood it is destructive. The alcoholic's notion of love is destructive and selfish as long as he drinks.

On the other hand, if a man knows that he has a physical defect that is made worse by drinking and continues to drink, he can be sure of only poor health and a short life.

Therefore excessive drinking seems to be a denial of life, though the addict may not be consciously aware of it. It is often a living death, isolated as the alcoholic is from friends, pleasures, the beauty of the world about him, and the joy of healthy living.

In the next chapter, we shall try to analyze the personality of Allen and of all alcoholics. "If you expect to be healed you must first discover your wounds."

FOOTNOTES — CHAPTER 2

1. Dr. E. M. Jellinek at the Yale School of Alcohol Studies, Fort Worth, July, 1949, expended the theme suggested by his use of this apt expression.
2. See *Alcohol Addiction And Chronic Alcoholism*, E. M. Jellinek, Yale University Press, 1942, pp. 16-49. Also *Alcohol Explored*, H. W. Haggard and E. M. Jellinek. Doubleday, 1942, pp. 156-164.

3.

THE ALCOHOLIC—
WHAT SORT OF PERSON IS HE?

Hundreds of years before Christ, a man walked the streets of Athens, talking with young and old, rich and poor, prying into the secrets and problems of living. He had no pretensions and no prejudices: his mind was open to all subjects and to all persons eager to learn the central lesson of good living. That lesson was and is "The unexamined life is not worth living." "Let us be sure," said Socrates, "before we go on to other problems, that we know ourselves."

A man will think twice before he buys a car, a house, a pair of shoes or even a necktie, but it's surprising how he may never think twice about the most important thing in his life—the little acts, thoughts and desires that go to make up his personal happiness and stillness of spirit. These are the most important because what a man does, thinks and desires is what he is. If a man is a real human being he will find out that his life is personal and just a bit different, if not a lot different, from every other person; this difference, this personal identity, comes from within. That is why no man can buy sobriety or peace of mind. Anything that a man can buy is not really his own. Somebody may steal his car in the night, he may buy the best psychiatric care available, but the best attention that money can buy will not keep him sober, though it may restore him to health temporarily. "The best things in life are free." They do not cost money, for money only secures goods not our own. The best things are free because all we have to do is make up our minds to have them. With genuine thought and desire they can be ours. "Ask and it shall be given you, seek and you shall find, knock and it shall be opened unto you."

How can a man find out what he wants, what he can get, what he can hope for, to make his life worth while? A store clerk is powerless to help you, if you stand before him and tell him nothing. You cannot get what you do not know you want. Yet how many thousands of us are like the speechless customer before a bewildered clerk! We make a satisfactory deal with a store clerk when we tell him what our material needs are; we make a satisfactory deal with ourselves when we know not only our material needs but our spiritual needs as well. The psychiatrists tell us that the difference between a disturbed personality who recovers and one who doesn't is the difference between the man who knows what is wrong and the one who doesn't have a clue; they call it insight. He who has insight may recover; he who lacks insight remains disturbed until he gets it. The man who knows he has an alcoholic problem and must do something about it is a man who sees the dawn of insight.

In achieving insight all alcoholics will agree that the abuse of alcohol is their major defeat; around their addiction to alcohol revolve six defective qualities of the mind. An analysis of these six qualities should help the alcoholic, or anyone in danger of becoming one, to understand his problem better. The alcoholic is dependent, sensitive, idealistic; he is impulsive, intolerant and given to wishful thinking.

Dependent

The alcoholic will likely discover that he has been too dependent throughout his life on some person—perhaps his father, his mother, a brother, a sister or some admired friend. He may find that he has been afraid to make up his own mind because it has usually been made up for him.

Alcoholism has often been promoted by the vain effort of a pampered son to break away from the chains that bind him, but drink tightens rather than loosens the attachment he tries to break. In this tendency we find part of the cause of that label alcoholics so often get: emotional immaturity. They have failed to grow emotionally because somewhere in their background there were forces that made them feel insecure, incompetent and child-like when they set out to face a problem alone. This, too, helps to explain why they are essentially a lonely class of people. It also explains, perhaps, why they resented advice about their drinking habits; they resented reminders that they should grow up and act sensibly. The tragedy was that they simply could not grow up until they got insight into their trouble, the insight that they were far too dependent on someone, too sure that that "some one" would pull them out of their scrapes, no matter how bad they were.

Drink clearly aggravates the problem of dependence. If I am dependent on you and I get drunk at the wrong time I am even more dependent on you than ever. No amount of rude awakenings will change the alcoholic, however, until he gets the proper insight. Once the pattern of dependence is set, say in childhood or youth, it takes a long time for the alcoholic, no matter how intelligent he is, to see himself for what he is, a deeply dependent person. This he may not see, though he has been fired a hundred times from jobs and cast aside just as often by fed-up friends. Probing deeper into this childish quality, one may see how it effects one's sex life and sets up a pattern of fear in the mind of the alcoholic.

As a result of the sex act, a human being begins life as part of his mother. As an infant his mother remains the closest object of affection and of usefulness to him in his needs. He can easily become spoiled and pampered, waited on and catered to, unless he is taught to be self-reliant and to manage for himself. A pattern of dependence may develop and persist unless he senses and understands the need to grow up, emotionally as well as physically. This pattern may even persist in married life where the wife actually plays the role of a substitute mother. The pampered person knows only how to be loved and to be possessed, on the level of a child. On the other hand, a child may be too often ignored and rejected by a stern parent. Unlike the spoilt child, the rejected one becomes defiant and aggressive, determined to master rather than be mastered, to possess rather than be possessed. He thinks of love objects as conquests to overcome in which he is the victor. Here you find your Don Juans and seductive sirens whose love experiences are selfish, child-like contests aggressively to be waged and won.

What is the common quality in the childishness of the submissive and the aggressive types? It is insecurity, a form of fear. All human beings strive for security; when it is threatened they become fearful. The whole personality becomes the scene of conflicts and tensions when either the submissive or the aggressive person begins dimly to realize that he has nothing to offer but pleas for attention. He is insecure because deep within himself he feels the need of self-honesty and the urge to grow up. He will remain tense and insecure as long as he fails to understand the meaning of mature love. Neither the desire to be loved nor the desire to be possessive completes the full-fledged love relationship. Love, on a mature level, embraces gentleness and tenderness both in giving and receiving, in all manner of life's situations as well as in the sex act. There is no place in mature love for passive dependence on a mother or mother substitute in a wife or in alcohol or in both. There is similarly no place in mature love for one sided exploits of mastery.

In both the passive and the defiant alcoholic there is an immaturity, a childishness which will persist until it is seen that adult love is a mutual relationship in which man and wife both give and receive freely of themselves, in genuine affection shorn of the long forgotten desire to be owned by Mother or to be the strongest kid in the neighbourhood. One thing I wish here to make clear. The alcoholic is not to suppose that he should not have strong friends, strong loves. That would be fatal, for the alcoholic is a naturally friendly and loving person. The problem of attachment is stressed only because it is injurious to the alcoholic if he leans or depends excessively upon the attention of others. His friendliness and love need to be disciplined into both giving and receiving.

Sensitive

Hand in hand with the alcoholic's insecurity is his touchiness. In his suspicious mind he feels persecuted. In a tense, defiant mood, he is ever on the alert to abuse from others. Do you recall, if you are an alcoholic, how anxious you were when your wife left a telephone number with you, or a message about someone who called to see you, how you wondered "What have I done now?" And you would brace yourself, get into a defensive mood, and prepare to launch an attack on your imagined oppressor. This sensitive, persecuted attitude was made worse after each fresh session of remorse, after succeeding hang-overs, until you became guilty about most of your actions whether associated with drinking or not. This guilty feeling made you sensitive, touchy and set you worrying often about what others think. In calm, sober moments of self-assessment it's amazing to learn that few people bother to think about you at all! Other people have their own troubles, their own headaches: they have no time really to bother about you; when they do, the problem is usually theirs, not yours.

Idealistic

Listen to tavern conversation late on a Saturday afternoon to learn that the alcoholic is a fellow with grandiose ideas.

Major Hoople would look like a meek performer in the midst of such verbal aggression. One chap is going to reform the government, another has a plan for a new weapon that some stupid expert is too short sighted to give the Defence Department; the local news reporter has put all artists and writers in their respective places. An old scholar sails "the wine dark sea" and explains how Homer just missed greatness. A musician scorns Mozart and is just finishing, he tells you, a symphony with a soul. An office clerk is buying a place in the country next year because his landlord appears to be irritated about payments past due on his city apartment.

The alcoholic can't stand reality; he flees to the world of fantasy where he can be what he wants to be, on his own terms.

Insecure, anxious, fearful and tense in the real world, the alcoholic seeks defense and protection in drink. He inflates himself in grandiose talk to ward off the ugliness of reality. But something else happens in that tavern conversation if one happens to hear it in other phases. The talk shifts from the aggressive abuse of others to abuse of oneself.

In his expansive mood the alcoholic was hostile and aggressive towards other people, their shortcomings, their stupidity, and their lack of understanding. In the grandiose phase, however, he could be generous and pleasant to those who would listen to him and for whom he would buy drinks; these, in turn, would expect his attention when they felt like airing their plans and dreams, and recounting to him their problems with difficult people and situations. But this grandiosity has two sides. The drinker inflates himself so much that he naturally becomes more sensitive to the dangers of deflation. Since he has made so much of himself, he is that much more likely to be bruised or offended. It is to be expected that he will turn his criticism against himself to soften the sting of anticipated abuse from others. So you may hear the alcoholic (often when nursing a hang-over) telling a comrade that he is worthless and miserable, a poor cad for neglecting his wife and poor old mother. He may relate, to his own bewilderment, that he wouldn't hurt his dear old mother or wife for anything in the world. "Yet," he says, "I seem to get drunk just at the time when they want me most to be sober. Mother will cry and my wife won't speak to me." What, he will ask, "is wrong with me that I do such things to them I love most?" The answer, though it would shock him perhaps to know, is that he commits these acts to gain attention either through pity, love or punishment. He comes to expect even punishment in his efforts to gain attention. He will suffer pain, strange as it seems, to bolster his distorted personality. There is a fusion here of the desire to hurt and the desire to be hurt in the unconscious wish to aggrandize himself. In his moods of self-pity, in the hang-over or well in his cups, he will reveal the other side of the grandiose quality; he will turn his aggression against himself. But whether directed inward or outward, it is an immature quality of the alcoholic vainly asserting his identity. By hurting, or by being hurt, he will seek even uncomfortable situations to satisfy his unconscious craving for attention. It reminds one of an infant crying for food as if to say, "Mama, here am I, isn't this awful?"

An alcoholic, whose mother was often distressed about her son's drinking, left home to take a job elsewhere. His drinking did not stop but the habit was less violently handled in his new situation. In telling me his story, this young man was amazed to learn that the violence of his binges at home was closely related to his dependence on his mother. He left my office so angered that I thought I'd never see him again. But he came back, and in a calm voice, told me he finally understood what I meant. It was not that he wanted to hurt his mother for the sake of hurting her, but to get the attention from her that he unconsciously desired, he would hurt both her and himself!

To be grandiose means not only to inflate oneself, but also to deflate oneself and to look for punishment, if necessary, in order to be the centre of attention. The dictionary covers it simply, "producing, meant to produce, imposing effect." As to means of producing the desired effect, the alcoholic can find a curious variety of techniques. as we have seen.

Impulsive

The alcoholic "wants what he wants when he wants it." This tenacious quality gets him into more trouble than any other single trait of his personality. The long term view, the patiently executed task, are ideas hard for the alcoholic to understand. To go easy, to do a little at a time, to live each day as it comes, to pause and choose between two modes of action, to think a problem through calmly; these qualities of the mature person are seldom seen in the alcoholic. Certainly his decision to have a drink is, more often than not, an impulsive decision. He is tense and worried or elated and happy. At either extreme of mood he decides on the spur of the moment; "A drink? Well, why not? When could a person deserve one more than I do right now?" About two minutes pause, a milkshake, and a thought for the hang-over might well shelve that first drink time out of hand.

In general behaviour, he tackles problems with a tense haste, anxious to complete rather than to become absorbed in them for their own sake. It is said of many alcoholics that they never finish anything; they become easily discouraged when the task does not respond readily to their treatment. Sometimes the alcoholic will impulsively envisage a project upon which he engages with a fervor and high enthusiasm, a project of perfectionist size which dwindles to a commonplace task in the light of actual conditions and possibilities of fulfilment. It is hard for the alcoholic to "come down to size." He abandons the project. Before he started drinking, he might have worn himself out in the same enterprise. Now the only compulsion he respects is his drinking.

To the impulsive alcoholic it seems contradictory rather than factual that the mature person lives just one day at a time and yet looks well into the future to see a task as a slow accumulation of little things well done for their own sake. The worthwhile accomplishment is not done impulsively and compulsively; it is done slowly with full regard for and interest in the little details and changes which daily go into its gradual completion. This is a tough lesson for the alcoholic to learn.

Intolerant

Hand in hand with the tendency to be impulsive is the tendency to be intolerant. Do you remember, if you are an alcoholic, when you were on a keg and you couldn't tolerate a drunk? Or do you remember the times you were drunk and disdained the "drys"? It is a commonplace fact of psychology that a person with some serious defect is, by nature, driven to direct the attention of others away from his fault. So the alcoholic is often guilty of a rigid mind, and an intolerant attitude towards others. He is so aware of his own defect that he unconsciously seeks faults in others, faults that he thinks he does not have himself. The alcoholic becomes rigid in his thinking and intolerant of others. He is always seeking a scapegoat on whom he can pour abuse and criticism to relieve the guilt and insecurity of his own troubled conscience. The alcoholic easily develops prejudices in finding a scapegoat in petty attacks on other religions than his own, persons of other races and other classes. That, by the way, is why A.A. is careful not to engage in controversies over religion, race distinctions or social classes. Controversy is bad for an alcoholic. He is inclined to carry the controversy too far, to the point where it may degenerate into petty strains and unreasonable hatreds.

Wishful Thinking

This is the kind of thinking that alcoholics know all about. They are experts at it if they are honest enough to admit it. Wishful thinking is arranging to do what you want to do and making it appear reasonable. An alcoholic relates that one of his dodges was to come home with a heavy supply of liquor and tell his wife he was preparing for some friends he was expecting. This was usual on Saturdays as the liquor store was closed on Sundays. Every special event, birthday, holiday, wedding, funeral, was good for a little wishful thinking. The amusing fact is that the alcoholic fooled no one but himself. But wishful thinking did not stop at excuses to get liquor; it extended often into his entire pattern of thought so that every action, every decision revolved around the core of the alcoholic compulsion.

Every alcoholic can tell his own story about alibis. He has made up so many of them that he has forgotten more than he can remember. The alibi complex is closely related to wishful thinking. He decides on an action that suits him and then builds around it every plausible excuse he can imagine. The hang-over has had more fantastic names than anything else I can think of; it has been called flu, dysentry, sore back, toothache, lumbago, pneumonia, kidney trouble, constipation, diarrhea and migraine. Like the other faults I mention, this one about alibis reaches into the alcoholic's conduct where alcohol is not concerned. He finds himself using alibis for everything. He has blamed other things and other people for his own mistakes. He has even played sick, to avoid disagreeable engagements or duties.

The six qualities discussed in this chapter may be called by other names, depending on the concrete personal situation. Defiant, aggressive, resentful, stubborn are four labels that can as well be used in describing some alcoholics as any of the six used in this context. The significant fact is that, whatever labels best apply, there will be found, invariably, a pattern of emotional disturbance in every problem drinker.

The Little Dictator

The tense and defiant feelings at the root of alcoholism are seldom consciously known to the alcoholic. The conscious mind may say, "Things haven't been going well, I must do something about my drinking." But those tense and defiant feelings in the unconscious induce the alcoholic to say, "Of course I can handle the situation if I really want to, without having to stop drinking."

So an alcoholic is often prepared to admit that he has a drinking problem. But, in the bottom of his heart, he defiantly believes he can handle his problem, and wishfully looks to the day he can drink like a gentleman.

By the way, a gentleman or sensible mature drinker is no more aware of being a social drinker than he is of being a social eater. It is only the problem drinker who clings tragically to the hope that he can learn to drink moderately.

The conscious admission of the alcoholic that he has a drinking problem is often brought about by social disapproval, by the annoyance of his boss, by financial difficulties. Thus the alcoholic may grudgingly admit his weakness. He submits. He does not of himself desire wholeheartedly to stop drinking.

Any person helping a "submissive" alcoholic must tactfully and gradually bring this fact to his attention. There are many degrees of submission, some far removed from total surrender, some close to it. In any case the prime purpose of the helper is to induce but not force the desire to stop drinking, and to make it the most sincere and the strongest desire of the alcoholic. When this crisis is well precipitated, the helper's role in the treatment is half over. Much of the remaining treatment is the work of the alcoholic himself with the friend or therapist as an interested observer and interpreter.

The force that blocks off the alcoholic from insight and self-knowledge and from a sincere desire to stop drinking is what may be called the little dictator. All the qualities of the alcoholic's personality come under his influence.

The little dictator, present in every alcoholic, keeps him from believing he is powerless over his problem.

Almost every alcoholic finds it hard to believe that his trouble is beyond his control. Consciously or unconsciously, he long resists the fact that he is suffering from a disorder he is helpless to manage. No one knows better than he that this iron "will power" has time and again failed him in his greatest need. Yet he continues to pamper and worship the little dictator, responsible for his alcoholic downfall.

No alcoholic can hope to recover from his disorder and achieve relaxed sobriety until he can say wholeheartedly, "I surrender, the little dictator is overthrown. I know now that I cannot handle alcohol. All my reservations and my inner delusions about drinking normally, all my nostalgic regrets about the good old times, are gone. I am through."

Very often the alcoholic begins as one who submits but does not surrender. He submits to abstinence because his wife is distressed, the children are neglected, the boss is angry, the community looks at him darkly—and so his pride is hurt. He submits to abstinence but he is still under the sway of the little dictator. He is still defiant, way down deep in his heart and mind. He is still saying, "By God, I'll show them." In this attitude, in obeying the little dictator of false pride, he is acting in just the same way as a wilful child refrains from candy because Mummy has threatened him with the disgrace of punishment if he does not obey.

Submission won't work. It makes the alcoholic tense and defiant, and builds up a beautiful excuse for a "slip", if anything happens to go wrong.

If the desire to stop drinking is sincere, he has to surrender, heart, soul and mind with all his strength.

He finally learns that all external supports, such as his wife or mother, children, family, money and prestige are what they are for him because of what he gives to them. No woman can love a man, no child can respect his father, no money can produce happiness, and no position can furnish a reputation until the person seeking these great goods gives his abilities and affections without stint, without reservation. Therefore a man sooner or later sees with mature eyes that the love of his wife, the affection of his children, the heavy bank-account and the reputation of his job or of his family cannot give him sobriety and self-respect. He begins to wake up and come to his senses when he realizes that all these wonderful external supports and blessings are what they are because of what he gives to them. He no longer leans on other people and other things. In heart, mind and soul he stands naked before the world, with all support withdrawn and all defiance gone. He declares unconditional surrender.

There are no more alibis to use as make-shift truces. Besides the futility of leaning on external supports, the alcoholic also learns that his will-power which he thought to be a safeguard against heavy drinking, was the very cause of his alcoholism! This force he called his will-power turns out to be better named false-pride. This tyrant, this false pride, is a tool of the little dictator, the cause of all the alcoholic's trouble, of his tensions of mind and body, and of his defiant struggles with society.

This little dictator has ruled every alcoholic, if not many other human beings as well. He must be overthrown if complete surrender is to take place. His overthrow, and the alcoholic's surrender and recovery go together. The surrender cannot scientifically be charted. It cannot be brought about simply by conscious effort on the part of either the person helping the alcoholic or the alcoholic himself. But definite steps can be taken to oust the little dictator.

An amusing example of the little dictator is found in this alibi:

"You see, I just can't help my drinking. The doctors say that the alcoholic is powerless over his problem. Well, that's me. I've been telling my wife about it. She doesn't nag me quite as much as she used to. I'm a sick man. I guess there's no hope for me. Made that way. Something in the blood. No cure for it so far as I know."

This man thinks he likes himself the way he is. Actually he is afraid to think of life without alcohol. The prospect terrifies him. He defies outside help—or ignores it. He refuses to go the whole way and learn that the alcoholic can recover—with outside help. The little dictator keeps him from seeking help beyond himself.

False pride, among other things, is short-sighted and fearful. When the will-power gag wears thin and ceases to register, the alcoholic may turn about face and, in desperation, use the helpless addict alibi. Either way, he is a victim of the little dictator and he wallows in wishful thinking.

4.

ALLEN'S STORY

Two friends of mine—alcoholics—went to see the film, "Lost Weekend". When they came out of the theatre, Don said to Tom, 'I'm through. I swear off booze for life.' And Tom nodded his head and appeared to agree with Don. He said, 'I'm through, too. I swear off movies for life.'

"Like Tom, I avoided reminders of my weakness. I didn't like to look at pictures that told me the truth about myself. I thought I had my own life to live. I was my own salvation. All my decisions were reached by myself. All my happiness or misery was of my own making.

"This, I think, was false pride. For me it had three tendencies. I refused to take blame for anything unpleasant, I sought more respect than I deserved, I would not admit that any person was better than I. Maybe I thought I believed in God. But I didn't really because I was God.

"Slowly I discovered that the short-sighted person cannot see into himself, cannot believe in himself. The person who sees well, inside and out, rarely stumbles.

"You wonder what I mean by short-sighted?

"The three tendencies of false pride, to be defensive, to seek attention and to be self-sufficient to the point of arrogance, all three are short-sighted. They don't go far enough and they don't go deep enough.

"The person of false pride is short-sighted. He becomes insecure, anxious and fearful because he does not see far enough into himself. He really hates himself. An odd statement, isn't it?

"In drink, I groped for a sense of power and glory that I did not see in sober living. The effort was mad as every alcoholic knows. Failing to clear my view in booze, I went all the way and blotted out. The blotting out was as futile as the vain effort to see better, because I survived. To live after a binge is to endure the hell of the hang-over, to endure the pain of seeing in fresh alert human beings something I might admire more than myself. I could respect neither myself nor others. I became cynical, sour, critical, sensitive. Yet I wanted to be liked; after a few drinks I could be sociable, attentive, complimentary, talkative, sentimental. I felt compelled to gain approval and make others like me.

"Now this desire to be liked covered a sense of uneasiness that I tried to hide in drink. This uneasy feeling had no basis in fact but was largely imagined; I suspected that other people were thinking and talking about me far more than they did; no one cares really, but the short-sighted alcoholic like myself imagines often that he is the concern of people when actually he is farthest from their thoughts; they have their own troubles and problems—the other person usually doesn't matter. Though I was never sure, I suspected this even when drinking and sometimes got drunk to attract attention. Failing to get the attention I deserved, I developed guilt, I became fearful, afraid that others would detect my weaknesses and shortcomings. Then resentment set in. I resented the efforts of others to help and advise me; I resented the acts and opinions of others in the circle of my acquaintances and was given to criticizing and belittling people I knew. At any cost, I had to keep defended. Defended? Yes, against myself whom I couldn't see and didn't know.

"When I tried to justify everything I did, taking no blame for anything, I failed to look at my weaknesses because I never liked what I saw when I took sober notes. When I tried to find satisfaction in alcohol to get that sense of power and glory, I failed for a long time to see that I was destroying my mind and body, destroying everything that all human beings wish to preserve.

"As I continued to abide by my own authority, to see no power greater than myself I went deeper and deeper into confusion, became less and less sure of myself until I could not tolerate myself indefinitely as a sober man.

"I felt I had to get drunk, either when depressed or when happy. Both the depression and the happiness were more than I could stand. I was afraid the first would persist and the second would disappear. I couldn't trust myself. I hated myself. I began to drink to pass out.

"It took some time for me to see that I was getting nowhere. My firm resolves, my thinking out of problems, my control or 'will-power' failed to bring any change for the better.

"Many well-meaning friends used to say, 'Why, for goodness sake, did you get drunk last night, of all nights, when so many counted on your being sober?' They would rarely add, 'Haven't you any backbone, haven't you any will-power at all?' But that was perhaps what they were thinking. Less friendly people have put it in stronger terms than that.

"I used to think 'will-power' was a sort of miracle-worker. It could make you do anything that struck your fancy. It could even make you do what you really did not want to do! All this puzzled me as I tried to understand it better. Finally it just didn't make sense whatever. How often had I beat myself against a stone wall! Breaking myself to pieces, one defiant desire trying to destroy a still stronger desire. With a conflict like that going on, the only sensible course to take was to try to find out what caused the conflict. I tried then to know myself better.

"I came to see that my desire to stop drinking, *up to this point*, was not my sincere wish, but simply the pressure of interests controlled by my false pride. That's why the fight had been so bitter, why I'd always come out on the losing end.

"So I decided to accept myself with all my weaknesses. I stopped trying to make people think I was other than I really was. This decision had a profound effect on me. I see now that my escape *into* alcohol and my defiant efforts to escape *from* alcohol were equally vicious. Both were attempts to be something other than I was. I had been fighting against my real interests. The 'will-power' I used in my struggle with the alcohol problem was the very cause of all my troubles!

"No wonder I felt bitter and defeated. How could I possibly change my own distorted goals with the same crooked vision that set them up?

"A very simple truth came to me. It is so commonsense that I hesitate to mention it. But I must talk about it because it helps me to see it clearer. I either go on growing or die. If I grow, I must cultivate just what there is in me. There's no good in trying to fight myself. I have to grow according to my own nature. Surely this goes for every living thing, every human being, not just for me—unless I'm a lot more queer than I yet know. So I came to respect and to explore the simple principle of personal growth.

"My sight is improving. I look at nature everywhere around me. All things that grow must have proper soil and sunlight or they perish. Good growth is what the farmer wants in his crops. Good growth is what a human being wants in his own life. Every human being knows that he cannot remain a child forever. He grows up into a reasonable, truthful and kind person. If he does not, he remains stunted and cannot take his place among mature men and women. I need all my faculties to become a mature healthy person. It is just that simple. To arrest personal growth in the excessive use of alcohol is to stagnate and die, in body and in mind. In both, for that matter, because I cannot really separate them.

"Is there anything more natural than the desire to live a complete life, to be truly human, and to respect the same desire in everyone else? Is there anything more natural than the desire to live completely, more natural than the *duty* to be a complete human being?

"I am trying to improve my understanding not only of myself but of others too. When I am sincere, I see it becomes rather silly to criticize or find fault. To understand that everything I see and hear and feel follows a natural course is to be aware of conditions and causes that can explain what I see, hear and feel. Everything has its explanation, don't you think, if we knew enough. Do I grumble if the weather is unpleasant? Do I take offense if a person annoys me? If I do, why?

"I suppose the weather bureau could explain why we have rain at a certain time because of given conditions. I suppose the psychologist, if he knew enough about me, could explain why I often act and think as I do. My attitude towards the weather or people is apt to be distorted if I do not try to understand them. And if I understand them, how can I say they *should* have been otherwise? The only way I can have it otherwise is to try to change the conditions. I can't change what I see to be already a fact. I can only hope, if I think a change can be made, to alter the conditions if possible so that I can meet the situation in a better way the next time I face it. I can't change the weather and I can't change people to suit myself. But I can change my own outlook. If I co-operate with people and try to understand them instead of swearing at them, our encounters will make good sense.

"As I think more about personal growth, I see how naturally self-respect goes with humility and these, in turn, with respect for my fellowmen. The more confident and whole-hearted my self-respect, the stronger will be my concern for my friends and acquaintances. If I cannot respect myself, I cannot respect others. This I found out in my drinking days. When I was insecure, grovelling, unhappy; when I was remorseful, full of self-pity and afraid of the day ahead of me, I simply could not feel kindly and think clearly about others.

"Every once in a while I have a session of self-acceptance. I sort of jump out of my skin and look at myself from the sidelines. I don't always like what I see. I see attitudes that look mean; these I can change if I try. But I also see limitations that cannot be changed. Nothing can be done about my intellectual or emotional endowments. I can make the most of them, but I cannot exchange them for those of some one who is not me. I cannot wipe out my background, my physical or mental make-up by a snap of the fingers. Why pine away in wanting what is not? I accept myself. It is humbling but it is quieting. Gone is the old urge to fight a losing battle.

"In these odd sessions of accepting myself, I learn humility and I gain confidence. I have only begun. A new life is ahead of me, if I do not forget the simple insights of the past year. The greatest lesson in this new outlook is one that I tend to forget. A flash of insight is worth little if it is not borne out in action. If what I believe is not charged with feeling and put into practice, then everything I say is wordy and worthless. If I rest content with my neat picture of adjustment, I'm afraid I can't stay sober. But I think I see what lies ahead of me and what there is to do. I have only to do it. The prospect is not a challenge. I am through with challenges. It is an adventure. I cannot doubt that it is worthwhile."

(Allen's story is not complete here. We shall meet him again in the chapter "Alcoholics Anonymous", where he explains what lies ahead of him and what there is to do.)

5.

THE ALCOHOLIC'S INSIGHT

Nᴏᴛ wanting to face life soberly arises from fear. As this condition becomes habit, the alcoholic realizes that he is unable to stay sober. From not wanting to be sober he becomes unable to stay sober. As the habit grips, the fear mounts and the drinker finds it harder to stop drinking.

So it is the pattern of fear in each alcoholic that must be traced in any long term program of recovery. This pattern will be singularly his own in the fusion of events that make up his background and his reaction to it.

Anyone helping an alcoholic will respect him as a person ahead of abstract lectures on the social, economic and moral evils of the drinking habit. I have yet to see the alcoholic whom, in the grip of his misery, you can impress with the broad facts. It is the man himself you have to reach, in the downright concrete experiences that touch his personal life. Throughout these experiences are traced his pattern of fear.

These experiences are governed by his false pride which combined with his growing habituation to drink, make of him a man afraid. This fear builds tensions within and aggressions without. Hence the "time bomb" reaction of the periodic drinker. Little nameless anxieties gather until he can stand it no longer. His social and business activities have failed to stamp out the growing panic that seizes his apparent composure. Then comes the explosion. Drinking bouts of days, weeks or months are not enjoyable. Any periodic drinker will tell you so. The binge is a negative measure to release tension and to dull the sharp edges of fear.

Allen found that false pride is expressed in the tendencies to be defensive, attention-getting and self-sufficient. This self-absorption creates fear. The alcoholic either destroys this fear or it will destroy him. To do so, he must look deep into those three qualities as they distort or frustrate his attempts to get well.

What is it to be defensive? What is back of it? The alcoholic with his perfectionist ideals is guilt laden and rigid. He has an idea of himself as he thinks he ought to be, an idea in conflict with what he vaguely suspects to be his real nature. He may disdainfully ridicule the lessons he learnt at his mother's knee, but those lessons lie deep in his unconscious. They emerge in self-pitying binges and sometimes in his dreams. In fact those deeply buried lessons take the joy out of everything he does, though he may not consciously know it. In the bottom of his heart he still accepts all the "don'ts" he was taught in childhood. So he is defensive. Joking, drinking, shrewd business dealing, sex—all are wicked. He does not abstain from them, but they are spoiled for him by the suspicion that they are degrading. The central desire of his whole nature is that of being caressed by his mother—either in love or in reproof. The main thing is the caress, even if sometimes it is earned through guilt.

But this pleasure he may no longer have in his manhood. So the alcoholic, childish and sensitive, resolves that nothing now really matters. Many of his activities become confused efforts to regain the lost maternal tenderness he knew as a child. When he marries, it is often a mother substitute he seeks in his wife. Disturbed by the give and take formula of mature married life, he turns from it disillusioned and disgusted. His drinking grows worse as the bottle replaces his wife as the mother substitute. As he plunges into imagined sin, disappointed with life, he reaps real misery in his remorse and self-pity. This is the result of rigid moral training which makes of the alcoholic a self-righteous, sensitive, mother-attached child. This outlook is as often hidden under the rough cynical exteriors of the hardboiled drinker as it is found openly in the drinker who expresses his misery in tears and nostalgic stories of the "good old days."

A frank detached view of this condition within oneself may at first be greeted with resentment. As it grows familiar in honest self-appraisal it will be seen as a personality trait to be directed in new channels if it is not possible to abandon it altogether and replace it with the hope that he can grow up.

Attention-getting is a technique of those who are in the habit of admiring themselves and of wanting to be liked. It is common among alcoholics. It is a normal trait, disturbing only in excess. After all, one cannot be grovelling and everybody enjoys being liked.

But when we go so far as to lose our capacity to feel love for others we are headed for trouble. If vanity is carried too far there is no real interest in other people and therefore no genuine satisfaction to be had from love. When the attention-getting alcoholic is sure of someone's affection he loses interest and has no further use for him. Other people and other things become means to the cramped interests of vanity. The person whose sole concern with the world is that it shall pay him attention is not likely to achieve his desire. He is never satisfied. He drops interests quickly when they cease to feed his ever-hungry craving for attention. This constant hunger leads time and again to alcohol where for a brief period the alcoholic's personality cravings are satisfied first in fantasy and then in oblivion.

The source of the craving for attention in the alcoholic is often a lack of self-confidence. Its cure lies in the principle of personal growth, the deepening of self-respect. Genuine self-respect arises from the outgoing efforts to value other people and things, not as means to personal vanity, but as adventures in which one loses his morbid self-concern, and can say honestly "This is wonderful. Where has the time gone?" The man or woman who grows in self-respect is never bored, never listless. There are countless adventures in the run of a day outside the narrow scope of his vanity to be taken in and enjoyed. He is sure of himself and goes on to explore the world around him in friends, hobbies, his work and his family. Maturely self-respecting, the recovered alcoholic has converted his grandiose dreams into a study of things and people as they are. He learns that his impulsive desires have to be cut down to the size of real things and active interests. The energy that went into his impulsive and grandiose schemes is levelled and spread out over an increasingly large number of interests that can be really satisfied and enjoyed. His *attention-getting* is changed to *attention-absorbing*.

The alcoholic, often self-sufficient, is intolerant of other opinions. He sees himself in wishful thinking as a man of power and influence. Like attention-getting, a certain measure of self-sufficiency is natural and normal. In excess, it marks a departure from reality, and makes a man appear foolish among those who have heard his views and greet him with amused disdain as his impossible projects collapse, one after the other. If he is spared the ridicule of his acquaintances by keeping his dreams of power to himself, he is the victim of a self-imposed unhappiness. If he is so far gone as to delude himself with his fancied greatness, he yet cannot fail to notice that he impresses no one except the professional bum whose feigned admiration he may have for the price of a drink.

The morbid tendency to be self-sufficient, like the craving for attention, can be traced to a lack of self-confidence and to the painful memory of a humiliating experience. Poverty in youth, spurned love, imagined awkwardness, failure to compete in sports, in studies, or in the social graces, may induce a person to over-compensate in dreams of power and even to accomplish much in some scheme designed to "show them" that he is a worthy object of admiration, that he can hold his own in an area that counts for much in the world of getting and spending. But for every Byron, Poe, Lamb or Alexander, miserable in his greatness, there are thousands of equally unhappy alcoholics who never get through their dreams to reality.

A success or failure, the power-driven alcoholic is never happy. If successful, there are still fields to conquer. (Discovering there were no new kingdoms to win, Alexander the Great wept and drank himself to death.) If a failure, his blocked ambitions make him miserable, critical, intolerant both of those who achieve what he is denied and of those whose ambitions never rise above their abilities. He is reduced to exchanging yarns of wishful thinking at the bar with an alcoholic like himself. After the third drink, both are talking at once.

How many alcoholics, in their self-sufficiency, have stubbornly resolved to show their wives and friends that they can become moderate drinkers, though no alcoholic has yet done it! Intolerant of what has been said and written thousands of times, many brave souls have sought and are still seeking to demonstrate that they are exceptions because they are stronger and more intelligent than ordinary drunks.

The only formula for these deluded people is to learn thoroughly the tragic lesson of wishful thinking. If there is a glimmer of willingness to stop drinking, his physical habituation, his "allergy" or body sensitivity—call it what you like—quite apart from all his personal disorders and fear, is enough to convince the alcoholic that he must completely abstain. The psychologist, William James, hits the fallacy of wishful thinking directly when he says it is simply a question of calling a thing by its right name! Let the alcoholic who aspires to be a moderate drinker never forget that the following situations are wrongly named:

1. "I do not want to waste good liquor that my friend has kindly passed me. I do not want to be rude or unsociable. I won't get drunk at this party. Just pleasantly high."

2. "I've never tasted this brand before. No harm to try just this one little drink. One drink never hurt anybody."

3. "This is a holiday. I'll relax and have a few. This will be my last. I'll quit tomorrow."

The right name for all problem drinkers in situations like these is simply that of being a drunk—being a drunk—being a drunk.

To choose the wrong name for drinking situations is to "slip." And a "slip" is a serious setback for the alcoholic who wants to get well.

The alcoholic, defensive, attention-getting, or self-sufficient develops a one-sidedness that makes of him a man afraid. His one-sidedness would be less tragic if he were able to express it. But even here he is thwarted, and fails to get the satisfaction he seeks. He turns to alcohol to distract himself. He is afraid to go after what he most desires. Perhaps he has failed in the trying and he lacks the drive to try again. The pain of sober effort is too much for him. In his fear he becomes alcoholic. Failing to have what he wants, he will forget it in drink. He will make his life bearable and he will dull his fear by becoming less alive. Drunkenness is partial suicide.

Now it should not be hard to convince the alcoholic or anyone else that happiness is desirable. I am assuming that the reader would rather be happy than miserable. This goal can be attained by all of us, if only we can become convinced that we are not the victims of weak will power. "A person can do anything in the world he wants." But this sweeping statement means nothing until we can agree on the meaning of will power.

When insight such as Allen's is achieved it becomes easy and sensible to believe a man can do anything in the world he wants. Every want or desire is felt to be a real need that can be met and satisfied. There are no vain fantasies, no vain struggles with "will power". A man with insight into his personality, with a knowledge of his limits and the courage of his capabilities will measure his life in accordance with them. He will not try to do what he is unable to do: he will not dream of goals he can never reach. He will do what he wants because he can have what he wants. He has taken his measure in a real and sober world.

The Myth of Will Power

A superstition about the drinking habit needs to be destroyed. If you decide to stop drinking, all you have to do is to set your mind on it, exercise your will power, and the desired results will be assured you. This is the myth of will power. This superstition is as false as trying to walk with a broken leg. A man with a broken leg has to undergo treatment. He has to suit himself to conditions imposed by the doctor before he is fit to walk again. It is no different with the alcoholic. He has to recondition his personality before he can be happy and well without alcohol. Conditions have been formed in drinking days which produced alcoholism. Drinking habits are likely to occur as long as those conditions exist. You might just as well order a camp fire to go out without removing the conditions causing fire as to order yourself to stop drinking. The fire will go out if you remove the causes of the fire. The alcoholism will cease if you modify the causes of your drinking.

Though will power is a misleading fiction, choice is real and effective. You may choose one course of action among a number of possible actions, but you cannot choose to do the impossible. If you are an alcoholic, you cannot choose to drink moderately. Nor can you decide, through will power, to stop drinking. You cannot fight your strongest desire through mere resolution. If you try, nothing but distress and pain result, and in the end, your strongest desire will assert itself in one way or another. You are free to act, but you must act to be free. If you choose to stop drinking, you must, at the same time, do something about your positive choice, the desire to be sober. Well . . . what is there to be done?

After a man is convinced that he would be better off without alcohol, he should not dwell on ways and means to not drink. To concentrate on not drinking is a negative kind of behaviour, and only serves to keep the pain of prohibition uppermost in one's thoughts. In removing the causes or conditions of drinking a new line of action and of outlook on life is required. This new outlook or reconditioning paves a new road over the old one and thus replaces the old tendencies with new activities. The desired end, sobriety, is reached by new activity instead of by the philosophy of "don't" and "watch out". Obsessed with the idea of not drinking, the drinker travels the old familiar road that leads again to drinking. The alcoholic, therefore, will seek to do something new and positive that has more to offer than either his drinking tendencies or his old way of life. This positive action will lead him to his desired goal, adventurous sobriety.

It is hard to think of anything more different from his old ways than the urge to help someone else recover from alcoholism. In this effort he cannot think of his own misery and frustration because his energies are directed outward on the welfare of another. This action has much to do with his own personal struggle, and it determines, oddly enough, any real success he has in solving his drinking problem.

Most important of all, the alcoholic will come to see that his desired goal is not a remote prize. His goal is in his daily activity. Means and ends are wrapped up together. He helps other alcoholics as a means to his own sobriety. And he uses his own sobriety as a means to help other alcoholics. The next important act is the one he will do when this one is completed. With such an outlook the alcoholic ceases to dream about impossible and remote goals. He lives in the present, deeming the here and now the most vital adventure of his life. In this way grandiose ideas are deflated and the alcoholic lives in the real world, facing each situation as it comes. As a man trains the habit of living realistically in the present, treasuring each action for its adventure value, and ever seeking new chances to help others recover from alcoholism, he hasn't time to pause and wonder about his own personal problems. His thoughts are absorbed in his new pattern of living. He will soon stop asking "How am I doing now?" as a check on his morals and the righteousness of his new sobriety. He stops asking this question because he is training a healthy habit, good in the living of it. It does not need the support of a moral sanction any more than a successful engineer or doctor needs to examine the effect of his work upon his character. Healthy human beings confident in the productiveness of their efforts seldom take time to assess the moral worth of these activities to themselves. Value of this sort comes spontaneously with healthy outgoing action. It is a pleasurable by-play, not a good to be sought for its own sake. When moral worth is sought as a separate prize men become self-conscious, morbid, negative. They become ineffective, unhappy and tense.

The alcoholic wastes energy in trying to fight his drinking habit head-on, by a negative resolution such as "I will not drink." If he succeeds with this method, for a while, it is like saying, "A disordered man who drank now does not drink." He remains disordered and will drink again. He is not on the road to recovery until he says "I want a sober life. The only way I can have it is to want something stronger than the desire to drink. To do that, I have to look around and within me in search of desires and activities that give me greater pleasure, greater good, better health than alcohol gives me. Besides that, I need help from a power greater than myself. I cannot do this alone. My will power has brought me to grief too often. I do not trust it any more. Will power is fear. It nearly destroyed me. Yes, now I have it! Will power, false pride, morbid fear—they all add up to death. But I want to live! So I must overcome fear, by wanting to live more than I want to die. I surrender to life. As I surrender to life, I surrender to God."

6.

SURRENDER AND THE FOLLOW-UP

IN Chapter Three, I used the term *little dictator*. Here I shall use it again to represent that deep complex composed of false pride, lack of insight, fear, unconscious resistance to recovery, will power, and those six qualities of the alcoholic described in Chapter Three. The *little dictator*, though a complicated process of activity, will be easily recognized in the dialogue that follows. The other actor in the dialogue is *Insight*, the subject of Chapters Four and Five.

The L.D.—"If I want to use my will power, (I am a pretty strong minded person, you know) I can quit whenever I like. I can take it or leave it alone."

Insight—"You have lost money during the past year and you will soon lose your job—and perhaps your wife. You sprained your arm in that car accident last week because you were drunk. You got "high", as you call it, the night before the biggest deal in your life. In the morning you missed your appointment. By the way, you hardly ever go to a party unless you are drinking. If you are sober, you look as though your best friend died. Your will power seems to make you very unhappy. Just what is your will power anyway? I'm not ridiculing you. I really want to know."

The L.D.—"Only weak people ask for help. I suppose I have a bit of a problem with my drinking. But I can manage this myself. Just imagine anyone admitting he is an alcoholic!"

Insight—"Sick people often need outside help. You are sick

but you don't know it and if you did, you wouldn't admit it, the way you are thinking now. It takes an honest man, and a brave man, to find out what's wrong with him. You are honest and brave, too, if you want to be. You are also intelligent. You really haven't far to go. But you are a little afraid of yourself. False pride is short-sighted. It always falls short of the facts. By the way, weren't you arrested for the third time last week for drunken driving?"

The L.D.—"What in hell are you talking about? Lately you've been saying altogether too much. Give me a chance once in a while to say what I feel. And mind you, I feel very strongly about what I do with my life. I defy everybody. Why shouldn't I get drunk if I want to? Supposing I do? Whose business is it but my own? Sure I drink, and sometimes I pass out. I don't want anyone preaching to me. I have my own life to live."

Insight—"I see you don't want to make terms with me. But at least you're listening to my side of the story. I represent healthy living. You're still afraid of it. It's funny, but when you defy life, you run away from it. When you settle with me, I take over. There is no compromise. The surrender is complete. I am no prude. I am no moralist. I am only interested in mature living. Within the range of my vision, there is freedom, all kinds of room in which to grow and flourish. I'm not as bad as you think."

As long as the alcoholic is governed by the little dictator he will not get well. When insight goes deep enough to seize his whole personality, something begins to happen. But before anything happens, he experiences the futility of his deceptive thinking. He sees, though unconsciously, that will power is a joke, that false pride is ignorance of the facts, that fear lurks in his defiant gestures and flights from reality. To talk of will power he realizes is plainly silly. To speak of the "weak" people of A.A. as he once did, now mortifies him. He remembers talking like that to an A.A. member on the train recently, while he proceeded to get drunk. Near the end of the trip, he was sneaking drinks in the lavatory. Mustn't let that drunk see him guzzling! The A.A. member called a taxi for him when he got off the train.

Finally, he sees that all his reasoning falls on deaf ears. There is no one now to tell his stories to. Everyone concerned with him has heard his tales a thousand times. He cannot defy them any more because he realizes at last that they don't want to fight, and they are not trying to run his life. They have stopped reasoning with him. That's all.

Something like this experience of insight (likely unconscious) occurs before the surrender. He is beaten. He is on his own. All his supports are gone. He is powerless over alcohol. That he knows if nothing else. What is more vital, he feels it. The surrender occurs. It just happens. It cannot be scientifically charted from insight to occurrence. Its dynamics are a mystery. It may happen suddenly. It may come gradually. But happen it does, as one can see in the release of tension, the absence of defiance, the new presence of humility and composure.

But to feel the deceptions of the little dictator and all he stands for is, I think, to pave the way to the surrender process, mysterious though it may be in its happening. These deceptions cannot be revealed by some one *to* some one else. They are experienced actively in some way by the alcoholic himself, just as the state of surrender involves an active acceptance of life. Surrender means work *with* and *in* life, positively and creatively. It has to be distinguished from submission. In submission, the alcoholic passively accepts sobriety and the terms of mature living, but defiance lurks in the unconscious. It is as though the submissive drunk were saying "I'll have it my own sweet way in the end. This is only temporary."

After the act of surrender, "the positive phase" sets in. The "positive phase" is an expression used by Dr. Harry

Tiebout* to denote the alcoholic's new found serenity, "internal peace and quiet". Surrender means that the fight is over, that the pain of struggle or tension is gone.

What can we say about the positive phase, the follow-up of the surrender.

There are four results of the positive phase, worth noting for their value in dealing with the problem of "slips".

(1) The alcoholic has ceased to be confused. His tense "will power" is seen as useless and wasted energy. With this conviction he reflects "Yes, my drinking was what I wanted, or I would not have drunk. It was crazy, I see now, to suppose I could stop through the agency of will power before I really wanted something to take the place of drinking. Now I want sobriety more than drinking. The energy formerly wasted in will power I now devote to my new found desire, sobriety. This involves daily effort."

He now avoids drinking because *for him* there is greater good to be had in not drinking. He sees that all the school lessons of his childhood about alcoholism were plainly negative and useless. If anything, they enticed him to try the forbidden sin! The teacher told him about the damage done to the drunkard's stomach, his nerves and his morals. How much more effective it would have been to learn about the joys of healthy living and the unequalled binges of the sun, fresh air and sound sleep! Not enough people know, he reflects, that the greatest luxury in the world is a good breakfast.

His thinking is positive now—a question of what to do, what to feel, what to create. His old will power had always legislated what *not* to do. Life has been made up of inhibitions. The stress was on restraint and inaction. Now he is free.

(2) Quietly, the alcoholic begins to feel new strength.

*The surrender concept is inspired in part by the lectures and articles of Dr. Harry Tiebout. I do not wish, however, to make him responsible for all of it, as I have introduced concepts not included in his treatment of the problem.

"The moral life," he says, "is not a life of restrictions. It is a life of mature choices and of growth. If my nature responds favorably to something, if I *like* it, then it is good. I do not desire sobriety because it is good. It is good because I desire it." There is nothing negative here. It is response, it is life, it is action.

(3) Genuine personal desire rather than the coercive views of others makes up the nature of a man. "A man thinks as he lives—he does not live as he thinks." After the alcoholic chooses abstinence as a good more desirable than drinking, his thinking shifts from a wet to a dry pattern. His thinking takes its cue from his newly found desire to be sober. He stopped fighting when he surrendered. He now goes along with the strongest desire of his being, sobriety. As there is nothing to fight against anymore, there is nothing to be negative about.

(4) The alcoholic finds himself. This discovery is important. After his long struggle between unhealthy indulgence and guilt, between what he was and what he felt he should be, the alcoholic enjoys the peace of insight. He sees that it is natural to be maturely self-regarding, to grow in tune with his personal desires. People differ. What he is inclined to do may be distasteful to someone else. One man's meat is another's poison. He grows tolerant. He will live and let live.

These four results of the state of surrender or "positive phase", need to be lived over and over again in the alcoholic's thinking and feeling. When they are forgotten, tension may again take hold, and "slips" may occur.

The positive phase, in the alcoholic's recovery, wonderful and encouraging though it may be to him, is not heaven. Life moves and changes—the positive phase of the recovered alcoholic is no exception. If the alcoholic knows that the desires and thoughts supporting his positive view of life are subject to change, he will be a wiser and a stronger man. He will not really grow personally until he sees his personal problem as one involving more than himself. The positive phase will not be sound until he understands his surrender as a surrender to life, not just to abstinence.

And how may we describe his surrender to life? No, it is not a grovelling attitude. The alcoholic need not pretend "I am the worst of men and deserve nothing of life's joys," What woman would be pleased to learn that her husband found in her an ideal chance for self-denial? To be selfish up to a point is the necessary ground for true happiness. The recovered alcoholic can see in his abstinence the saving of energy for other adventures, not a self-righteous and gloomy denial. And here the most crucial fact of all enters the picture. Self-denial is the very opposite of complete surrender to life! Surrender to life is not a truce, not a defiant submission. It is a going-along-with, a teaming up with all the natural healthy forces that express themselves in the alcoholic's surroundings. The whole opposition between the alcoholic and the rest of the world, implied in the doctrine of self-denial, ceases when he grasps the meaning of life's interests for him in the scenes he knows. So his surrender to life is not just a surrender to abstinence. He surrenders to the living scene in which he moves. The persons and things in and around him claim his attention. If he does not respond he is alone. And a lonely man is an unhappy man. *The misery of self-denial disappears when the alcoholic, in surrender to life, develops genuine interests in persons and things outside himself.* He loses his fear of life and engages in it whole-heartedly, once the surrender is honest and complete.

The alcoholic can look for the danger signs of a "slip" when he finds himself looking morbidly inward. His most cherished desires have to be satisfied in something else or with some one else. Strong personal growth is assured him when he fully senses that his own best interests are fused with those of other people and with adventures in which he is not alone but plays a part. "No man is an island unto himself."

Setting out on a new life of sobriety, the most encouraging fact the alcoholic can know is that *becoming well is more desirable than being well*. He can view his disorder as a means to a more creative life than he ever knew before. This principle of becoming well, this concept of personal growth, he adopts as the heart of his new way of life. He never stops growing, he never stops "becoming well". He is calmly aware of new adventures with the dawn of each new day, he never knows it all because another experience is just around the corner and he is willing to learn. But he does not rush. He is not excited. Time is on the side of the alcoholic who has stopped drinking, of the man who has cast aside his fear. Humble and open-minded, convinced now that the whole truth can never be known by any human being, he surrenders his dreams of mastery. Like millions around him, he slowly settles into the adventure of living and learning. He "becomes well" until he dies.

In this process the alcoholic learns that he has many quiet pleasures ahead of him. It is reassuring to find out that he has really great power for meaningful life. Anyone as sensitive as an alcoholic can tune himself to freedom rather than to fear, if he lets himself go. When formerly he sought to escape from fear through drink, he by-passed the good things as well. *The depth of his former fear becomes now the strength of his capacity to live deeply and well.* The proof is not far to seek. Ask any alcoholic who has made a genuine recovery. Long forgotten interests are revived, and new ones come into being. People are seen in a new light. He sees and understands much as he did before he drank with this telling exception—he is no longer tense, he is no longer afraid. All the energy sapped by his fear is now expressed in positive thinking and doing. It is a question of direction. The positive thinking is learning to accept himself.

In his former confusion he knew little about himself. He knew neither his limits nor his talents. He tended to ignore the former and glorify the latter. He drank to blunt the edges of self-criticism and to inflate his grandiose schemes and dreams. So long as he thought and felt this way he did not really want to recover—that would have been to forfeit his dreams and accept his limits. The whole network of wishful thinking has to be cut away, strand by strand, until he sees himself as he is. The first strand to destroy is the idea that he can control his drinking. This tenacious little thought will sooner or later bring him to the plain and homely fact that he either quits altogether or goes on to more and more misery. No man dies by being cut off. Thousands of alcoholics have quit and are healthier than ever they were. Another brutal little truth is that no man ever improves his drinking pattern. There is no such thing as being just a little alcoholic and staying that way. Alcoholism, like a pregnant woman, grows. Unlike a pregnant woman, it flowers in death.

If the alcoholic fails to accept himself he will have trouble. Though he stops drinking for a while, he may drink again because he has failed to understand the fears and the body sensitivity which lead him to drink. The sequence is self-ignorance, fear, drunkenness. If you know and accept yourself, you eliminate fear, and drunkenness will be seen in its true light. To continue drinking thereafter can be nothing but downright suicide.

But self-acceptance and self-knowledge are not enough. Dr. J. D. M. Griffin, a psychiatrist who was kind enough to discuss with me the material of this book, presented the most formidable question I know in the alcohol problem. "Are there not," he asked, "many alcoholics who accept and know themselves quite well but who continue, nevertheless, to get drunk?" The answer to this question, I think, lies in the act of surrender *before* the follow-up of self-acceptance and self-knowledge. The act of surrender happens in the alcoholic himself. No one else can surrender for him. The person helping the alcoholic recover can do much to *induce* the desire to stop drinking, but he cannot hand him over this desire and the surrender which follows it.

In initiating recovery, self-acceptance and self-knowledge are secondary to that all important desire. Though the desire to stop drinking may gain strength through insight, much of that mysterious initial insight is *unconscious*. Insight in the stage preceding surrender is *feelingful*, with deep sources not known clearly to the conscious mind of the alcoholic. *It has to be of this deep dynamic quality in order to reach and oust* the defiant resistance to recovery. This resistance is as deeply lodged as the forces which remove it.

Clearly, then, self-knowledge and self-acceptance in the *active* alcoholic will simply be forces on the conscious level that protect and pamper the underlying resistance to recovery. Intelligent drunks on Skid Row can offer challenging philosophies supported by Omar Khayyam, Horace, Schopenhauer and Sartre. The sociologists and psychologists with neat schemes of adjustment have nothing to sell the inveterate drunk who can say "I don't like your stuff" and proceed to match them, jewel for jewel, from his intellectual storehouse of wet but bright ideas.

After genuine surrender, action follows in the "positive phase" as Dr. Tiebout calls it. It is in this "positive phase", sober for a year or more, that the alcoholic on the conscious level can begin seriously to accept and know himself. But in the light now of sober living, not within the drinking pattern. There is an enormous difference between knowledge of the "wet" sort and insight of the "dry". Get a man living right; let him, then, begin to think right. A man's thinking follows his desires, no matter how much intelligent assent he may congenially give to something he does not really believe in and feel.

It is, then, to sustain and keep the positive phase active that makes self-acceptance and self-knowledge important. They do not necessarily start an alcoholic on the road to sobriety. But they certainly are essential in keeping him on that road, once he has started out.

The alcohol problem has an advantage over a great many other personality disorders because it has a name and the main trouble can be spotted right away. The alcoholic knows what his surrender centres on. It is the plain fact that he is drinking too much. I know that much can be said in favor of the views which stress that "drinking is not a problem". It is comforting, maybe, to believe you are not an alcoholic when you are. But I doubt the worth of such a delusion if you are really anxious to get at the root of a problem of which the symptom is as disturbing as the cause! The alcoholic's major trouble is his excessive use of alcohol. This he knows right now, though he does not yet suspect anything about the fear, the tension, or other psychological imps that lurk in the background. In his alcoholic misery he is not concerned about changing jobs or finding his proper niche in life. This comes after the surrender, not before it. Adjustment in vocation is certainly essential in *maintaining* happy sobriety.

The alcoholic, we may suppose, sees himself first of all, as a person who drinks too much. The alcohol problem is therefore much more definite than many other human problems. It is a disorder that lends itself well to the surrender approach. When his defiance and grandiosity are crushed, and he feels beaten, the alcoholic can say "I am powerless over alcohol. I will stop fighting it, because I want sobriety more than drinking. I will turn to the sober pattern of living."

Now the differentiation may appear to be raw, but it is wondrously effective. The alcoholic looks at life now in two patterns, one wet, the other dry. That is the simple psychology of the alcoholic, and it works, because for him the whole truth of living lies in that distinction between alcohol and no alcohol.

Naturally the problem is not solved at that point. Within the dry pattern there are fine lines to be traced and distinctions to be made, in the whole adventure of adjustment that awaits the newly recovered alcoholic. But the biggest hurdle is cleared when he abandons the drinking pattern and surrenders to the dry way of life.

Besides positive thinking, there is positive doing, the outlet of energy formerly devoted to fear. There must be productive action as well as productive thought if the recovered alcoholic is to stay solidly in the "positive phase" of recovery. It is not enough to quit drinking and to think straight.

To know better does not always mean we shall act better. Yet we cannot do without good thinking. Blind feeling may cause more harm than good. "I meant well but I guess I didn't think" is as common an apology as "I wonder what went wrong. I had it so well worked out." In the first case the action is impulsive, unthoughtful. In the second case the action is too reasonable, too mechanical, and thus inhuman and cold.

Somehow we have to bring out thinking and doing together. The plea for self-acceptance and self-knowledge falls flat unless we are prepared to do something about it.

The alcoholic is subject to sudden rushes of strong feeling. He either expresses himself thoughtlessly and impulsively or stores up these feelings until the tension snaps and he gets drunk. As these feelings are stored up, he develops fear and becomes hostile, silently angry. He is all alone because he does not share these feelings, he does not take them out in friendships, consuming interests and deep affections. The alcoholic grows lonely and bored. It is not surprising that the release in drunkenness runs in two extremes, the one passive, dull and inert, the other manic, boisterous and aggressive. The two extremes are equally a protest against aloneness, fear and boredom. Often the two extremes occur in one person on the same binge.

The solution here seems to be to find outlets for these feelings, activities that will not allow this energy to gather and break uncontrolled in an alcoholic flood. Aloneness, fear, boredom. What kinds of activity can replace them? Music, the theatre, sports, reading, hobbies—best of all, for the alcoholic—fellowship and love.

Psychology sets forth the worth of self-acceptance and

self-knowledge. Life tells us, just as importantly, about love, "the sense of the heart". The alcoholic can learn much from both, and so bring his thinking into line with his doing.

The alcoholic who stops drinking and shows a feeling of kinship, born of his own misery, for a fellow alcoholic, need never be afraid of fear, of boredom, or of loneliness. In this feeling of empathy, he will find himself acting confidently and positively. He knows what he is talking about. He communicates the lessons of his self-acceptance to his fellow alcoholic and tells him about a healthier life. He gains by giving. He profits by love. In sharing his thinking, he acts, and in acting he strengthens his thinking.

So far as I know, there is nothing more effective in the follow-up treatment of alcoholism than the simple therapy of one drunk helping another—to stay sober, and to enjoy sobriety.

7.

ALCOHOLICS ANONYMOUS

To A.A. and its spectacular success goes the credit for being the most efficient means at present for coping with the alcoholic problem.

What is the secret of the success of A.A.? Many call it a miracle. Many say it is the wisdom of the ages condensed into less than 200 words in language that all can understand. Miracle, wisdom, science, religion, it works, and 300,000 men and women have found sobriety in the A.A. way of life.

Alcoholics Anonymous is a fellowship of men and women who share their experience, strength and hope with each other that they may solve their common problem and help others to recover from alcoholism.

The only requirement for membership is an honest desire to stop drinking. A.A. has no dues or fees. It is not allied with any sect, denomination, politics, organization or institution; does not wish to engage in any controversy, neither endorses nor opposes any causes. Our primary purpose is to stay sober and help other alcoholics to achieve sobriety.

The A.A. program of recovery is incorporated in the 12 steps. The A.A. book of experience, Alcoholics Anonymous, and other literature, including the 12 points of Tradition, are available through any group or General Service Headquarters, P.O. Box 459, Grand Central Annex, New York 17, N.Y.[1]

The Twelve Steps

(1) We admitted we were powerless over alcohol—that our lives had become unmanageable.

(2) Came to believe that a Power greater than ourselves could restore us to sanity.

(3) Made a decision to turn our will and our lives over to the care of God as we understand Him.

(4) Made a searching and fearless moral inventory of ourselves.

(5) Admitted to God, to ourselves and to another human being the exact nature of our wrongs.

(6) Were entirely ready to have God remove all these defects of character.

(7) Humbly asked Him to remove our shortcomings.

(8) Made a list of all persons we had harmed, and became willing to make amends to them all.

(9) Made direct amends to such people whenever possible, except when to do so would injure them or others.

(10) Continued to take personal inventory and when we were wrong, promptly admitted it.

(11) Sought through prayer and meditation to improve our conscious contact with God as we understood Him, praying only for knowledge of His will for us and the power to carry that out.

(12) Having had a spiritual awakening as the result of these steps, we tried to carry this message to alcoholics and practice these principles in all our affairs.

With this new basic philosophy, the new A.A. member sets about to reorder his life around four main ideas—the *Self, Society, Service* and *God.* The difficulties and strains of the self are covered in the first seven steps of the A.A. program. In these seven steps the A.A. member is busy putting himself in order. He learns humility, honesty, self-acceptance and fair-play. In these seven steps he examines himself as thoroughly as possible. With the help of God he acquires wisdom and practices kindness. He develops a sense of humour, especially the ability to laugh at himself, for the alcoholic usually takes himself too seriously. He probes into his sexual conflicts and other personal problems. He develops inner security and self-confidence. He destroys fear.

In the first step of the A.A. program there is surrender, a long accepted principle of psycho-therapy in gaining insight into one's problems. Dr. Harry Tiebout, a famous psychiatrist and friend of A.A., stressed at Yale School (1949) that inducing the state of surrender is the first and most important feature of his treatment. After the act of surrender takes place, he can actually see his patients relax, physically as well as mentally; their tensions ease after their defiant and grandiose ideas disappear, after all other support is withdrawn, after they see they are completely hopeless and helpless on their own power. The first step of the A.A. program is a simple statement of this surrender. No one can recover from alcoholism who does not experience the act of surrender.

After the surrender of the first step, the alcoholic learns the lesson of humility in the second and third steps. His old tense defiance is further broken down when he gives himself over to the guidance of a power greater than himself.

The self-honesty and self-knowledge achieved in the fourth step become the tools for uprooting the vicious qualities which either brought him his trouble or developed in the course of his drinking career—childishness, sensitiveness, grandiosity, impulsiveness, intolerance and wishful thinking.

In the fifth step, *fear* is ready for even more release. After the surrender of the first step, the humility of the second and third, and the searching analysis of the fourth, the alcoholic now unburdens all excess weight. It is a disposal of emotional garbage that has been carried for years, each year growing heavier than the last. He throws away his guilt and anxiety and fear by admitting the exact nature of his wrongs in a very intimate and unobtrusive way. He does not proclaim this act before the world. He admits his wrongs to himself, to another human being, and to God as he understands Him. Two of his worst faults, intolerance and grandiosity, are completely reshaped when this step is taken.

In the sixth and seventh steps he finds the spiritual insight which gives him his greatest strength. He realizes more and more that no man can handle the problems of human behaviour on his own power. He must continue to seek help but he must *want* to do so.

The first seven steps taken by the alcoholic provide him with what he most needs when he goes on the program, *personal recovery*. They seem to be designed to hit directly at acute personal distress, and therefore chiefly concern the *self*.

In the eighth and ninth steps the alcoholic takes *action*, in society, in his relations with other people. Now he approaches his fellow man in a spirit of co-operation, not of *defiance*. Finding his place in society had formerly meant a challenge to him which he felt compelled to meet aggressively. There was something to beat, something to fight. With this aggressive attitude, there was always the fear of failure and in his panic resorted to alcohol. In the eighth and ninth steps, aggression is converted into goodwill. He learns to go along with society, rather than to defy it. He learns that it is far easier to follow the traffic through the green light and to stop when society flashes on the red signal. To defy society and go one's way, regardless of others, is to court tragedy and death. In the eighth and ninth steps the alcoholic achieves prestige, self-respect, love, fellowship and a concern for others—all the qualities which express productively the alcoholic's urge to be aggressive and defiant.

In the tenth step, he sees himself now not only as an individual but as an individual in society. The 10th step is a reinforcement of the fourth. He continues to take personal inventory but now the inventory includes the eighth and ninth steps, steps that take him out of himself into the world around him. The tenth step brings self into society in an amiable partnership. A sincere working of the tenth step teaches him that he must constantly check on himself and on his relations with others. He can no longer say as he once did, way back in the warm glows of his early drinking, "Everything is rosy now". He can be happy and contented only in the humble knowledge that he is capable of taking just one day at a time. He can never be sure that everything is perfect; when he thinks like this, he may have a serious relapse, for any man is ready for his greatest fall in the very moment of his deepest pride.

In the eleventh step, there is the gentle but firm reminder of God and the fact that the A.A. program requires every member to do something about Him. Interpretation, fortunately, is wide open, because the alcoholic dislikes regimentation. He must find God in his own way, if at all. He can support the religion of his choice, but the merit of this choice is that he goes to it now with renewed faith. On the other hand, he is free to understand God outside the area of doctrine, if he sincerely and honestly finds Him from the depth of his own convictions. Even Jesus said "It is not I but your faith which hath made thee whole."

A.A. cannot set forth a doctrine of any sort, be it religious, scientific, or social for that would be to exclude certain sufferers whose human needs are as great as those of the exclusive set.

I suppose the only deep basic belief in A.A. amounting to a dogma is that life is worth living and intensely valuable. And if life is worth living, that goes for the next fellow as well as for the alcoholic concerned. Belief in God is an admission of humility and of limits, and keeps the alcoholic from ever supposing that he or any other human being can explain the universe in terms to suit everyone in the same way. Now this humility is far from negative. The A.A.

program to stay alive must keep its eyes and mind open to every insight coming from other sources. Let me quote Bill W. from his Yale talk of 1945:

"Let's reach into other people's experiences. Let's go back to our friends the doctors, let's go back to our friends the preachers, the social workers, all those who have been concerned about us, and again review what they have above ground and bring that into a synthesis. And let us, where we can, bring them in where they will fit."

The twelfth step is the synthesis of self, society and God in service. The test of A.A. principles takes place in living deeds, for without them the program collapses. The A.A. member learns, when all is said and done, that what keeps him sober is helping other alcoholics stay sober.

As A.A. is an intensely personal fellowship, preferring human experience to scientific explanations, it is better to let one of its members speak for himself. It is Allen again, an alcoholic who has found that the A.A. way of life embodies everything that meets his needs. Much of the material in this book comes from him. His views are his own. Each A.A. member can interpret the program as it suits him best. What Allen says, therefore, is not necessarily the view of any other member, but he is an example of how the A.A. program can be flexibly followed to suit every sort of person.[2]

"For a long time my desire to stop drinking was not honest. As I see it now, it was giving up something that down deep in my heart I didn't want to let go. I stayed dry in a martyr-like way, giving up something that was part of me for the sake of somebody else. Then I saw that life is really more exciting without alcohol. The desire for sobriety became the strongest desire of my being.

"I know now that I am powerless over alcohol and my life unmanageable, if I continue to use it. There is no need to fight now. I no longer *want* the drug that was killing me. A man only fights for what he wants. I want sobriety more than anything else in the world.

"Though I no longer want alcohol I need help to stay sober. Torn for years by a habit-forming sickness, I could not recover by myself, though I tried everything within my power. It is my belief in a power greater than myself that keeps me sober.

"I do not understand God. All I know is that healthy living must be part of His scheme. If not, there would be no life. I was not healthy when I drank. God, I think, must be back of all sane healthy living. When I pray, I ask Him to help me grow healthy in mind and body. I know, too, that He cannot do this for me unless I do my share. I abandon my will and life to this belief.

"I make out a moral inventory on the basis of what Bill W. once suggested in one of his talks. I examine my life in the light of three problems—Sex, Security and Other People. What are my sex problems? How secure am I in my conscience? How honest am I in my obligation to my family and in my business dealings? What are my debts to other people, in money or in other ways and how can I improve my relations with them?

"To admit to God and to yourself the exact nature of your wrongs is to have made a thorough job of the fourth step.

"But more difficult still is the humility and courage it takes in the fifth step to tell another human being all the errors you can think of in your whole life. I did not remove my fear and worry, two causes of my drinking, until I told a friend my complete life history.

"God needs me as much as I need God. I could not know His care and ask Him to remove my defects of character until I decided that I wanted to remove those defects. Those defects disappear if I am sincere when I say "Lead us not into temptation but deliver us from evil." I must work on this prayer every day. If I don't I find that I am not always ready to have God remove my defects of character.

"Forgive us our trespasses as we forgive those who trespass against us." In these powerful words I get my clue to the meaning of the seventh step, "Humbly ask Him to remove our shortcomings."

"I come to see that God forgives me exactly to the extent that I forgive others. I can expect that He will remove my shortcomings only if I cease to criticize and hate those who offend me, and if I resolve not to resent those whom I most offend.

"In the first seven steps of the program I have been mostly concerned with my personal problems. In the eighth and ninth steps I move into the realm of other people, alcoholics and non-alcoholics. I harmed many people in my drinking days. It is not hard to make a list of them. In making amends to them it has worked out well in almost every case. Rarely have I met ridicule or scorn. Rarely have I been snubbed. One gesture was ignored and that hurt. But as I think it over, I see that I make a bad situation worse if I continue to pester this unresponsive victim of my old selfishness. He wants nothing to do with me. After all, can I blame him? So be it. But I must go on with these efforts until my slate is as clean as possible.

"The eleventh step continues the third as the tenth continues the fourth. The whole program lives. There is nothing final about any one of the steps. The more I live and watch others in the same adventure the surer I am that a human being never stops growing.

"As I have a fear of being disliked, I suppose there will always be people who seem to dislike me and whom I offend. There will be those who watch me darkly in anything I say or do and I, in turn, will watch others critically, as long as I remain sensitive.

"But as I continue to take personal inventory and admit when I am wrong I find that people are much less critical of me because it takes the wind out of their sails. I beat them to it. Then, too, it is hard to be critical of others with the knowledge and admission of my own defects clear in my mind.

"As to improving my conscious contact with God, there

is one that I am working on now. It is about my relations
with other people. All my contacts with God take place in
this human world. I have never been out of it except when
I was drinking. This new contact with God shows me that
human nature is a lot like everything else in nature. If I
ignore the rain or the snow I may catch cold. This is nature's
way of "hating" me. If I ignore the feelings and views of
my fellowman when I come in contact with him I may catch
the emotional cold called resentment. This is human nature's
way of hating me. And I learn to hate my fellowman, by
failing to understand him. The demands of my fellowman
on me are at least as important as the demands of the
weather.

"About all my thinking and living I see now that I tend
to build excuses and reasons for my own designs. It is hard
for me not to be a wishful thinker, but something helps me
now when I suspect my thinking is crooked. I look directly
at things and people again and again. I try to sense their
meaning not for me but for what *they* are. I have no right
to hate a person or a thing if I do not understand it. If I am
confused, I try not to let it bother me. Gradually I find that
things and people speak for themselves if I look accurately
and keep my mind open. I guard against the old impulsive
tendency to make snap decisions. Whatever it is will turn
out as it should if I do not push the result too hard. I try
to apply this to my family, my business, my associates, my
whole life.

"Many A.A. members have a hard time with the spiritual
side of the program. I think this trouble arises from the belief
that 'spiritual' means something mysterious, far-fetched,
'out-of-the-world' though really it need not mean anything
of the sort.

"As you look through the eleven steps leading to the last
you notice that not one of them says anything about pills
or food or books; not one of them is *material*. They are all
spiritual. Some new members have come to the group saying 'Well, what do we do now, where's the cure, what do

we have to do?' They soon find out there is nothing in the program you can touch, taste, smell or take in your hands as you grasp a bottle of medicine. Even the words they hear mean nothing until they are understood and felt.

"As I see it, it is impossible to go through the eleven steps leading to the twelfth without having a spiritual experience. That, I suppose, is why the original framers were so sure of themselves when they wrote, 'Having had a spiritual experience as the result of these steps,' instead of 'We hope something spiritual will happen to us.' They are certain that anyone honestly working the program will have a spiritual experience. If he does not, something has gone wrong, something has been missed or neglected.

"The next words make up what A.A.'s call 'twelfth step work'. Carrying the message to other alcoholics brings results that pills and medicine failed to bring. When you compare the man you see at his first A.A. meeting with the same man weeks, months and years later, you see the practical effect of the spiritual experience he has gone through. He is the same body but the easy manner, the clear eye, the sincere greeting, these show through his neat clean appearance. He is sober, but spiritual change is more marked than the physical improvement. You might say that his better appearance really comes from inside: his change of heart has erased the frowns of shyness and the wrinkles of fear. Here is the material witness of the spiritual awakening. Here are the real goods in human flesh. Neither reason nor money bought them. I think the word 'spiritual' covers it best of all.

"To practice the principles of the twelve steps in all my affairs I see to be a life time's job. As there are less than ten percent of all alcoholics on the A.A. program the rest of my days could be spent in carrying the message to only a small fraction of them. In this service, if I am sincere, I need never be bored. Thousands of adventures await me. What time there is to spare can be put to the service of the non-alcoholics."

A description of the A.A. program is not complete without its Twelve Traditions. These traditions, practical out-growths in working the twelve steps, have been found so valuable that A.A. groups have fallen into difficulties of all sorts whenever they have ignored them. Most A.A. groups therefore stress their traditions as much as the Twelve Steps. The traditions are so clearly expressed they need no explanation but themselves. Here they are in abbreviated form.

The Twelve Traditions

1. Our common welfare should come first; personal recovery depends upon A.A. unity.

2. For our group purpose there is but one ultimate authority—a loving God as he may express himself in our group conscience. Our leaders are but trusted servants—they do not govern.

3. The only requirement for A.A. membership is a desire to stop drinking.

4. Each group should be autonomous, except in matters affecting other groups or A.A. as a whole.

5. Each group has but one primary purpose—to carry its message to the alcoholic who still suffers.

6. An A.A. group ought never endorse, finance or lend the A.A. name to any related facility or outside enterprise lest problems of money, property and prestige divert us from our primary spiritual aim.

7. Every A.A. group ought to be fully self-supporting, declining outside contributions.

8. Alcoholics Anonymous should remain forever non-professional, but our service centres may employ special workers.

9. A.A., as such, ought never be organized; but we may create service boards or committees directly responsible to those who serve.

10. Alcoholics Anonymous has no opinion on outside

issues; hence the A.A. name ought never be drawn into public controversy.

11. Our public relations policy is based on attraction rather than promotion; we need always maintain personal anonymity at the level of press, radio and films.

12. Anonymity is the spiritual foundation of all our Traditions, ever reminding us to place principles above personalities.

The great wisdom of the A.A. program is to be found in its complete understanding of the alcoholic personality. The entire Twelve Steps and Twelve Traditions take full account of the alcoholic's tendencies. The program does not try to destroy these tendencies; it accepts them and redirects them.

The principle of anonymity, in which names of members are to be respected and withheld from the public, if members so wish it, is a natural right so long as certain citizens, who control our economy, continue to be disdainful and morally critical of the alcoholic. But the true meaning of anonymity in A.A. is an anonymity of service. Nothing so well redirects and transforms the alcoholic's grandiosity as the doing of good deeds for fellow sufferers in distress, without material reward and without publicity.

"Live and let live" says in a few words more than many lectures can reveal about tolerance. It is a slogan directed against enemy No. 1, resentment.

Another slogan, "Easy does it", is a constant reminder to the alcoholic that he cannot absorb the A.A. program in a day, a month, a year. He can stop drinking immediately he takes the first step. But it takes time to know and work the rest of the steps and the twelve traditions. Time is on the side of the alcoholic who stops drinking.

From the entire A.A. program the community at large may learn much. Alcoholic or non-alcoholic, wet or dry, regardless of race or creed, can profit from the universal principles of A.A. because A.A. opposes no one. It is a simple program with but one clear aim, to live more abundantly each according to his own lights and needs, and to be conscious of the same aim in every human being. Its classic prayer is one for the whole world, "God grant me the serenity to accept the things I cannot change, courage to change the things I can, and wisdom to know the difference." As long as A.A. continues to say this prayer and put it into practice the movement will never die.

Religion, Science and A.A.

A.A. has drawn from philosophy, religion, psychology, and medicine for its insights. It puts these together where they fit in human experience and places them before each of its members to interpret in his own way as best he can. No external pressure, no rules, no "shoulds", no "don'ts" are found in the program. The members proceed on the basis of their capabilities. The grace of God is their common inspiration.

Though A.A.'s draw heavily upon the Christian message, they do not take sides in theological controversies. As A.A.'s they are not committed to any creed. A.A. is not a creedal religion, though it stresses, as John Dewey does, the religious feeling and the spiritual experience. This attitude, by the way, is congenial to alcoholics. By nature they are suspicious of authority, no matter how cogent and embracing the authority may be. In the A.A. program they have something to which they can respond in their own way, on their own time, from the depth of their own convictions. As they become more mature, they see, of course, that they cannot remain the individualists they thought they were. They come to recognize the rights and feelings of others. Yet they come by this insight of their own accord with the help of God to whom they have freely given themselves. Still, He is their God in a very selfish kind of way.

Members come into A.A. with purely selfish motives. Let a man say he is quitting alcohol to please his wife or daughter, or his boss and they will reply that he won't stay sober or suspect that he is not sincere. No, everyone of them will admit that he is quitting alcohol for his own sake, for the sake of good living, before he can hope to make a success of the program. This desire must be the strongest desire of his being; it is admittedly selfish. They soon face the paradox of ultimate truth, the plain fact that they stay sober only by helping others stay sober. Their selfishness merges into unselfishness.

They find that the peace of spirit they sought is gained through service. They have enough to do in making this service available to alcoholics, but the twelfth step suggests that they practice their principles of tolerance and kindness not only among alcoholics but in *all* their affairs, among alcoholics and non-drinkers alike. They learn finally that God is much more than an alcohol therapist, though He certainly seems to be most efficient among drunks.

But A.A.'s are not evangelists: they are not moralists. They are not on the path of the man who wants to drink. They are only concerned with the man who wants to stop drinking and cannot do so alone. For many of them the simple twelve steps and twelve traditions are enough. Nothing more is required to make the message meaningful and effective. Yet the founder once told me that the A.A. program must run as deep as the soundest roots of psychology, medicine and religion. These roots, embedded in rich personal experience, inspired the original members to write the twelve steps. Otherwise they would be as the seeds scattered on the ground that grow and flourish a while but quickly die.

The twelve steps, every one of them, teem with Christian meaning. That is clear on even a casual reading of the program. From the first, humility and honesty, to the last, service to fellow sufferers, the gospel message supports the program is every word of its simple structure.

But as meaningful as this is, thus to have the support of the gospel, I believe it is more meaningful to see the A.A.

program as one to which every alcoholic can subscribe, Christian, Jewish, agnostic, yes, even the atheist. Every alcoholic who sincerely desires to stop drinking qualifies for membership in A.A.

Suppose a Jew were writing these words. Could he not say that the program is patterned on the teachings of the rabbi Hillil? Could he not stress that the whole program, humility, kindness, tolerance, self-knowledge, enlightened self-interest, service to others, fellowship, anonymity, is drawn from these sayings attributed to Hillil, a contemporary of Jesus?

"My abasement is my exaltation, what is unpleasant to thyself, that do not to thy neighbor; this is the whole law, all else but its exposition. If I am not for myself, who is for me? And if I am for myself alone, what then am I? Separate not thyself from the congregation. Judge not thy neighbor until thou art in his place. He who wishes to make a name for himself loses his name. He who works for the sake of a crown is lost."

Suppose a Mohammedan were explaining A.A. That is most unlikely, as Islam forbids the use of alcohol. But it is conceivable that a Mohammedan could join A.A., for Islam means literally submission to the will of God. If he did, he could subscribe to the program as consistently as a Christian or Jew, and were he to bring in his religion, he could justify Mohammed if he wished to do so.

Suppose an agnostic or atheist were writing about A.A. That is indeed likely, for many A.A.'s joined the fellowship in just that category. All that is expected of any alcoholic who desires to stop drinking is an open mind. A man is not long in A.A. before he sees a Power greater than himself in operation. The atheist soon admits the philosophy of "man for himself" is futile and false: he soon sees that God, if nothing else, is a simple name for the contagion of love, even though he finds it hard to form an idea of God beyond the one so simply framed in the twelfth step—"carry the message to other alcoholics and practice these principles (the principles of humility, honesty, tolerance and kindness) in *all* our affairs."

As to the spiritual experience stressed in the twelfth step, it can happen to anyone, regardless of creed or faith, who genuinely follows the program. It may be a sudden vision as it was with the founder. With most of them it is a conversion in the sense of a slow change, though conversion it is, without doubt.

William James' "Varieties of Religious Experience" is a book treasured by the early members of A.A. In this book conversion is explained in a way acceptable to those who are skeptical of a term that imposes doctrinal obligations. Conversion in the psychology of James is seen as a reconditioning of the motives for living, the drawing from deep wells of energies whose riches were ignored in the superficial life of material needs, petty rivalries, and false gain. To contact these hidden reservoirs is to reach God. A man reaches Him often in his most dire needs. The work of James touched off the hope that science and religion are one inquiry, not two in conflict with one another. This gave the early members of A.A. something to grapple with. The result was a firm belief in God, but God as each man experienced Him in his own life.

A.A.'s have the open mind on this human turn-about. They see that it may come in a flash, and precipitate itself suddenly from a background of misery and dejection. They see, too, that it can come gradually as it does with most of them, as insight slowly dawns and they view themselves and world about them with sober though not always mature eyes. This emotional immaturity, however, has features they prize, such as the faith of little children, their sincerity, adventurousness and naivety, their unreserved and honest life. But the childishness which induces them to get drunk, they set out to analyze the better to destroy it. Like children they are sensitive to pain and like children they are dreamers. Their skins are so thin and so easily bruised that they unconsciously seek to strengthen themselves in drink and cover up in numbness. That applies to the aggressive as well as to the timid; both flee from fear to the false security of drink that momentarily toughens and later leaves the wounds more raw than ever. The alcoholic is driven to criticism and rebellion because his fearful mind dislikes the voice of society which says, "You are grown up; you are no longer a child with someone to run to with all your troubles. You have duties and you must perform them." The active alco-holic therefore either defies, or flees from the conventional world. In defiance there is divorce, crime, unemployment, poverty. In flight there is sickness, alibis, mental institutions, perhaps suicide.

So A.A.'s welcome the insights of science; psychology has been of priceless value to them in their self-analysis and understanding of the sober mature world. Not only the work of Wm. James, but the science of Freud, Jung and Adler is found in the A.A. program, acting as a catalyst between the needs of personality and the deepest insights of religion. That many members of A.A. do not recognize the scientific labels known to psychologists is not important. What matters most is that the facts they represent are operative in the movement.

The most vital, though the most neglected, feature of the genius of Freud was his use of the person to person relationship. Remorse, morbid guilt, fear and worry are removed through the releasing agency of a confidential personal relationship. (Freud's psycho-sexual theory is important but often over-stressed and misinterpreted.)

The group therapy of A.A. has improved on Freud by removing the doctor-patient or the "I know and you don't" attitude, and replacing it with the patient-patient or "We're all in the same boat" attitude; it also helps to supply the basic needs of all human beings, affection and mutual understanding. It's worth is incalculable when contrasted with the limitations and failures of the authority—dependent situation, so often controlled by fear and ignorance.

Through this participant principle of A.A. an alcoholic can say, "This man is just like me. He has the same problem. He and many like him have solved their problem. I am in the same boat. There is no harm here. No one is trying to make me over. This man, this fellow-alcoholic, is helping himself by helping me. He is as sick as I am. I see that I can be among people of my own kind. There is nothing to hide, nothing to fight, and everything to gain."

From Jung comes the insight, scientifically confirmed in case histories, that many people with serious personal problems need a religious outlook on life. "Among all my patients is the second half of life—that is to say, over thirty-five—there has not been one whose problem in the last resort was not that of finding a religious outlook on life." Jung's patients were disturbed primarily because they lacked a unity of purpose in their lives; they needed the integration which the best insights of religions have, throughout history, given to their followers. A.A. is alert to this fact. Its program is not just a cure for alcoholism, it is a way of life.

Freud made sex the basic drive in life. Jung extended this view to include the sex, ego and herd instincts. A.A. members can classify their problems, as Allen did, under three headings, similar to Jung's classification, sex, security and society. The value of another classification of Jung's, introversion—extraversion, is also known among A.A. members. The introvert tends to brood and withdraw into himself; the extravert, on the other hand, is impulsively outgoing and may neglect the things of the mind. In the A.A. program both these types get the insight they need, and the chance to express it. The introvert does not repress his natural inclinations to think. The difference now is that in the A.A. program of service he has company and he can put his ideas to work. The extravert, similarly, need not repress his natural urge to be active. As an A.A. member, however, his actions are now directed by a much needed emotional control. He has now a way of life. Without this core of deep purpose, his former attitudes led him to confusion.

Adler contributes his theory of compensation to the A.A. program. In every group, the principle of compensation is constantly at work. Men and women who never before in their lives spoke in public, come forth and express themselves confidently. Many members, friendless, alone, and insecure find in A.A. the fellowship, love and respect they desperately need.

The much discussed complexes of inferiority and superiority, authored by Adler, find their balance in a vigorous expression of the A.A. program. Feelings of inferiority and superiority, in excess, are signs of insecurity, a weak ego. This weak ego is strengthened in A.A. The battered fearful personality of the alcoholic is rebuilt in the wholesome atmosphere of good will, kindly feeling, and mutual respect of the casual A.A. meeting. Those who criticize A.A. on the grounds of its emotionalism should remember these vital facts (1) Modern society tends to be calculating and hard. If a group, like A.A., feels like taking the brakes off its emotional repressions, this perhaps is healthy rather than ominous. It is compensation for activities necessarily renounced in the daily struggle for existence. (2) As members grow in A.A., the initial emotional energy required to start them on the program spreads out in activities of service. Alcoholics are emotional by nature. When their conflicts resolve, this trait is an admirable quality. No group savours real pleasure or enjoys each other more than a crowd of congenial alcoholics who have stopped drinking. (3) Every member of A.A. knows that within and behind his emotional nature, there is the constant demand of honesty. It is in the single requirement of admission to the fellowship—an honest desire to stop drinking. The plea for honesty continues throughout the twelve steps of the program. The member who is not honest will not stay sober. As long as A.A.'s remember the central demand of honesty and truth, they need never fear nor resent the criticisms of those who mistakenly label the movement as over-emotional.

The synthesis of religion and science in the A.A. movement is capped, for many, in the belief that God is the author of science as of everything else. A.A.'s learn to be open-minded, to welcome insight from any source that can enrich and support their way of life.

With the help of psychology and medicine, they learn that their problem is not just a moral one. They learn with some relief that they have not been moral monsters of weak will, people who deliberately chose gross sensuality and degradation. They learn rather, that they are sick in body and mind and that much can be done to help them by a sober insight into the constitution of their troubled minds and weakened bodies. Psychology furnishes the mental picture; medicine, the physical picture. A.A.'s call alcoholism an obsession of the mind coupled with a body sensitivity. They explore this obsession in the fourth step of the program each according to his own lights. They are also made constantly aware in their meetings of the body sensitivity. That first drink is fatal and overrides every other consideration, no matter how good a man the alcoholic might otherwise be. Medicine continues to explore this sensitivity. A.A.'s stand by and listen attentively. But they believe modern psychology and medicine, though highly valued in their program, are but parts of the whole.

The A.A. program embraces much of the best thought and inspiration of western culture.

There was Socrates who said that the unexamined life is not worth living; Plato who believed the world of the senses is but a shadow of the realm of Ideas whose crowning Idea is the Good. There was Aristotle who stressed self-realization and moderation. Where one could not be moderate, abstain. The Stoics and Epicureans preached frugality and the value of things of the mind.

Christ shattered the world with his paradox that broke down the calculators of morals, the truth that love grows as it is divided. Love in Christ became a world principle and ceased to be a romantic notion. It catalyzed self-respect with humility and kindness. It brought together mature selfishness and fellowship. Saint Paul enriched this concept of spiritual love.

Saint Augustine intimated the futility of the pledge. He showed that time is most really an attitude of mind. Well do alcoholics realize this when they remember that pledges to stop drinking were dreary periods between drunks. Enforced periods of dryness for a month, a year, or ten years were periods that cut into their alcoholic lives. They were a series of deaths. So A.A.'s work on a 24-hour basis. They work on the great insight of Christ "sufficient unto the day is the evil thereof", and support it with Saint Augustine's shrewd analysis of the nature of Time. No one can bargain for the future, it is never here. A human being can manage only one day comfortably at a time.

St. Thomas revived Aristotle's principle of self-fulfilment. It is a man's duty to become what it is in him the best to become. Pride, says religious tradition, is a major sin, the greatest obstacle to true self-fulfilment. It is pride that keeps an alcoholic from taking the first step of the A.A. program.

St. Francis was a living example of the activity of love. "It is better to love than be loved, it is better to understand than to be understood."

Luther, Knox and Calvin, among others, stressed the grace of God, an expression constantly on the lips and in the hearts of all sincere A.A.'s. But it is the grace of God linked with service to others—a reminder that they must recognize no barriers, no class distinctions, in the exercise of this service.

A good thought comes from Spinoza. A man's strongest desire will sooner or later express itself. A.A.'s set out to make the desire to stop drinking the greatest desire in life. Hence their slogan "First things first".

These are a few examples taken from the wealth of western tradition to show that the principles of A.A. are not passing fads.

All A.A. meetings close with the Lord's Prayer. This is evidence that A.A. is not simply a scientific program, not simply a collection of gems of wisdom, not simply an emotional outlet. A.A. is all these and something more, in its faith and its humility.

The prayer closing each meeting is a prayer that can be said by men and women of every creed and race. The God of A.A. is God as each member understands Him.

FOOTNOTES — CHAPTER 7

1. A.A. defined, the Twelve Steps and the Twelve Traditions are drawn from *The Grapevine*, monthly Journal of Alcoholics Anonymous, New York.
2. See the excellent book, *Alcoholics Anonymous*. This book is regarded very highly by A.A.'s. It describes a variety of experiences out of which the fellowship has grown and now flourishes.

8.

PERSONAL GROWTH—THE BASIC ISSUE

WHAT is personality? It is what we do, say and appear in the presence of others, as much as what we are by ourselves.

When our activities are forbidden, ridiculed or rejected by others we must, to be ourselves, find some other way of fitting into the pattern of life about us.

We want to adjust to the scene in which we move, without having to conform to the authority or views of others. We want to be ourselves but if we fail to adjust, we are misfits. A misfit should not be confused with an individualist. Keep our integrity? By all means. Pursue our personal desires? By all means. But if we have a personality problem that threatens our well being as well as that of others, we are misfits. The world is full of them. The motto of misfits might well be, "A sincere desire to destroy fear and to live maturely. From sickness to health. From flight to surrender."

Fear disappears when we surrender our false pride. To surrender our false pride is to relax, resolve to be open-minded, accept ourselves, know ourselves, and start to grow again. Live and let live. Surrender to life.

The basic question everyone must ask himself is "Do I want to live maturely?"

The drinking pattern, its analysis, the scientific suggestions for breaking it, the great service of Alcoholics Anonymous—all assume that love of abundant life is stronger than the half-dead, half-alive values of the sick alcoholic. The reader may now feel that the same basic question faces many sick people who are not alcoholic—serious neurotics, and countless other misfits. The question "Do I want to live maturely?" does indeed face everyone, alcoholic or non-alcoholic, whose misery and half-hearted efforts at living stem in part from the man himself. Partial living is immature, frustrating, tense. It is better to be fully than partially alive. But let's return to our topic, the alcoholics.

When the alcoholic becomes convinced that he is powerless over alcohol he must follow up his surrender with an even stronger conviction. Life with alcohol is unendurable. Life is worth living only if he totally abstains. So long as the attitude is one of sacrifice, the alcoholic will never achieve adventurous sobriety. The attitude must be a desire for richer living in the belief that the alcoholic life is, in one way or another, suicidal.

The alcoholic is powerless over his problem. The alcoholic is suicidal, whether he knows it or not. These two facts are clear to anyone who has been through the experience. They are also clear to anyone who has studied the problem and made a careful study of the drinking pattern.

One requirement of the alcoholic is asked in order to insure recovery. That is a sincere desire to stop drinking. And what for the alcoholic does the desire to stop drinking mean? Positively, it means the desire to live. Sobriety is life.

So far so good. But there is still the bleak fact to face, that the alcoholic is powerless over his problem.

After deciding in favor of mature living, the misfit has no choice now but to find the help he needs in a power greater than himself. What is this power? Psychology says it is insight and A.A. says it is God. What is the quality common to the insight of psychology and to the Great Power of A.A.? Though the psychologist and the A.A. member differ in many respects, both agree that the power greater than any one person is the power of service. Though psychologists differ in their views about their science, all agree that the mature person is one who understands not only his own needs but also the needs of others. This insight remains barren unless it is put into practice. The twelfth step of the A.A. program makes it clear that service to other alcoholics and the practice of kindness, humility and honesty are two principles acceptable to the God of all members, though their ideas of Him may differ in countless other ways.

When the alcoholic stops drinking, inspired hopefully by an honest desire to quit, he is for a time confused. In this state he is on the receiving end of service. If he has deep personality trouble, he may require a psychologist or psychiatrist. He is sick and like all sick people he needs care. Perhaps he is not so disordered as to require professional attention. If not, it is almost certain that he will gain recovery through A.A. Now after insight has been gained through the help of a psychologist or the fellowship of A.A., or both, what is it that guarantees recovery?

What has next to be done after the alcoholic has regained his health, cleared his mind, and reshaped his personality? He will try to do the same for someone else, not by preaching, not by "shoulds" or "musts", not by rules and orders, but by voluntary action when the person needing help seeks it.

This seems to be the root principle underlying the psychology of alcoholism and the fellowship of A.A. One of the reasons why alcoholics helped by a psychologist or psychiatrist join A.A. is because they have there a constant opportunity to do the service that keeps them sober.

Every act of service is a power greater than the man performing it. What control does any man have over the little nameless turn he does for his fellowman in distress? He has no control whatever. He is simply the vehicle of a power that will persist after he is dead and gone. This power is productive and creative, awake to the distress of every human being who wants help. It has only to be sought and it will be found. Another kind of act greater than the man performing it is the power of destruction. But the alcoholic has already tried that. Alcoholism, he knows from bitter experience, is a power greater than himself—a force not of service but of destruction. He has had enough of that. It nearly destroyed him. He turns now to the greater power of service. Many men of strong faith call the productive power, God; the destructive power, Evil. Whether through the insight of psychology or the Great Power of A.A., every alcoholic in the honesty of his conscience will declare in favor of what his sincerity tells him. No one would wish it otherwise.

But in the end, every recovered alcoholic enjoying sobriety, will tell you that he is happier without alcohol than with it, that he is glad he is alive because ahead of him he sees a life enriched by a new understanding of himself and of others. This new understanding of the needs of others, he will tell you, is the surest guarantee he has of staying sober.

Sooner or later the alcoholic recognizes his body sensitivity as the factor which makes him forever unable to drink normally. In addition to that, the insight available to him through psychology or A.A., well understood and practiced, will ensure happy sobriety.

The same sort of insight is needed by all those who seek the way of healthy living. Most needful are the young people in school, the nervous and neurotic who do not know what is wrong with them, all those who, though not alcoholic, have many problems of other sorts either now or in store for them, in the days to come.

All of us need to know about the dangers of false pride and of petty interests. We need to know the value of self-acceptance of mature selfishness, of personal growth and the nature of our genuine desires.

This insight everyone needs, though many are in no danger of becoming alcoholic. We may fall into all sorts of other disorders if we fail to understand ourselves and our relations to other people.

The alcoholic who answers the basic question with a decided "yes" can recover and his "cure" will be something like this. I quote from one who is working on it. There are many like him in A.A.; the recovery of thousands like him out of the ranks of other "misfits" can be as certain as that of alcoholics. Even healthy people might use this philosophy!

"Our time on earth is so brief we should do everything we can to lighten the burdens of fellow sufferers. Love them. Give them hope. Pull them out of their despair. It's no good wasting our time in blame and criticism. Let's think only of the needs that beset our lives. We are all on the same road. Let's try to make each other a little happier. The well adjusted have a lighter load to bear but we all journey to the same end. Let's help them, too, whenever we can. The best that may be said of us when our days are over is that no act of ours was the cause of the suffering of others. If a fellow human being in distress caught a ray of hope or a flash of insight we were ready with light and sympathy to encourage him on his way.

"There will be time to stop once in a while, lest we grow too tired and too tense. Time out to relax and stretch, to view life less seriously and have a good laugh at ourselves.

"Laughing destroys our self-pity. When it's clean, it's like praying. We learn our limits and take heart. We surrender to life."

BOOK II
SOBRIETY

1.

WHY BE SOBER?

In the opening chapter of this book we looked at the situations which prompt people to drink. Here we will learn why they decide to be sober.

Nobody discards an experience of value until he learns that the experience is worthless. If it is found to be worthless, he looks for something else that will do the job more effectively.

But we are all human. We tend to hang on to old habits for a long time after we know them to be defective and unrewarding. We need a lot of convincing to abandon the drinking pattern. After all, many of us once had great fun and adventure in the nostalgic drinking days of years gone by. We wonder if we can recapture those lost golden hours and hope desperately that we can have them again.

We want to be very sure that the drinking pattern has lost its value before we can even try to be sober.

So the first approach to sobriety is negative. It is negative but important because it explains why we must clear the ground for something new. (The positive approach to sobriety is discussed in the next chapter.)

The first approach to sobriety can easily be understood if we examine the facts as they occur in the drinking history of every alcoholic. There are three sets of facts:

    (1) The differences between reasons for early drinking and the causes which govern addiction.

    (2) Addictive drinking from start to finish.

(3) The kind of person an alcoholic becomes, *no matter who he is*, and the problems in store for him.

If you can hope to have again those golden hours of drinking, after you have honestly absorbed these facts, then God bless you and have one on me!

But if you decide that drinking no longer has any value for you, don't despair. In and around the facts you will see that there are valuable lessons and clues that can easily be put to creative use. The expensive education of addictive living is not lost. Your alcoholism can be of priceless value to you as you learn what you were, what you are, and what you become. You can just as easily move towards sobriety as you can move deeper into addiction. It all depends on how desperately you want to be free.

Pleasure Drinking and Addiction

There are three important differences between the reasons why we started drinking and the causes which govern addiction.

(a) Early drinking is symptomatic. It is a sign of our emotional needs—a craving for pleasant, friendly relations with other people, to feel better in order to enjoy these personal experiences, and to benefit from adventures we are afraid to try in sober behaviour. On the other hand, in addiction all these experiences are either destroyed or spoiled. The addicted drinker cannot honestly say that alcohol helps him to be friendly, to feel better, or to engage in productive adventure. Addiction illustrates *compulsive* behaviour, a pattern of drinking that is followed with no regard for the early reasons for "having a few". Addiction is a disorder in its own right. Early drinking is symptomatic.

(b) Early drinking is an unfortunate response to deep natural needs. The needs themselves are quite natural and justifiable. The response to them in drinking is unfortunate to those of us who are potential problem drinkers, but what we are striving for is nothing to be ashamed of. Addictive drinking, however, is not a response to those deep natural needs. Addictive drinking is sick drinking. It is sick because there is no rhyme nor reason in it, in the area of choiceful behaviour. You have sometimes heard a sincere friend say, "I can't understand why I slipped. I really wanted to stay sober." This is tragically true. Your friend can't understand what happened because the slip was caused by factors which eluded his conscious control.

(c) In early drinking, there is some choice in the drinker's behaviour. He can choose to drink only on week-ends for enjoyment, he can choose to stay sober for important engagements, he can choose to spare his family and friends embarrassment. But in addictive drinking, choice is either destroyed or greatly impaired. Chemical and psychological changes are clearly registered in his drinking and dry behaviour. Together, these factors govern the drinker's behaviour in the addicted stage and cause the condition known as loss of freedom.

After loss of freedom, there are three factors to note clearly in addiction.

(a) A physical sensitivity is now present in the drinker. One drink is enough to start a blood alcohol level that blindly urges the whole person—intelligence and all—to experience the feeling that a higher blood alcohol level will bring. So the urge to drink more is often irresistible. Very often there is a self-perpetuating urge in this sensitivity inducing the drinker to drink more in the same way that a ball rolling down hill supplies its own power in a natural momentum. There is no rhyme, no reason to such drinking. One just goes on and on.

(b) In early drinking, the drinker found that he could relieve his disturbances, and could use intoxication to behave in a way *opposite* to the way he would behave in sober life, because of his tensions or anxieties. For example, depressed in a sober state, he could feel high and happy, if drunk. Hostile in a sober state, he could become friendly if drunk. But in addiction, an intoxicated state usually only *worsens* his sober difficulties. If depressed when sober, he becomes more deeply depressed when drunk. If hostile when sober, he becomes more aggressive, even violent, when drunk. And if elated when sober, he becomes expansive and sentimental when drunk, but in a way he usually regrets, when events are recalled in the hang-over.

(c) In addiction, the drinker becomes socially dislocated. When he started drinking, years before, alcohol served as a socializer, enabling him to mix "well" with other people. But addicted, he screens himself out of the circle of his friends, until finally he can get along with no one—not even himself.

Once a drinker has become addicted, he can *never* return to the pleasure of early drinking. This is not a private opinion. It is the verdict of science.

The Five Phases of Addiction[1]

(1) *Pleasure Drinking*
Self unity—at peace with oneself.
Socializes easily—at one with the world.
Few serious hang-overs.
Rewards seem to exceed bad reactions.
Feels comfortably "high".
Anxiety, shyness submerged.
(All of the above merely temporary and brief.)

(2) *Problem Drinking*
Memory lapses.
Sneaks drinks.
Preoccupied with alcohol.
Gulps drinks.
Guilty about drinking behaviour.
Avoids reference to alcohol.
Memory lapses increase.

(3) *Resistant Drinking*
Loss of freedom.
Alibis.
Social pressures.
Grandiose behavior.

(4) *Resigned Drinking*
Prolonged "benders".
Marked ethical deterioration.

(3) Marked aggressive behaviour.
Persistent remorse.
Periods of total abstinence.
Change in pattern of drinking.
Drops friends.
Quits jobs.
Alcohol-centred behaviour.
Loses outside interests.
Suspicious of friends.
Marked self-pity.
Geographic escape.
Change in family habits.
Unreasonable resentments.
Protection of supply.
Neglect of proper nutrition.
First hospitalization.
Decrease of sexual drive.
Alcoholic jealousy.
Regular morning drinking.

(4) Impaired thinking.
Alcoholic psychoses.
Drinks with persons below his social level.
Drinks rubbing alcohol or the like.

(5) *Helpless Drinking*
Loss of alcohol tolerance.
Indefinable fears.
Tremors.
Can't do simple operations like winding a watch or tying a shoelace.
Obsessive drinking.
Vague religious desires.
Alibi system collapses.
With help, he may still recover or destroy himself.

Now please look at the description of pleasure drinking. This is the period in which we derived pleasure and satisfaction from drinking. It represents our early drinking period in "the good old days". This experience is gone forever. We cannot turn back the clock. So we will not vainly try to recapture an experience through alcohol that has become inaccessible to us because of the four phases that have wiped it out—the four phases which follow early pleasure.

Still, there is a valuable lesson to learn from the memory of our early drinking days. In it we can find the reasons why we drink in the first place. These reasons will give us sound clues to the procedure required by our recovery.

1. All phases, excepting phase one, are adapted from Dr. E. M. Jellinek's famous "doodle".

I find I must try to experience inward peace, to get along with other people without fearing or resenting them. There will be no hang-overs if I do not drink. As to dry drunks, they will pass. All I need to know is that a dry drunk, an "emotional binge", cannot last if I take the proper steps to improve my physical health, and to avoid situations which cause elation, depression or anxiety. Sober, rewards will speedily exceed bad reactions. And I will begin to feel comfortably "high" when I get rid of my fear and loneliness. I learn that my fear and loneliness, my anxieties, shyness and sensitivity will cease to be a problem when I have the faith that my recovery has to come to me *through you.*

We can use to great advantage the lesson to be learned from the phase of pleasure drinking, the first period of our addiction. We *relearn* something we already know. We recognize old needs in a new light, and satisfy them deliberately in sobriety.

In problem drinking, physical distress of various kinds may go along with emotional upset. The physical troubles include asthma, fatigue, obesity, duodenal ulcer, colitis and constipation. Emotional troubles are often closely related to physical disorders.

If a problem drinker suffers from one of the physical disorders, induced by emotional trouble, such as asthma, fatigue, obesity, duodenal ulcer, colitis or constipation, he often thinks that drinking will relieve it. This is a great error. The physical disorders we have mentioned, when they have emotional causes, are brought on by a person's need for self-protection—usually in over-sensitive persons. Alcohol may indeed bring temporary relief because of its anaesthetic qualities. But you have only to question an ulcerous alcoholic who, if he is frank, will tell you how short-lived is the power of alcohol to bring him relief from his discomfort. He will tell you too, how painful it is to get drunk—to get enough alcohol into his system to dull the pain of his rebellious stomach, and how distressed he feels in the hang-over, with a return of ulcerous pangs worse than ever. The same applies to the other physical disorders. Alcohol is no cure, but, in the long run, a worsener of the drinker's physical condition.

As problem drinking grows worse, the drinker may be urged to overcompensate for his sense of inadequacy in splurges of work, social activity and new achievement. In this stage he is bothered and worried by the question "How does my drinking affect my activities, my self-esteem, and the approval of others?" He supposes that his main problem is to show himself and others that he is competent, aggressive and capable of doing as well as, and indeed better, than the usual run of people. He proceeds in the wrong direction but is not aware of it. What he needs is not a sense of mastery, but rather, a satisfaction of much deeper needs.

But as long as the drive to achieve deceives him, he will face an unpleasant conflict. This conflict consists of the effort to adjust to life—the life of prestige and of achievement—set against the deeper compulsion to drink. False pride, fear of failure, and ignorance of his problem combine to worsen the conflict, and to deepen his alcoholism. Two main blocks stand in the way of recovery:

(a) Inability to understand the whole process from early dependence on people, the meaning of the shift from dependence on people to dependence on alcohol, and the tenderness taboo with its pattern of loneliness and fear.

(b) A mistaken pride (and fear) which stresses human aggressive goals to the neglect of personal goals. The problem drinker mistakenly supposes that he must increase his capacity for power and prestige. He neglects the personal needs of relaxed freedom, of satisfying creative activities, and of the give-and-take of affection.

These two blocks cause a conflict in the problem drinker. It is a conflict between fear of life without alcohol and the aggressive standards imposed on the drinker by society at large, a society much influenced by the tenderness taboo. For example, "will power" is an aggressive word denoting force, popularly used by many people. Hence the drinker will grit his teeth and say "By God, I'll show them." The influence of aggression is also revealed in patients who are anxious to gain intellectual mastery of their problem, without responding to the deep need to change their feelings or way of life.

The problem drinker moves into the full-fledged phase of *resistance* when the two blocks to recovery divert him into a side road of new protests. The new protests are a resistance to real recovery and a resistance to the plights of Skid Row. He is afraid of sobriety, and equally afraid of the disgrace of Skid Row. In the spirit of "By God I'll show them," he renews his splurges of effort in competitive aggression. In these splurges he grows intolerant, arrogant, defiant and hostile. Fear, directed outward in this way, becomes hatred, resentment, and sometimes elation. Such disturbed emotions may well be the cause of the following physical disorders: hypertension, migraine, hyperthyroidism, cardiac neuroses, arthritis and diabetes. Drinking does not relieve these disorders—it only makes them worse than ever in the long run.

Also, the drinker in the stage of resistance may suffer from other physical disorders resultant upon excessive use of alcohol, such as peripheral neuritis, fatty liver, cirrhosis, pancreatitis and possible brain damage.

In the phase of resistant drinking there are, among other symptoms, two of special importance to us. These are *loss of freedom*[2] and the alcoholic's *basic conflict*.

Loss of freedom refers to inability to drink satisfactorily, and inability to cope with sober behaviour by oneself. The drinker crosses the line from early drinking to addictive drinking when he gives evidence of *loss of freedom* which refers to evenings of mild indulgence as well as to "pass out" periods, because *moderate sessions can never be planned with certainty*. As often as not, a planned moderate session will end in a binge. So loss of freedom does not mean that the problem drinker will get drunk every time he imbibes.

2. The term *loss of freedom* replaces *loss of control* in Dr. E. M. Jellinek's studies.

It just means he can never be sure. His control is unreliably relative. He is unable to drink satisfactorily and he cannot cope with sober behaviour by himself.

The *basic conflict* is the battle between the desire to control drinking and the compulsive urge to drink. Failing to gain recovery at this stage, the drinker, after aggressive splurges of defiant effort, moves into stage four, the phase of acceptance.

In the phase of resigned drinking, his fear of life without alcohol is greater than his fear of death from drinking. But you cannot dismiss fear with fear, you cannot fight fear with fear. Thus, though relieved temporarily by accepting his addiction, it is not long before new fears set in which are nameless and vague, sometimes called free-floating anxiety. The fear of life without alcohol, though it enables him to accept his addiction and to ease the worry of death from drinking, only serves to cloud his life with anxiety and to destroy his alibis. The only excuse he has for drinking now is that he is hopelessly addicted. His alibi structure started to crumble when he gave up the effort to control drinking.

Besides the nameless fears ushered in by his overpowering fear of life without alcohol, come guilt and feelings of persecution so strong that they are sometimes *paranoid*. Paranoid feelings are observed in the drinker who suspects everyone wants to harm him. He may even believe people in the next room are talking about him, when, in fact, nobody is in that room at all!

From his hostility and guilt, there arises a state of depression, even of despair.

In this stage of resignation, the drinker may shift from alcohol to sedatives and narcotics. He soon becomes a very lonely and a very desperate person. He is not far, now, from the final state of addiction—complete helplessness.

Locked in the isolated state brought on by the stage of resigned drinking, the problem drinker has the exact opposite of the pleasure experiences he prized in his early days of drinking. Now he is lonely, depressed, resigned to his fate. He has lost his freedom to enjoy life. When pleasure turns into a necessity, it ceases to be pleasure. When escape turns into a necessity, it becomes slavery. Thus, escape and pleasure, two of the main reasons for early drinking, are completely lost in the stage of acceptance in addiction. The drinker, in deep addiction, is completely without an intelligent reason for drinking. Yet he is so completely dependent on alcohol he cannot stop, knowing there is no longer any rhyme or reason for drinking.

From the stage of resigned drinking, he moves into the final phase of addiction—the stage of helplessness. Now we see clearly that the problem drinker has travelled the whole road back to infancy, physically and mentally. Like a child, he is unable to make an intelligent decision for himself. Physical habits resemble those of the small child, either awake or sleeping. There is lack of continuity in thinking and feeling such that contradictions abound in his statements. Time and space are poorly understood because the memory is defective, and general behaviour reveals brain damage, either permanent or reversible. At least the child can grow. But the drinker, in the helpless stage has no hope of improvement while he continues to drink. Recovery is impossible without the help of an intelligent person who is kind and interested enough to persuade him to take treatment.

The Kind of Person an Alcoholic Becomes

I want to describe the typical problem drinker's six general tendencies in the early years before he starts drinking, and how these worsen as addiction deepens.

Mild	Deepening	Serious
dependent	childish	anxious
sensitive	persecuted	paranoid
idealistic	grandiose	elated
impulsive	compulsive	obsessive
intolerant	rigid	depressed
wishful thinking	fantastic thinking	defective thinking

(The above chart represents the worsening of personal disturbances as addiction deepens. The drinker in early addiction has a set of disturbances which may well be similar to those of many people in society at large. But in the trait *sensitive* there is included also his peculiar physical sensitivity to alcohol. Around it are clustered the other traits which either induce or foster the physical problem. These six traits are influenced by social customs, personal background and the desire for (a) reduction of discomfort and (b) the search for pleasure and freedom—that "free and easy" feeling.

Please note in column three the last trait, *defective thinking*. Here, well advanced into serious addiction, the drinker reveals a combination of psychological and physical disorder. The original mild disorder of wishful thinking follows a natural path to eventual brain damage unless checked by a recovery program.

But there is nothing to worry about in the trait, *sensitive*, though it too, reveals a combination of psychological and physical disturbances. There is nothing to worry about provided we stay sober. Actually we can use the trait, sensitive, to great advantage in our sobriety programme, as we shall see.)

All human beings exhibit a *dependence* on other people from the day they are born. So it is perfectly natural for everyone to experience the problem of getting along with parents, brothers, sisters, friends and acquaintances. But the potential problem drinker is in a special class of dependent person because he is dependent in a three-fold way which distorts his growth. His dependence is not a mutual give-and-take relationship; it is a crutch-like leaning which robs him of his personal identity. He is dependent on alcohol and on his own unknown feelings. Also, more than he admits, he is dependent on the views and indulgences of other people. Thus dependent, he gradually grows *childish* and at last he becomes chronically *anxious*, drinking or dry.

This basic trait leads towards his *sensitivity*. He is easily

hurt, even early in childhood, and he may respond excessively both to fear and to joy situations. Such dependence
on the feelings makes him more dependent on other people
than one observes in the normal run of children. A disturbance in the feelings causes him to run to parents for protection, or to flee from them in anger or fear to the solace
of still other persons—a friend, sister or brother. In any
case, a loneliness develops, a loneliness bred in fear of having to shift for himself. If such a child fails to find emotional
help, his loneliness grows all the deeper for having to shift
for himself too early in life. The "self-made" man, for
example, though resourceful and brave, often neglects the
fact that human nature exacts a high price for putting a
person on his own before he has lived an average childhood.
The price is emotional intoxication and loneliness. Emotional intoxication results from his failure to understand
his own feelings.

If, on the other hand, the potential problem drinker is
over-indulged, his childhood too long delayed, the result is
the same, emotional intoxication and loneliness—after the
child experiences the truth that we human beings cannot
indefinitely expect others to take over our problems. As
drinking grows excessive, the alcoholic will feel *persecuted*
and he may even become *paranoid*.

The other side of sensitivity is physical. Not much is
known about the potential drinker's sensitivity to alcohol.
But we are certain that it is there, either in a potential form
or in the actual way we are constituted chemically, from
away back. Whichever it is, it is reasonable to suppose that
the psychological sensitivity and the chemical one support
one another as growth continues in an excessively dependent pattern.

What are the experiences which lead to the potential
drinker's third general tendency—*idealism*? Every candidate
for alcoholism or for drug addiction early shows a strong
idealistic tendency in his youthful behaviour.

What is it to be idealistic? It is to have a rich imagination, and there is nothing wrong with that. If people were not imaginative, we would have no art, no science, no religion, no hope for the future, no changing of undesirable or hazardous threats to our happiness and well-being. Man is a social animal and much of what makes him an advanced social creature is due to the capacities of his imagination. So it is good to be idealistic.

But if, in youth or early adulthood, this idealistic tendency is ridiculed or blocked, it will find devious and sterile outlets. If the idealistic person is also sensitive, as the potential addict is, he will recoil from the block that stands in his way, or from the ridicule he may confront. In this recoil, his idealistic tendency will lose its foothold in the real world and soar into thin air. He becomes *grandiose*. He will find expression of his idealistic tendencies in fantasy—a dream world of his own.

Thus it is that potential addicts have within them the tendency to grow romantic and sentimental, even though they may not always appear to be so in their everyday behaviour. Actually, some of us, in the effort to cover up our sentimental and romantic feelings, cultivate either a tough and hard-boiled attitude or an indifferent and blase "look" in our everyday behaviour. Behind both these masks, a shyness grows, and, at last, a sense of inadequacy joins the shyness.

Many people in our culture suffer from the effects of the tenderness taboo but potential problem drinkers—those of us who eventually become alcoholics—suffer from it more severely and more damagingly than others, the others who have no drink problem.

The tenderness taboo is a social clamp on expressions of affection—that interchange of personal goodwill that has no angle but itself, no "deal" but the enjoyment of ourselves as persons in our own right. Every human being has a deep capacity, and therefore a deep need, to give and to receive affection without any other thought but to respect the dignity and freedom of one another. This capacity and need does not strive to control, possess, impress or direct another human being. On the contrary, its purpose in human life is to give you a sense of being yourself, confident and adequate to do what you like and what you can do best. Also, these interchanges of affection give you your sense of freedom, freedom from fear, freedom from loneliness, for loneliness breeds fear, and fear, in turn generates deeper loneliness.

Now, what is it that blocks an otherwise healthy idealistic tendency, turning it away from productive use in the real world, and diverting it into the deep sentiment and romantic turns of fantasy? It is the tenderness taboo. If only we could have given full vent to our sentiments and romantic feelings, the damage might still have been avoided, or at least reduced! But no, we were deeply impressed by the opinions of those less sensitive than ourselves, less in need of affection than ourselves, tough, well-adjusted persons, who, though needing affection just as we do, found it practical and worthwhile to develop a strong *ego*, at the expense of deeper personal needs. To have a strong ego is to be tough in a tough world, to take nothing for granted, and to take the raps of reality without flinching. This is good armour, but how can you get close to people with a wall of armour around you?

When the young potential drinker tries alcohol, he experiences a sense of pleasure and joy in its use. So he returns to it, time and again, as the solvent of his problems and way to his happiness. Drinking puts him at peace with himself, he socializes easily, and feels comfortably "high". Anxiety and shyness are removed, and he indulges in grandiose fancy, a dream world where he conjures up situations to suit his repressed wishes. He may, at last, even grow *elated*, at the prospect of some great plan, or in a state of excitement prior to a binge.

Early in the drinking pattern there appears the onset of problems. He dimly perceives that his dreams and wishes are only in his fanciful mind, that in the hang-over there is no real evidence of his having done what he imagined last night he wanted to do. Or, if he had ventured to do what he desired, he discovers that his ideal plan came off badly. Even now, when he is sober, he has the tendency to be *impulsive*. (Tendency four on the chart.) Unknown to him, there stirs the need, under the clamp of the tenderness taboo, to express himself. But he is not sure just what he should do to be himself, to express himself. So the urge to be aggressive at first takes the form of impulsive spurts of energy in poorly directed actions. Now he looks around, and finds most people concerned with the pursuit of money, power, and sexual or sensual experiences. He, too, makes spasmodic efforts in these directions. Intelligent, and often driving, he may well be successful in business, in acquiring prestige, in sensual conquests. His spasmodic efforts may, under vigorous discipline and pressure of pride, take a routine form levelling off into a fixed habit. Thus it is that problem drinkers are often successful in material terms of achievement.

But still—the impulsive, unharnessed urge to be himself, to express his real self, lies deep under the crust of form, convention and habit. This urge finds an outlet first in excessive drinking, then later in problem drinking. Just a drink or two are not sufficient to let the impulse really go. An impulsive gesture in sobriety is even less able to trigger off the full force of the inhibited feelings repressed by the tenderness taboo. But if this impulsive tendency is not well understood, it can arise in the sober state, rationalize the drinker into having "just a few" and then, as though by an uncontrollable force, the drinking goes on and on. After a time, the impulsive activity becomes *compulsive*. The drinker has lost his freedom. He is addicted. Quite apart from the physical sensitivity to alcohol, vital though it is, addiction means a deep, blind devotion to an impulsive force more important to the problem drinker than any other value in his life. Such devotion takes behavioural form in the prizing of intoxication, and his drinking need can become *obsessive*.

In my opinion, this is a deeply important experience in the problem drinker's life. In addition to all the causes which show that he drinks to avoid unpleasant realities, because he is immature or afraid, alone or inadequate; because he is unhappy under the pressure of the tenderness taboo—in addition to all this, he drinks also for the positive pleasure-giving experience of intoxication. This obsesses him. So he prizes intoxication, not only for its value as an escape, but also for its capacity to make him believe he feels better. He likes being drunk because intoxication briefly and temporarily brings him two achievements in one operation—(a) he seems to solve his problems and (b) he is able to be himself, happily, as he thinks he wants to be. The cost to him of this operation seems high, insanely high, to the non-drinker. But, to the problem drinker, who does not think or feel like the non-alcoholic, the value of intoxication is something you cannot measure in sober terms. For example, a man when drunk in the state he most enjoys lives in a sort of "eternal now" oblivious to worries of the past and to concerns of the future.

The hell of it is this: As he more and more depends on alcohol as the answer to his problems and the way to his happiness, he gets into more and deeper distress when he is sober, and as a sober man he is often compelled to think in sober terms, whether he likes it or not. And worst of all, intoxication no longer has the 'glow" it used to have. It is much less pleasurable, and the hang-over is worse than it was when he was drinking, years ago. Because he is more unhappy now in the sober state, the usual pursuits of sober people are less attractive than they ever were. He becomes disillusioned about money, about prestige, and even about normal sensual thrills, as they are valued by people in society at large. But out of necessity he is still interested in them.

Without realizing it, he reverts to youthful rebellion against the values of sober living. Insecure in the sober day-by-day living of most people, his sense of inadequacy deepens, he grows lonelier than he ever used to be, and he feels sensitive to the slightest sign of abuse or criticism. This is the origin of his tendency to be *intolerant* (tendency five on the chart), an intolerance that grows naturally in self-defence. Intolerance breeds *rigidity*. This you observe in his almost incredible sense of order and neatness directed at the world outside himself. It seems that he is trying to find in the outside world what he cannot find in himself. Guilt arises from this misgiving—the suspicion that he cannot put his feelings in order. He becomes *depressed*.

The disorders which result from an over-sensitive need for self-protection, e.g., a sense of inadequacy, a feeling of loneliness, self-pity, and a desperate return to childish methods of dealing with problems, induce the operation of tendency six, the use of *wishful thinking*. (Actually, wishful thinking is at work from the very beginning of problem drinking.) Drink temporarily dulls awareness of these problems but the hang-over brings them back, more difficult than ever. Wishful thinking loses its plausibility, and grows *fantastic*. At last he cannot even believe himself. Then disorder may become chronic, drinking or dry, and, in the end, his thinking is plainly *defective*. He loses real sense of space and time, of logical processes. Brain damage is evident as well as gross psychological disorder.

Summary

The positive goal of this entire analysis of the drinking pattern is to stress the value of containing the pattern wherever you find yourself within it. If you take the required measures to arrest your addiction at the stage you last experienced, you can know creative sobriety. Of course, there is much more to sobriety than just knowing the nature of your problem. After we arrest addiction, there is still ahead of us the interesting adventure of a creative sobriety program.

The basic reason for early drinking was that we were not satisfied with the way we felt in sobriety. We wanted to change the way we felt. We did not feel quite right without a drink. There was a growing sense of inadequacy. So we drank to feel better, to be ourselves as we longed to be. "Feeling better" enabled us to get along with other people, and to enjoy adventurous experiences that we were unable to find in sobriety.

There is absolutely nothing wrong with such personal needs. The whole problem lay in the method we chanced to find in drinking as a solution to these needs. Alcohol met our personal needs for a while. But drinking did not prove to be a satisfactory way to feel better, to get on with others, or to gain adventure. Addiction set in, not because we wanted it that way, it happened to us. And then we found with dismay and fear that our old friend alcohol had turned into a treacherous enemy.

After we became addicted, we got sick instead of feeling better, lost friends, instead of deepening friendship, and were trapped in the boredom and pain of hang-overs instead of experiencing adventure.

Still, if we really want a worthwhile creative sobriety we have to think again about what we were striving for when we thought alcohol could meet our needs. *These will be the goals that we shall strive for in sobriety.* Let us look at them in the next chapter.

The goals of creative sobriety involve a search, for each man must understand his needs and longings in his own way. In the next chapter we will observe this search in the pursuit of common ground and common goals among a group of recovering alcoholics.

2.

THE SEARCH FOR A CREATIVE CLUE

A GROUP of alcoholics, sober for several months, gathered together from time to time in search of a continuing sober program. They speak for themselves. A therapist chairs the meetings. He opens the discussion.

"There is only one reason why we are here today. We are all alcoholics, and I assume that everyone wishes to recover, wishes to do whatever it is necessary to do to achieve sobriety."

Most patients agreed they were alcoholics, after casual but detailed queries. Alcoholism was described as a kind of drinking which interfered with one's life seriously enough to cause alarm, to convince the drinker that he had lost his freedom to drink. This conviction varied in depth from patient to patient, accompanied by resistances usually observed in group sessions with alcoholics.

"Don't you think a man drinks because he worries too much?" Hilton asked.

"Yes, and also because it is snowing," said Lindon, deflating the alibi.

"Or raining?" Sully asked.

"Yes, or because a friend just died, or is about to get married," added the therapist.

"Well, now, with me it was a tonic. You see, my nerves were bad. My doctor gave me some pills, then some white thick stuff in a bottle. Then he suggested I try a little drink or two before bedtime." The men could not be sure whether Lindon was serious or carrying the joke.

"Lin took it for medicine, that's all," suggested Clemens.

"Wait now, let me get this straight. Lindon took whiskey for medicine. Now he's here to take treatment for the effects of the medicine! What is this, anyway?" Arthurs was with it, joke or no joke.

"This first session is an exercise in drastic honesty," said the therapist. "This urges us to deflate our complacent feelings, our old notions about trying to control drink, to make excuses, to defend our excesses. Most of you know all about the alibi. I'm just reviewing a little. We'll have no room for fresh insights if we even suspect that the drink we thirsted for brings us what we need. We have to become really empty, to see that life, for us alcoholics, rings hollow, that our thirst has to be quenched by something other than alcohol. To get honest with ourselves is to become empty, empty enough to realize that alcohol cannot fill us, and to begin our enquiry with the basic question, 'What really is the meaning of our thirst?' Isn't it true and simple to say, first of all, that we drank because we were thirsty?"

"Oh, sure! I just thought that maybe worry might be back of it all." Hilton was serious.

"There is a lot back of it all. But let's start with thirst, that urge or craving of the problem drinker, the thirst of the alcoholic. Let's work out what we can about the meaning of thirst."

"I like that approach, if I understand you right," said Sully. "Everything I've read about the drink problem stresses psychology and medicine, but says little about how it *feels* to be thirsty, and then to be drunk."

"I know what you mean," said Alvin. "You plough through pages of explanation—chemistry of alcohol, its effects on the liver, on the higher centres of the brain, the wretched state known as the hang-over, the loss of your job —you can go on and on—the distress of your family, but nothing, just nothing about the real thing."

"And what is the real thing?"

"The glass going to the lips, the feeling of the drink in

your mouth, the tingle in your throat, and that warm glow in your stomach." Alvin was intense. "Then the delicious shudder, all over your body, sort of untying all those knots from head to foot. Like Sully says, the experts tell us nothing about the shiver and the burn and that feeling all over that's so hard to explain—the feeling you get when you're high."

"What is it you find wrong with the scientific approach?"

"Now, doc, it is not for me and Alvin to say there's anything *wrong* with what we've read. I guess it's just that it's not enough."

"What, for example?"

"Well, it's all cause and effect. That span, or gap, in between the cause and effect or somewhere—I don't know—anyway, what does it mean, the plain fact of needing a drink? Sure, let's look at the meaning of thirst but let's do it our way. I have got nothing against science. I, we, want something more, something we can understand. We're not chemists, not psychiatrists, not preachers, not social workers. Still, we need to know, in our own way, what drink means to us. If you see what I mean, maybe you could develop that thirst-idea of yours in a way that alcoholics can feel."

"Uh-mm," reflected the therapist. "Well, so long as you recognize that we need science somewhere along the line, I think we can go ahead on your basis."

"We know that, doc. Before you arrived on the scene, everyone here was pretty well dried out, and we appreciate what medicine and science can do to put us on the right road."

"Yes, but there will be other important facts, other values in science for us to know besides the use of science in recovering from acute alcoholism."

"You mean there's a medicine we can take to control drinking?" Arthurs was hopeful.

"Your guess is just the opposite of what I had in mind. The fact that an alcoholic can never learn to drink moderately is an observation amounting to a scientific certainty.

So far as I know, no study has yet demonstrated that an alcoholic can become a social controlled drinker. This brings us back to our point; let's get after the meaning of thirst. Thirst surely is central in our discussion, and surely it is the physical factor in our thirst which makes it impossible for alcoholics to drink moderately. But, there is more to it than that. Sully, you and Alvin, and the others seem to be with you, you start it off the way you like. I'm with you on this, though I must admit you've changed my course a little."

"Well, we say a fellow is thirsty, don't we? We say he craves a drink, we don't go into all this business about worry, or anxiety, or complexes. We say he's thirsty, he needs a drink. Alvin and I have talked a lot about this." Sully nodded to Alvin.

"Yes, sure, that's right."

"That means he's dry, eh?"

"Yes."

"All right, he is dry, he is thirsty for a drink."

"Yes, yes, I agree, he is thirsty for a drink." The therapist was interested.

"For a drink? Doesn't he want to *feel* something? Is it just a drink?"

"Uh-mm," nodded the therapist. "He wants what the drink will do for him, to give him the desired feeling, the life he is looking for."

"The drinker who is dry, or thirsty, desires the opposite of what he feels. Dry, he wants to banish dryness; thirsty, he wants to be filled." Alvin read Plato.

"That sounds right enough."

"Now then, is there any way a thirsty drinker can understand his craving or longing for drink without somehow knowing that he can slake his particular kind of thirst?"

"Of course not. He has to know that a drink will relieve him. If he did not know that, he couldn't crave it."

"So he does not desire or crave what he feels when he is dry?"

"That's absurd. He wants to feel different. He wants to do something about his craving. He wants to satisfy it."

"But he does want something?" The group wondered where Alvin would take them.

"Naturally."

"He does not want what he feels. He is dry. He is thirsty. He is empty, and he wants to be filled."

"Yes, yes, what are you driving at?" The therapist was curious.

"Well, it isn't his mouth, it isn't his throat, it isn't his stomach, it isn't his nerves, it isn't any of these which know fullness because they are empty and dry, or parched and quivering."

"I see what you mean, Alvin. But they *expect* to be eased when he takes a drink."

"Yes, but the only way a drinker can know that he will relieve his dryness, and soothe the stomach and nerves is by *remembering* that a drink helped him before. Tell me, how possibly can we know that a drink will help us unless we remember it?"

"I don't see why we went through all this talk to reach such an obvious conclusion."

"Because it shows," said Alvin, "that our thirst is an expression of the whole person. It is not just a pang of physical need. The meaning of thirst is not just physical. The simplest way to say it is 'The drinker, all of him, is thirsty and longs to be filled.' The problem drinker's thirst for alcohol is a concrete expression of a deep craving, a deep unsatisfied desire of the whole person, or as much of him as you could call a person."

"The goal of every alcoholic is always the opposite of the way he feels when he craves a drink. Is that what you mean?"

"Yes, that's the idea."

"And the thirst which leads to the opposite of his thirst shows that he remembers in some dramatic way what it feels like to be filled."

"That's what I mean."

"I see your approach and I like it," said the therapist. "I'll try to put it together. The fact that the drinker *remembers* how to quench his thirst shows that the initial impulse and the thirst arise as a signal of the memory. It can be a signal to meet a trivial need, or a need of the whole person. If it is a trivial need, you know that it arises in a moderate drinker, the fellow who can take it or leave it alone. If it is a personal need, you know that it arises in an alcoholic— you have an urge that has to be met, there's no putting it off. It pleads for a substantial change of all your feelings."

"Sure, that's it."

"Now, just what are those personal needs—that you call our thirst?" asked Lindon.

"We are going to stick to feelings we all recognize. So let's ask Sully and Alvin to give us their views of those needs, the needs which are indeed the alcoholic's special thirst or craving, or urge, or longing. But let's make it clear that we will speak of those needs as they were in the early days of our drinking."

"Uh-mm. Well, I needed more confidence in myself," confessed Sully. "If I was sober at a party, I wouldn't speak to people I didn't know very well. But with a few drinks, I could approach them and engage in all sorts of topics. I got a real lift out of drinking before I became alcoholic. I felt better too. Then after about a year's drinking, I could never enjoy myself anywhere unless I had something to drink."

"Yeah, that's right," agreed Alvin. "When you first start drinking and for a while afterwards, there's no awful craving like you have after years of it. I mean that desperate physical need for a morning eye-opener. At first, there is just a vague but strong desire to drink for the fun you get out of it. Well, you just feel better all over. It's hard to explain, that feeling. But I remember it, everything looked brighter, everyone seemed more friendly and kindly, you just seemed to be a better person after a few drinks. Then the whole idea was to keep that glow, not to get real drunk, but to take enough every hour or so to keep the glow."

"Like I said, didn't we drink to get rid of our worries?" Hilton was in it again.

"Well, no, not at first," Sully replied. "Maybe later we came to believe that drinking would cure everything, and we became good in excuse-making. But at first, we drank, at least many of us did, in the hope, time and again, that something big and wonderful would happen to us, and for the pleasure of the lift we got out of it. Of course, after you're well stoned, your worries do disappear. But I think that's secondary to the positive lift of well-being and the feeling of new adventure you get in the early days of drinking, before you realize you're alcoholic."

"I'll try to sum up these views. Later, the rest of you will want to express your feelings about thirst. To keep it simple, we drank to be better persons, to strengthen our self-respect and confidence, to be friendly, and to have people like us. The 'glow' Alvin mentioned is a feeling of increased well-being, physical, social, spiritual. It is interesting that strong alcoholic drinks are often called spirits. The different expressions of well-being could be gathered together in the simple word 'personal'. So I suggest that the meaning of the alcoholic's thirst is personal."

"What about the moderate drinker's thirst? Is it personal too?" Clemens asked.

"No," said the therapist. "The moderate drinker does not have the same urgency to meet the variety of needs which we group together in the word 'personal'. He may want to relax a bit, he may simply savour the taste of a good wine with meals, or a cool drink on a hot day. Drink may well be part of a man's way of life as a pleasant frill. In the alcoholic, drink is itself a way of life, or becomes so, a central need of first importance, ahead of everything else."

"Is that what you mean by the spiritual need of alcohol?" asked Hilton.

"Yes, the alcoholic eventually prizes drink as the most

important experience of his life. In that sense, alcohol fills a religious need for the potential alcoholic."

"Wait now. I thought we were going to stick to early drinking situations, before we became alcoholic," Alvin wanted to stay on the original track.

"Pardon me, Alvin. You're right. I find it hard to keep the periods distinct and separate because they merge into one another gradually, almost without your noticing the changes. Let me put it like this. In early drinking, the need for company or friendship, the need to be liked, and a strong sense of adventure and wonder are the needs which later develop into a sort of religious obsession in the addiction stage."

"Do you mean that there is something religious about friendship?" Arthurs was incredulous.

"Yes, I do. But that can wait on our discussion ahead."

"Well, as far as we've gone," said Sully, "it looks as if there was nothing terrible or wrong about our thirst—our personal thirst—in the early days of drinking. There were strong needs there that somehow had to be met. We wanted to see and be seen in a better light, we wanted to feel better and to be friendly. We were looking for something better than we knew in the every day world. Nothing wrong with that, is there?"

"No. I think it is natural and right to try to be a better person, to feel better, to act confidently, to be happy with other people, if possible, and to seek new adventures."

"And that is the meaning of our thirst, is it?" asked Lindon.

"Yes, more or less so, in the early days of drinking."

"What a pity! If only we could have stayed out of trouble, and didn't have those damn hang-overs." Clemens looked mournful.

"Or lose our jobs," said Wendell.

"Yes, or our wives," reflected Milton.

"I miss my self-respect most of all," Alvin added.

"Don't you think we might manage a drink or two to take

like medicine?" It was hard to tell whether Clemens was serious or joking.

"As medicine?"

"Yes."

"Yes, to take when your worries pile up, just a few to relax your nerves". Hilton played along with the revived alibi.

"Here's the old run-around again. The boys want to be able to drink a little because they're sick. So we're all here for treatment of 'treatment'!" Arthurs was with it again.

"We can go back to the early pleasant memories and relive them. I want you to do just that," the therapist suggested. "But it's no use trying to fool ourselves. We can't repeat, we don't want to repeat, the vicious pattern which brings us to treatment as sick men. We can relive, in imagination, the meaning of our thirst. But to drink now, we all know, is not going to bring the results we once hoped for. To drink now is to bring the *opposite* results of what we first wanted. To drink now is to repeat a vicious pattern of sickness. This repeating of trouble is imitation, a blind imitation of behaviour that is called addiction. If it were a planned, alterable or controlled imitation, we would have no trouble. But it is an imitation that is imposed. It seizes and possesses us—it is an addiction."

"Just no drinks, period, no matter what." Clemens was resigned.

"That seems to be the pitch." Arthurs looked hurt.

The therapist thanked the men for their hints and clues and promised to prepare a talk on their discussion. In due course the talk was finished. Here it is.

The Mystery of Thirst

A man will be sober because he wants to be. And he wants desperately to be sober for the same sound reasons that he first drank (before he became addicted).

You never forget those pleasant feelings of the early drinking days. It is the memory of them which is one of the main causes of slips. The impulsive urge to take a drink after you have been sober for some time, or even the deliberate planning to try drinking again, is born of this trick of memory. It is a trick of the human mind which tends to make us recall pleasant times, and to ignore the misery which always follows them in the behaviour pattern of problem drinkers.

Let us face this fact. We can never wipe out the memory of those early pleasant drinking occasions. But we are resolved now to be sober, because in sobriety we have the only condition of everything else in life worth knowing and enjoying. What about it, then? There is only one course to take. And that is to make use of the memory of those early drinking occasions in a study of their meaning.

What is the meaning of those early drinking occasions before we became sick?

(1) A search for one's real self, stripped of tensions, fears and pretenses. A drink or two, we used to think, helped us "to be ourselves". Everyone deep down, wants to be himself, as he supposes he is *at his best*. That is the origin of the view that one is more honest, more likely to express his real nature when drunk. And everyone who strives to be himself, without fears, believes that he can get along with others, if only one can banish shyness and shed the tendency to be sensitive and easily hurt. Thus we tried to feel better, in drinking, in order to be our relaxed natural selves—so we thought.

(2) We tried, not only to be ourselves, but to improve our relations with other people.

(3) We were therefore seeking fellowship, whether we were conscious of it or not. For fellowship means being yourself, in a pleasant and relaxed way, among other people.

These three needs or desires make up what we call *per-*

sonal thirst, and the aim of this thirst is personal growth.

Stephen Crane has well expressed these fellowship and idealistic desires in his novel "George's Mother". The illusion here is brought out in relief, in neglect of the misery of addiction.

They made toward a little glass-fronted saloon that sat blinking jovially at the crowds. It engulfed them with a gleeful motion of its too widely-smiling lips. . . . Jones was waving his arms and delivering splintering blows upon some distant theories. . . . They drew up in line and the busy hands of the bartender made glasses clink. Kelcey . . . began to feel that he was passing the happiest evening of his life. His companions were so jovial and good-natured: and everything they did was marked by such courtesy . . . They began to fraternize in jovial fashion. It was understood that they were true and tender spirits. They had come away from a grinding world filled with men who were harsh.

When one of them chose to divulge some place where the world had pierced him, there was a chorus of violent sympathy. They rejoiced at their temporary isolation and safety. . . . Kelcey felt his breast expand with manly feeling. He knew that he was capable of sublime things. He wished that some day one of his present companions would come to him for relief.

His mind pictured a little scene. In it he was magnificent in his friendship. . . . He was all at once an enthusiast, as if he were at a festival of religion. He felt that there was something fine and thrilling in this affair, isolated from a stern world, and from which the laughter arose like incense. He knew that old sentiment of brotherly regard for those about him. He began to converse tenderly with them.

. . . With an air of profound melancholy, Jones poured out some whiskey. They drank reverently. They exchanged a glistening look of tender recollections, and then went over to where Bleecker was telling a humorous story to a circle of giggling listeners. The old man sat like a fat, jolly god.

. . . Their feeling for contemporaneous life was one of contempt. Their philosophy taught that in a large part the whole thing was idle and a great bore. With fine scorn they sneered at the futility of it. Work was done by men who had not the courage to stand still and let the skies clap together if they willed."

Stephen Crane, deftly ironic, paints the picture of problem drinkers in the pleasant stages of intoxication. He elsewhere describes equally well the sordid aftermath in the hang-over, of which a few sentences will do. "When he moved his eyelids, there was a sensation that they were cracking. . . . He looked about him with an expression of utter woe, regret, and loathing. He was compelled to lie down again. A pain above his eyebrows was like that from an iron clamp. . . . He was aghast at the prospect of the old routine. It was impossible. He trembled before its exactions." Enough of that. Anyone who has been through it knows well the whole grim story. It is the pleasant moments of intoxication that will interest us here, as a clue to creative sobriety. Throughout Crane's neat sketch of the drinker's illusory paradise, vain and silly as it may appear—even to the confirmed drinker, who, sober now, will repeat the performance as though by compulsion—throughout it, one senses the fascination that drink holds for those who grope for more than the filling of human needs. We can condense these gropings to a few definite aims, if we believe it is worthwhile to try to understand the nature of the alcoholic's original personal thirst.

What are these aims, groping and perhaps unconscious, in the original drinking sessions? Tritely, first of all, the drinker indulges just to feel better, he is better disposed towards life. He drinks to be a good fellow, to be so regarded by others, and to get along better with people than he does ordinarily. Drink fascinates him because in this friendly attitude there is the prospect of high adventure, not to be known, he thinks, in sober living. So valuable does the experience of drinking become that it takes on the flavor of *religious feeling* in the illusion of fellowship, of accord with all that is exalted, of being himself as he fancies he ought to be.

It is a tragedy that drinking at last fails to quench his personal thirst.

Before we begin to examine ways and means to quench personal thirst in an adequate, safe and effective manner, we shall review briefly why alcohol failed to do it, though it seemed for a time to be just what we needed.

For a time—a few years, maybe ten or more—drinking seemed to satisfy our complex cravings. Then insidiously, but surely, there came the day when we had to admit that drinking no longer quenched this personal thirst. Worse, it began to bring the opposite of what we most deeply craved. By the time we sought treatment, alcohol made us feel worse, rather than better, it strained relations with other people, rather than eased them, we became miserable companions (even with ourselves) instead of "high" and personable.

What happened? We grew addicted to the use of alcohol. We no longer drank for the good reasons of our personal thirst, we drank because of our sick need for alcohol—once a drink was taken.

The onset of sick need explains why alcohol finally fails to satisfy us. Our original personal thirst demands creative growing expression. Alcoholism arrests personal growth. It is not creative. It is *imitative*.

All of us are familiar with the behaviour of children. We have been children ourselves—a fact we tend to forget— and as parents, teachers, uncles or aunts, we watch their progress with interest, amusement, and often impatience.

When a parent first notices the child repeating aimlessly over and over again some phrase or wisp of song, some ritual of behaviour, he may be dismayed at this childish repetition, and self-imitation. But a parent with many children or a teacher eventually learns that even intelligent children pass through phases of behaviour which look excessively repetitive or imitative. There is nothing to be alarmed about. Maybe the sound of a phrase fascinates a child so he repeats it over and over again, until automatically he pops out with it long after he has ceased to enjoy hearing himself say the words.

We know children have to grow in more than physical stature. They go through trial and error, they stop for a time, level out, and emerge again in a slower upper curve of learning. Within this process there are periods of imitation, or of repetition, but the goal is not to stay fixed; it is to move on to adulthood, to mature behaviour.

Even in adulthood, there are patterns of behaviour which are imitative, and these we call habits. They are short cuts in the complex action of human behaviour. But habits are expected to suit our age. We do not revert to childish techniques we have outgrown.

When we do, we get into trouble. And that is what happens in the imitative nature of addiction. Because alcohol first affects the highest centres of the brain, the source of the best adult inspirations, the learning process is blocked and impaired more and more. As dosage is increased over the years, we may naturally expect an arrest or fixation in normal personal growth. In this arrest, where little new experience is acquired, the drinker has no choice but to repeat, viciously, the less admirable traits of behaviour. As the process continues, the addicted drinker reverts to lower levels of behaviour, back further than adolescence and puberty. Now the situation is more serious than it was when the drinker bored and alienated friends by repeating stories and jokes over and over again the same evening. Now he loses control over elementary bodily functions as children do under the age of five.

So the imitative nature of addiction is not just the repeating of unpleasant hang-overs, worsening and increasing over the years. It is a reversion to childhood behaviour that it is the aim of education to overcome, and imitation of behaviour of the sort that children are expected to alter in the growing process. (But our original personal thirst craved for new experience, creative friendship and adventure.)

Addiction is an event which, in its imitative patterns, arrests growth, alienates friends, and turns adventure into vicious routine. So we seek a way out of addiction, because to remain within its grip would be to destroy ourselves. Imitation is not the true nature of the problem drinker. Imitation, like addiction, is not the answer to our personal needs.

The desire to be ourselves, to become ourselves, to grow in harmony with others, and to seek adventure or experience more meaningful than anything found in the common daily life—these are the demands of our original personal thirst.

We begin to plot the ways of creative sobriety when, after we have stopped drinking, we recall our early thirst and examine its meaning. This meaning was not known to us when we started drinking years ago. But we can know its meaning better now, after the experience of our failure to quench this thirst in alcohol.

The question now to examine is "How can I be myself, or how can I become myself?"

Related to this effort of being ourselves was the attempt, time and again, to try to feel better. We tried to feel better because essentially we were striving to be ourselves, without strain, fear, shyness, or cover-up of any sort. To be yourself and to feel better are two efforts which mean about the same thing. Each of us is trying to be the person he wants to be. Hence personal thirst.

> The black earth drinks and drinks again,
> The trees in turn drink in the earth,
> The sea drinks up the breezy air,
> The sun in heaven drinks the sea,
> The moon drinks up the glowing sun.
> Tell me, friends, why do you think,
> That I myself ought not to drink?

From this charming little poem, you could set out in defense of drinking. Though that is not my purpose, I am equally not concerned to condemn it. I am neither wet nor dry, in any militant sense.

Sobriety is a term of meaning, sometimes of a threat or fear, sometimes of hope and peace. But it is a word of meaning to those for whom it is a threat or hope,—to the problem drinker and people like him. So this is for the alcoholic, the drug addict, or anyone obsessed by human desires who fails to learn the real nature of personal thirst.

The drinking song which introduces our theme was written over 2,000 years ago by an anonymous Greek. He is making a plea for the privilege of thirst, the longing to be in accord with his friends, and to enjoy, beyond that, the ecstasy of union with the whole world. And yet, in this ideal harmony, he wants to feel his own identity, "I, myself". He registers his feeling concretely "Why do you think that I myself ought not to drink?" The fact that he is seeking approval of his action betrays some doubt that drink, whether of alcohol or some other intoxicant, is the only way to meet the urges of thirst.

The centuries pass, and the scene shifts from Greece to the land of the Hebrews. Man's search for his reality has grown from a vague longing to be in accord with the whole universe to a personal desire to be at one with God, who is mindful of him. "My soul thirsteth for God, for the living God; when shall I come and appear before God."

Then there comes a man, who urged by his thirst to know the living God, retreated into the wilderness where he fought temptation for 40 days. There he searched within himself for guidance, but the story tells us of urges of power, to glory. Is this the tendency if man is too long alone? But temptation was reformed and the way to God was charted. It was to leave the wilderness and move among men. He did not stay alone to fight the powers of evil, he came forth to move once more in the world, and communicate to fellow sufferers the nature of the adventure which brings peace.

He looked inward, long and hard, but that was but the preparation for the adventure which lay ahead. The urges of thirst are not met by negative battles with will, by efforts to suppress it. Thirst is in the nature of man. He must try to quench it with the best that is in him. By the example of the Galilean, you chart your way among fellow creatures. The inward search directs you outward into traffic with the world.

To the woman by the well in Samaria, during the adventure of his message, he said "Whosoever drinketh of this water shall thirst again, but whosoever drinketh of the water that I shall give him shall never thirst, but the water that I shall give him shall be in him a spring of water welling up into everlasting life. To be a better person must come from within. This "spring" is the dynamic knowledge of the difference between human needs and personal ideals, and it wells up to nourish both. But to leave the personal ideals athirst, to indulge only our human needs, is to dry up the spring, and leave cravings which seek outlet, desperately, in the various forms of addiction and obsession.

There are hundreds of allusions, in the literature of all languages, to man's basic thirst and responses to its urging.

Ben Jonson gropes for love in his poem, "Drink to me only with thine eyes." The demand is high, and he looks, perhaps, for too much in a woman, more than it's right to expect of her, no matter how fair, when he writes "The thirst that from the soul doth rise, Doth ask a drink divine."

Still, the poets persisted in seeking response to the soul's thirst in human love. Shelley, noted for his infatuation with beautiful women, sensed the Greek longing for harmony and accord with the universe, and used it to justify the urges of human passion.

> The fountains mingle with the river
> And the river with the ocean
> The winds of Heaven mix for ever
> With a sweet emotion;
> Nothing in the world is single;

All things by a law divine
In one spirit meet and mingle.
Why not I with thine?—
See the mountain kiss high Heaven
And the waves clasp one another;
No sister-flower would be forgiven
If it disdained its brother;
And the sunlight clasps the earth
And the moonbeams kiss the sea:
What is all this sweet work worth
If thou kiss not me?

In poetry, in song, in sacred literature, there is abundant evidence that thirst is basic, thirst not just for strong drink, not just for sex, but a thirst for God, for all that life can mean to a human being. In the complex process of seeking answers, many of us fall into traps, the traps of addiction.

Recovery from addiction or obsession of any sort is less recovery than it is new adventure. It is recovery only in the sense that the addict regains an attitude of wonder, the attitude of his youth, a faith in living which remains unquestioned until the misery of addiction causes him to question life, and doubt its worth. It is recovery, too, in the sense that the tendencies which make him sensitive to addiction are the same tendencies which can make for a vigorous adventurous life.

Many books have been written on the sickness of the alcoholic. It is time now to say something about the prospects of sobriety, not only for the alcoholic, who may doubt the value of being sober, but for any human being who, troubled and anxious, is caught in another kind of addiction or obsession or is on the verge of being caught. It is for anyone who is uncertain about how to satisfy the thirst to be simply a person, as he supposes he is intended to be.

But the troubles of many of us are so vague, so nameless, that it is well to place our stress on the alcoholic. In him we know we have a definite problem as a target. The symbol of the glass, or hang-over, and the experiences directly located in or around alcohol, serve as a ready reference for the complex troubles which surround, precede and follow them. Those of us who do not suffer from the ravages of drink may yet see ourselves in the alcoholic, for it is the theme of this book that alcoholism is one expression of a complex disorder shared by many of us who express the response to basic personal thirst in a variety of addictions or obsessions other than problem drinking.

Now to say that alcoholism is an expression of a widely shared disorder is not to say that alcoholism is *only* a symptom of something else. The disastrous opinion that problem drinking is only a symptom of a deeper disorder, though in a sense true, brings more trouble to the alcoholic than any other view I know. We should try, instead, to see that alcoholism stamps the whole man and expresses all of him. His relation to drink is his main concern, first, last, and always. Even his sobriety takes its departure, and embarks on its adventure, from the central station, his addiction to alcohol. When he forgets that, timetables are meaningless, for he does not really know where he is going if he knows not the point of departure. He is soon lost in a maze of alibis. What the alcoholic has in common with other kinds of addicts is *thirst*. For thirst, as the tradition of our literature shows, can be more, or other than, craving for drink. The various addictions result from tragically wrong routes to the meaning of life, taken by the sensitive and impulsive wayfarer in ignorance of their dangers, or in thrall of deceiving thrills. With a peculiar sensitivity, not yet well understood by science, the potential alcoholic is somehow introduced to strong drink, as much by chance as choice, likes its deceiving promise, and feeling it to be the answer to his problem and to his search, becomes addicted to its use.

The complex disorder of addiction, shared by many people, finds expression, in those peculiarly disposed to drink, in alcoholism. The way that drink tends to make them feel and behave is the problem here. One may argue that drink only aggravates or only precipitates a disorder, already there, or in the making, but it is clear that the alcoholic must try to live without alcohol. Many people tend to define alcoholism narrowly, and suppose that the disorder is limited to the mere problem of the ingestion of alcohol. Now it is true, above all, that the alcoholic must learn to live without alcohol. But to do so, he must practice more than the art of abstinence, and learn more than the nature of his sickness, important though these are. If he is to enjoy a sober life, he will seek to know more than the dangers of drinking and the misery it brings him, more than the negative values of sober living. To deepen his insights, to live in peace, and to enjoy his sobriety, he will want to know how creative, how positive his new way of life may become. He can be inspired and strengthened by the prospect of *adventure* in sobriety, with all its hazards, its freedom, its pleasure, and its zest.

Now adventure is very different from planned results. An adventure is what you experience in the act itself. You seek adventure, not primarily for what it means when it is finished, but for what it means to you while you are having it, enjoying it.

Adventure is well suited to the temper and outlook of an alcoholic. He drinks for the feeling he has while drinking, clearly not for the results it brings in the hang-over. After he becomes addicted, sick, remorseful, he yet reflects fondly on the good old times, the early days of drinking when adventure and rare zest were the main attractions to which his thirst drew him time and again. But the face of adventure changed when the drinker saw at last that the novel, the wonderful, the zestful were lost in a vicious pattern of mechanical dullness. A repetitive circle of blackouts, remorse, sickness, guilt surrounds the dismay of learning that the old adventure has become a mere imitation of behaviour distasteful to everyone including himself.

Genuine adventure is prized for the experience itself and the prospect of new joy in each new effort. The musician, the painter, the hunter, the lover are less concerned about the effects or results of their effort than they are about the efforts themselves—the act of making music, the act of painting, the act of hunting, the act of loving, and hoping with each new experience to create anew, to vary the past pattern, to savour strange thrills.

Though the adventures of drinking are deceiving when the drinker becomes addicted, though they change from adventures to compulsive imitations, the alcoholic is yet suited temperamentally to the prospects of genuine adventure. He is more attracted to the prospect of adventure than the practical man who always judges life by a series of results and consequences, and finishes with a paunch and a television set.

The alcoholic, in his early drinking days, sought to be in harmony with everything and everyone around him. He prized the amiable, the cheerful and the friendly. He strove to escape from the dull world of his everyday life where he could find nothing adventurous, nothing new, nothing wonderful.

So there are three sound reasons why the alcoholic is well suited to adventure. His past drinking is evidence that he prized feeling, rather than result, experience rather than consequence. He sought the foreign, the strange, the new and the diverting in his distaste for the humdrum, the safe, and imitative nature of daily life. And he sought to be in harmony with all around him, to identify with persons whom he would find threatening without the support of alcohol.

Contrary to those who believe that the alcoholic has to live a life completely at odds with his nature as a drinking person, I suggest that the alcoholic is well suited to a sober life, *if he seeks sobriety as an adventure*, not as the sure consequence of a treatment measure.

There is one deep significant difference between the harmony or at-oneness that the genuine adventurer seeks, and the similar harmony that the alcoholic longs for. It is in this difference that the alcoholic will find his clue for the prospect of adventure in sobriety. The true adventurer strives to see persons and things in their own right as well as in accord with himself. The alcoholic sees people and things only in their relation to his own deep sick needs.

When he began drinking, he was searching for something ordinary living could not give him. In addiction he loses all hope of finding this great golden experience. But in sobriety he resumes his search, and will be engaged in it as long as he lives.

. . . .

"I've been thinking a lot about thirst the way the group has been delving into it." Wendell opened the discussion. "You know, I used to wonder why I wanted a drink, got so I needed one, after sexual intercourse. It seemed that I needed drink to round out the experience. I don't know. And I had the idea too, that I should have a good edge before the experience. What do you make of that?"

"Glad you mentioned it," said Hilton. "It was the same with me. And with other experiences too, like closing a big deal, or looking forward to one. And no pleasure seemed complete by itself. There was a constant gnawing for vaguely something more, whether it was business, or pleasure."

"A longing, a thirst for something more. Did you find that drink brought satisfaction?" asked the therapist.

"For me, no. It was desperately needed, yet it brought no real peace," was Wendell's reply.

"It seems to me now," reflected Alvin, "that drink just happened to be the only way I could meet that strange longing, or thirst, for something I couldn't find anywhere, no matter what it was."

"The personal thirst of the alcoholic," observed the therapist, "certainly seems to touch everything important in life, from what Milton and Wendell say, or rather, it *tries* to touch and to reach whatever it is we can call important."

"How in the world," asked Alvin, "can we explain or

understand why we turned to drink after we knew that it could not fill our deepest needs, even made them worse?"

"That sound question can only be answered in what is called addiction, as I see it," replied the therapist. "We drank originally for the reasons we discussed, and then, one day, we woke up to admit that our need for alcohol was greater than the original personal needs which first endeared us to the pleasure of drinking."

"How would you describe addiction?" asked Alvin.

"I'd like to remind you, first of all, of what Milton said. That impressed me. He said 'Drink just *happened* to be the way I could meet that strange longing.' Addiction is something that *happens*. No one sets out consciously to be an alcoholic. Alcoholism happens to us, because we are the kind of people to whom addiction can happen."

"That's what loss of control is," remarked Alvin. "We don't seek to lose control, do we?"

"Not consciously. But down deep I think we did drink to loosen control. We don't lose jobs or friends because we want to. Those troubles come with loss of freedom to drink, the loss of control which comes with addiction. When addiction has happened to us, the compulsion to drink traces its vicious circle, not because we plan it like that, but simply because we can't help ourselves. What we failed to understand was this; we could not loosen control over ourselves through alcohol without also losing everything else of value. I suggest that we use the expression 'loss of freedom' instead of 'loss of control'."

"What about those early strivings which you seemed to think were natural, at least not evil or sick?" asked Alvin.

"Those early strivings—to be a better person, to feel better, to act confidently, to be well liked and to enjoy new adventure—all these gradually disappear as addiction grows worse. The need for alcohol blots them out, or makes them secondary."

"Did those strivings just happen to us, as you say addiction happens?" It was Milton again.

"Yes, more or less. Those early strivings are never well thought out, never well understood by the potential alcoholic. If they were, there would be far less danger of becoming alcoholic."

"Do you mean to say we didn't realize what we were doing in turning to drink as we did in the early days?" asked Wendell.

"We were conscious of a growing strong desire for alcohol, but we were not aware of its meaning, not aware of the meaning of our thirst."

"What is the meaning of our thirst in addiction?"

"You all know really," said the therapist. "But it is a little unpleasant to examine. The meaning of thirst, in addiction, changes from deep natural personal needs to a blind imitative pattern that we are unable to break. After the compulsion seizes us, binges occur regularly, there is daily excessive drinking, or both. The same process occurs over and over again, with damaging monotony, relieved only by a worsening of symptoms—guilt, remorse, fear, resentment, sentimentalism, physical sickness. The only remaining shred of the early strivings is sentiment—inappropriate laughter or tears, grandiose praise or grief, way out of proportion to real affection or sorrow. Sentences are repeated, stories retold like a broken record. All this is the opposite of what the drinker sought in the first pleasant days of drinking. No one wants to be a bore."

"Well, if he sought something in those first days, he must have had some idea of what he wanted." Milton pressed the inquiry.

"You have a point there. Every drinker has at least a vague idea that something new, something wonderful will *happen* to him when he drinks. Otherwise he probably wouldn't bother. But I suggest that he expects good things to happen to him, as though alcohol were a sort of magic. He does not expect that he will have to exert struggle or effort to get what he wants, as he knows he must in sober life."

"Doesn't he have a fair idea of what he wants, and then expect that drink will simply help him to get it?"

"Maybe so. There is some reason to believe that there is conscious striving for certain purposes, and also reason to believe that much of the striving is unconscious, or eventful. Anyway, after he is addicted, it is clear to any interested observer that his drinking gets less and less manageable, more and more blindly imitative. The addict imitates his own distasteful behaviour and that of fellow addicts, even to his own distaste in the remorse of the hang-over."

"Why should he imitate such behaviour, if it is distasteful? The word 'imitate' puzzles me."

"Because he is addicted. The imitation is compulsive and chiefly unconscious, a process over which he has no control. It is an imitation similar to the mimicry of a small child who repeats sounds with little idea of their meaning, and no thought of control. That's the sense I mean when I say the behaviour of an addict is imitative. The drinker's conscious imitation leads to a rigid pattern of imposed imitation. But conscious imitation may also lead to a flexible pattern of free imitation."

"I suppose," said Wendell, "you're going to say we should imitate, with careful planning, the actions of dry people, instead of letting ourselves fall into the rut of what you call the blind or imposed imitation of addictive drinking."

"If there was anything I loathed," said Sully, "it was the kind of advice I used to get to 'be like George or Harry,' some exemplary guy, who never drank, or if he did, he drank like a gentleman."

"To recover from alcoholism we have to start by imitating some kind of behaviour which will help as a model."

"The old temperance stuff again!" Arthurs was sceptical.

"Not temperance, but abstinence," the therapist suggested.

"All the same thing, if you really like to drink," insisted Arthurs.

"True enough. There is no such person as a temperate alcoholic. You abstain or you don't. But the approach here is not what we traditionally know as the 'temperance' approach, which of course means abstinence."

"Don't tell us we should imitate drunks! I'm always disgusted with them, when I'm sober. But that's silly. You don't mean that." Arthurs was resistant.

"That is just what I mean—with a difference. The first models for a recovering alcoholic are other alcoholics—recovered."

"That shakes me," said Arthurs. "I always figured that it was a good sign to feel disgust for the fellow drunk. Made me feel, well, 'isn't that awful, no one should get that way. Disgraceful'."

"The nature of our thirst, in early strivings, shows that we wanted to be better persons. If you hate a drunk, you hate yourself, you tend to lose respect. And it is self-respect the recovering alcoholic needs most to strengthen. After feeling disgust, you get drunk, sooner or later, if you tend to hate alcohol and alcoholism. It is a process of self-destruction."

"O.K. But I can imitate a recovered drunk. I don't have to feel sympathetic for the guy that stays on the booze."

"The guy who stays on the booze is always a picture of what we were, and can easily become again. He is you and I. To feel disgust for him, to hate him, is to turn against ourselves."

"Kind of a selfish attitude, isn't it, just to be thinking about ourselves?" Arthurs was fighting for something, or against something.

"Yes. But if you are selfish in a way that helps someone else, that's not so bad, is it?"

"No, no. But what can you do for a fellow who wants to keep drinking?"

"Show him that you are like him, but that it is not hard to be sober, if he really wants it that way."

"This attitude—this good feeling for a drunk—it is necessary?"

"Yes, I think so."

"But it is the recovered alcoholic, you say, whom we can imitate. We try to understand the active drunk, we try to imitate the recovered one. That's it, isn't it?" Sully took over.

"The two attitudes are closely related. You imitate the recovered man in order to help the active drunk. And as you understand the active drunk better, the better you can imitate the recovered man."

"What about the drys, or the moderates?"

"Let them wait. There's lots of time. Our lives will be limited if we stay only in the company of alcoholics. But, at first, I suggest, follow the pattern of recovered drunks. It is a severe task to imitate drys for the same reason that it is dangerous to hate drunks. In both, we are trying to be what we are not. In imitating drys, we ape people whose feelings, desires and needs are very different from ours. In hating drunks, we hate ourselves. In both, we destroy ourselves, we dissipate energy in impossible attitudes."

"I don't know. Why is it important to imitate recovered drunks when we know that a respectable 'dry' is a far sounder, a much stronger model?" Doubtful Arthurs was back in the picture.

"We need to remember our discussion on the nature of thirst, the meaning of thirst in the early drinking days. There we can find the reason why it is important to follow recovered alcoholics, and to feel sympathy for active ones."

"Ah, yes. But we found out that those early strivings led us into addiction. We don't want to repeat that, if we can help it."

"I keep thinking about the view that those early strivings were all right, nothing wrong with them." Sully was trying to reach Arthurs.

"It is just those feelings that the recovered man lives again, and strives to satisfy in sobriety. Those are the feelings we want to experience again, we want to understand and to undercut all the unpleasant memory of addiction and get back to where we started. So we don't fight addiction by the temptation to drink. We try to forget it, and go back to try to understand those feelings, which are the meaning of thirst, in the days before addiction."

"Isn't that an imitation? Surely it is." It was Alvin.

"Yes, but it is a conscious imitation, as distinct from the blind compulsive repetitions of the active addict. We see it in the behaviour of recovered men—this reliving of early strivings—but we see it as a conscious effort in the service of sobriety. So to imitate recovered drunks is to imitate men who are trying to meet their basic personal needs without alcohol. They are men like ourselves. So it seems to be good sense to take them for models."

"Isn't there the danger of repeating, or imitating bad qualities as well as good ones?" asked Milton.

"Yes."

"Well, maybe compulsive behaviour of a sort just as vicious as alcoholism can happen to us if we only imitate recovered alcoholics."

"It can," agreed the therapist. "For example, all alcoholics have certain tendencies in common. If we don't know what we are doing when we imitate, we may only strengthen the tendencies which lead again to drink. In our next discussion, we shall try to understand how an alcoholic wants to feel in order to maintain the adventure of sobriety."

3.

THE GOALS AND IDEALS
OF THE SOBER PERSON

SULLY reminded the therapist of the problems raised in the previous discussion.

"You said that conscious imitation of recovered alcoholics was a good practice in the recovery process, and later added that there is also danger in imitating recovered men, since they have tendencies which can lead to drink."

"But we need to distinguish between blind repetition, and consciously following a model."

Sully reviewed the discussion. "The blind repetition or compulsion is our behaviour in active addiction. Now what about those early strivings. Were they compulsive or conscious?"

"We got help here from Milton. He argued that the early strivings might well be partly conscious. When a fellow first takes to drink, he believes in its pleasure-giving quality, and in its value as a crutch. That much is conscious. But there is also an eventful side to it. I mean there is much in thirst that the drinker can't clearly explain. As he gets to be compulsive, he sometimes drinks when every other urge or warning says *no*."

"Yes," agreed Milton. "It's clear to me now that compulsive drinking can't very well be consciously controlled, though we might have had some reason for drinking when we started."

"So the pattern in following a model will be to try to

relive what we can recall of our early strivings, and try to see how well we understand them." Sully went on to complete his thought. "In recalling early strivings and what they mean, we do just what I suppose the recovered man does."

"That's important. You have struck below the surface. We need, not only to imitate surface behaviour, but to try as well to understand how and why the other feels and acts as he does. And this will be more than consciously to imitate the observable behaviour of a recovered man."

"More, in what way?" asked Milton.

"I could say a lot about that," Sully observed.

"Fire ahead, you started an interesting theme."

"When I was a child, I was filled with the sense of wonder. Every new experience was a joy, and my world grew rich."

"Do you, the rest of you fellows, know that Sully is a poet?" Clemens was amused and a little disdainful.

"Let him be," Arthurs suggested. "It sounds good."

"As I grew up, I was pressed to understand all I saw into useful channels—will it serve this purpose or that, will it harm me?"

"I'm no poet, but it was like that with me, too," admitted Arthurs.

"Long trained to heed useful things, I came to suspect anything which injures or offends. I began to lose my sense of wonder. Now I exploited situations and ceased to explore them. Habit, I found, like anyone else, and this is more than poetry, is at ease with the familiar, and wary of the strange. I turned away from people, as animals do from danger, or I exploited them until they turned away from me."

"People turn away from us because we make too many demands on them," said Alvin. "We pick on anyone who happens to be indulgent, until they get wise and avoid us. If they didn't, they couldn't call their souls their own."

"Yes, we tried to control people to suit our purposes," Sully continued. "Naturally they would resist us. In turn, we would defend ourselves against their indifferences by becoming hostile and critical. All this came about through neglect of that long forgotten sense of wonder. You say I'm a poet, but that does not make me different from the rest of you as alcoholics. If we could cultivate the imagination, as all artists do, not just poets, and believe, as they do, that persons and things are worth knowing in their own right, we might learn to appreciate our personal differences, even if we need to do so on the strength of our likenesses."

"We are beginning to get an answer to Milton's question, when he asked what more is there to recovery than conscious imitation of recovered drunks."

"All this," said Alvin, "ties in with Sully's idea and mine that it is worthwhile to understand this problem in our own way."

"And that is to be creative, not just imitative. I think we'd like to hear Sully complete his theme."

"With conscious effort I can approach you by trying to see if there were experiences in my life similar to those you knew. Maybe I'll have to imagine an experience like yours, if I cannot duplicate it in memory. I think of Wordsworth. Remember what he said about 'recollections of the moods of childhood'?"

"Yes," Alvin added, "and he also spoke about emotions recalled in tranquillity."

"Well, this is the theme I've been following, in our discussion about imitation. But there is more than imitation here. There is a big difference between an experience and the memory of that experience. There is a still bigger difference between an experience and the imagining of one like it, but never actually lived."

"What's the idea?" asked Arthurs. "Should we all be kids again? I thought the main deal here was to grow up."

"We can't recapture the acceptance of life, and the sense of wonder, as Sully described it, that we felt as children. Nor do we want to do so. But to recall those childhood experiences, to relive them consciously is not to be children again."

"We can't go home again." Sully remarked that this idea was developed in a novel by Thomas Wolfe.

"So the imaginative effort to understand, and feel those early desires, what we described as the meaning of thirst, is not to go back to childhood. It is, instead, to grow up. We either stop growing, or relapse into earlier phases of growth, if we give no thought or feeling to the meaning of our early life, especially as we were when we started to drink."

Sully continued. "The whole difference between childhood, and imagining it now, is the fact that something new has to be reckoned with. There's the other fellow to think about. I have to communicate with him by a conscious striving to be well disposed towards him. I was not conscious of that when I was a child."

"This brings us around more and more to what Sully and I wanted when we tried to say that we alcoholics need to understand our trouble in our own way." Alvin was stressing the common goal and the personal approach.

"I want to be fair," said Sully. "Since I've been here I've seen how valuable science can be in helping us recover. But, like Alvin, I still think we've got to see this whole problem our own way. Sooner or later we have to leave this clinic. We can't take the doctors and aides with us. There's something we've got to do for ourselves after we're discharged."

"Yes, and it is just that personal effort I want to stress. You see, personal effort is more than imitation, even when imitation is a careful plan to follow the best tendencies of recovered alcoholics, the tendencies which keep you sober. Personal effort is creative, not just imitative."

"We grow as we create," agreed Sully. "We remain stunted, or shrink, if we fail to be creative in the imaginative act."

"You mean we grow only if we are able to recall early experiences? That's a good one. It's like being a child again. What is this?" Arthurs asked.

"I agree with Sully," said the therapist. To recall early experiences is not to be a child. That effort of the imagination, which gives new meaning to those memories, is a grown-up act."

"Imagination? Say, did you ever see a fellow on the booze for days when he looked like he was about to fly north with a flock of mallards?" Arthurs was looking for a challenge.

"I can imagine it, even if I never saw it," replied Sully.

"Well, he's the sort of fellow who looks dreamy, but boy, you can have that for me." Arthurs recalled his hang-overs.

"Sure, and he may be thinking, not about mallards, but about those shiny black crows. You know, the ones that glisten with little greenish specks, the ones with the beady and hungry eyes."

"The doc is a poet too," observed Clemens.

"I know what he means," said Arthurs, "and I'm no poet."

"Well, all I'm trying to say is, we're sick when those weird and hideous images appear before us. There's not a drunk in the world who can't remember the horror of D.T.'s or of bad nightmares. But we don't create images like that. They happen to us. We need to distinguish what happens to us as sick people from what we create in the recovery act. Call it the difference between fantasy and imagination. The imagination is a great human capacity and very much neglected. Actually, without it, we couldn't be human. Without it, we certainly couldn't be personal."

"Will you give an idea of your difference between human and personal?" asked Sully.

"Money, power and sex are human goals. Freedom, creation and love are personal goals."

"Related to us, to us alcoholics, where do these two groups of values fit?"

"In my opinion, alcohol is the addict's fate in his search for something more than money, power and sex. But the tragedy is that he loses sight of the 'something more' in his addiction."

"Well," Clemens remarked, "if alcohol suits him better than riches, or fame, or sexual adventures, why isn't it sensible to settle for a life of drinking and let it go at that?"

"Because alcoholism is not a personal activity. It is an

addiction. It is the very opposite of what we mean by **personal**. A personal activity is chosen, you are free to choose. An addiction is an event, it happens to you, you can't help it."

"Still," Clemens went on, "alcoholism is a direct outcome of those early personal strivings that you urge us to regain from youth, and bring forward to relive."

"That's true. And that explains why the alcoholic turns so readily to drink, once he has tried it. It *seems* to give him the answer to that vague longing, that strange thirst that none of the usual attractions of life can give him. But what he fails to see is that his strivings require *action*, not magic, not something that just happens out of the blue. Everything about drink is passive, i.e., to the alcoholic. As he compulsively drinks more and more, the active centres of the body slow down. He reacts to everything at a slower and slower pace, until he reaches the familiar pass-out. While drunk, and still conscious, he depends more and more on nice things to happen to him, as one binge succeeds another. The unexpected windfall of some extra money, the chance presence of a beautiful and gracious girl who will tell him how wonderful he is, the prospect that a witty remark of his will earn the admiration of those who hear him—these dreams are all in the nature of something happening to him, as if by magic. Even his authoring of wit is an event which only an adequate intake of drink can produce. It is not an action he could soberly undertake. As for money and the beautiful girl, he thinks of them largely as means to the thirst for something new. The sober effort required to have them rarely occurs to him, or if it does he figures that they are not worth having."

"So I repeat," said Clemens, "why not settle for a life of drinking. If money, or power, or sensual pleasure are not his real goals, and if alcohol gives him the feeling of the something more that his thirst requires, what is there to recover from? He has what he wants, or the closest to what he wants that he can get."

"And I repeat that alcohol cannot be the answer, because it is not personal activity. Only personal activity can satisfy personal thirst."

"You'll have to explain better what you mean by personal activity," Clemens requested. "So far, it has seemed to me that alcohol well fits the drinker's needs, because it gives him more than money, power and sex can give him. I agree with you that the alcoholic thirsts for more than power, money and sex, and he finds this in the feeling that alcohol gives him."

"I don't know," observed Arthurs sceptically. "I don't agree with either Clemens or the doc, not completely. I think that the alcoholic, like anyone else, wants the great benefits of money, power and sensual pleasure. Actually, he finds them more attractive than most people do. So my opinion is that alcohol is a substitute for money, power and sex—a substitute for his failure to have and enjoy them."

"That's interesting, Arthurs. What do you think of our argument about personal thirst?"

"Well, it's all right, I suppose. But I would say that for most drunks, the desire to be a better person, to be well liked, to feel better and to sense new adventure—all the strivings that you call personal—all are bound up with the desire for money, power and sex. They go together."

"So the attraction of alcohol is that it gives the drinker the illusion that he is filling personal needs, that he has in drink what he hoped money, or power, or sex could give him. In that way, alcohol is a substitute for those three goals."

"Yes, that's the idea."

"There's nothing more?"

"No, that's about it, so far as I can see."

"If you had all the money you wanted, all the power, and all your sex needs filled, would you stop drinking?"

"Man! I wish I had the chance to find out," said Arthurs eagerly.

"Well, how do you imagine you would feel? Would you have any reason to drink?"

"Any reason is reason to drink," said Sully, "and if you haven't got one, you'll make one up."

"Well, you know," Arthurs continued, "a fellow might go on drinking just because he's addicted. I might really have everything I wanted if I had wealth and fame and the love of the women I desired. But we've been learning here about addiction, about the way alcohol kind of possesses or enslaves you. So maybe I'd go on drinking, even without reason, because I'm addicted."

"That's sound enough. But it does show, does it not, that there is more to alcoholic drinking than a substitute for those three great human goals."

"Oh sure, if you mean that there is also the fact of compulsive drinking to contend with."

"The fact of compulsive drinking is the main problem," said Sully. "It's not just an extra. It's the reason we are all here."

"What the argument amounts to now is this: Either we alcoholics thirst for more than the pleasure we get in money, power and sex, or we use alcohol as a substitute for them. In either case, we become addicted; alcohol not only fails to give us more than the three goals offered, it gives us much less—especially in the evidence of our poverty, our loss of self-respect, our frequent failure in love life. It also fails as a substitute for the three goals we've discussed so much. Because even Arthurs, who set forth the theory of alcohol as a substitute, admits that to satisfy the three goals might well still leave us addicted to alcohol."

"This is a fine how-do-you-do. What do we do next?" asked Arthurs.

"There's only one thing left to do. That is to go back to those early strivings, as I've tried to say all along, look at them and try to feel them, not as children, not in the youth that is lost forever, but as we are now."

"Maybe that's the course of action for all neurotics, not just alcoholics." Sully generalized his thought.

"I think it is. But the advantage of the alcoholic is that he has something definite to work on. It is his compulsive drinking, the event that gathers up all his trouble and misery in one kind of behaviour. So, in recovery, the alcoholic can centre his attention on his drinking, the nature of his thirst, and the way he can better satisfy this thirst than by drinking."

"What about 'the shiver and the burn' we talked about in our first sessions?" asked Alvin. "Doesn't that get lost in the excursion into our youth and in all this talk about money, power and sex and that mysterious something more that crops up time and again?"

"Well, what about it? I don't think we have lost sight of our stress on drinking. It certainly is not my intention that we should. If we are to recover, we have to find something to take the place of our thirst for alcohol, and to take the place of that 'lift' that alcohol gives us. To enjoy real recovery, we must somehow lose the craving for drink. We must desire something more than we desire alcohol. There's nothing wrong with the original nature of our thirst, provided we understand it, and do something creative about it."

"That's an important provision," observed Clemens. "Is that your distinction between an event and an action?"

"Yes, to understand our early strivings, or thirst, and to create a way to meet them, is an action. Simply to have them and to respond to them, more or less impulsively, is an event."

"And our discussion of thirst?" asked Sully. "You call it *personal*, if it is understood, and *human* if it just happens?"

"Yes. I'm glad you sharpened that difference. In our earlier discussions, we were inclined to describe our thirst as personal, whether understood or not. We did that because of the all-embracing nature of our craving—it touches everything important in our lives. But so does death. So it is a good idea to call our thirst personal when we try to understand it; human or eventful when we describe it as just happening in the drinker who feels a craving, or longing, and knows little or nothing about it."

"What about the power and the glory and the beautiful girls?" asked Arthurs. "You know, those three human goals that we talked so much about? They still look pretty good to me."

"Why shouldn't they? The alcoholic enjoys money, and a sense of power, like anyone else. And he savours the pleasure of sex and of sensual living just as keenly as the next person."

"Even if drink doesn't solve his problems surely we can still enjoy the ordinary pleasures of life," Arthurs observed. "We don't have to give them up, do we? Just think of it, think of it, we might as well be drunk or dead if we have to be hermits. For me, I want to be human before I get what you call personal."

"I couldn't agree more. It is human to want money, to have power, and to satisfy the senses, all of them. And alcoholics, if nothing else, are human. So go ahead, Arthurs, live and like it, I'm all for it. Only we have to watch out for what you yourself said earlier."

"About the substitute for human pleasures in drink?"

"Yes, that's it."

"All right. So I said alcohol was just a substitute for money, power and sex. What do we have to watch for? How do we do it? If we just stopped drinking, wouldn't our problems be solved?"

"I don't think so. I'd like to say 'never'. But that is too final. There may be the odd fellow, here and there, who just stops drinking. But it isn't common. It is very rare. Besides, mere abstinence does not solve the real problem of his thirst."

"What else is there now, really, besides the pursuit of money, the power it brings, and the ordinary pleasures of life? What else is there to have?"

"If there is nothing else, there is the constant danger of

addiction. As you once said, the alcoholic, being the kind of person he is, turns readily to alcohol if he is frustrated in gaining any of the human goals. You also admitted that if he were to gain his human goals, he might still be addicted to alcohol. Kind of a vicious circle, isn't it? He drinks because he can't have what he wants. And when he has what he wants, he still drinks because he is now addicted. We feel sure, at least some of us do, that having what we want, instead of killing the desire for drink, deepens it, if having what we want is money, power or sensual pleasure. Then, of course, we all know that some unexpected money was always earmarked for an extra supply. Any special power we acquired served our need for drink. And if we got as much drink as we desired, we lost our zest for sex and the normal sensual pleasures. The outcome was that alcohol ceased to be a substitute, and became so vital to us that we at last sacrificed everything the three human goals could do for us, except to be destroyed in the service of addiction."

"At this point, it is hopeless, just hopeless, that's all. I don't see a way out." Arthurs was glum.

"But there is. And you can still have those pleasures that you don't want destroyed. You feel like this, don't you? 'If I drink, I destroy myself. If I don't drink, I as much as destroy myself, because alcohol is a substitute of everything I prize most."

"That's about it. And more too. Because my view that alcohol is a substitute for human strivings means that those strivings can become addictions too, even if the alcohol problem were solved. Still I can't get away from it. Those human strivings, those normal pleasures, still look mighty good to me."

"Sure they do. Why shouldn't they? The way out is to try to find a substitute for their use, other than through alcohol, which still enables you to satisfy your thirst for them."

"That sounds hopeful except that you can't have your cake and eat it too."

"You can, if you keep making cake. We have to create

something new. It's not good enough to be just human, and to follow the ordinary impulses of human pleasure. This is the difference between 'personal' and 'human' we were talking about."

"All right, I see that. But what are the goals we should seek to be more than human, and yet be human too?"

"The goals are learning to be free, to create and to love."

"That recalls other discussions," Sully remarked, "and it sounds a lot like the sort of thing an artist believes."

"This is serious," said Arthurs. "I'd like a better breakdown of it all."

"Money, power and sex seem to be the goals of most so-called well adjusted people. The trouble is, the alcoholic is not well adjusted. I'm inclined to believe that he has an advantage here, when 'to be well adjusted' leaves much to be desired in the struggle to be a person. Anyway, if these human goals do become the alcoholic's objective, he sooner or later returns to drink. That has been the drift of my opinion. The alcoholic has a deeper sense of incompleteness, a greater thirst than the moderate drinker or 'dry'. Money, power and sex fill human needs, and, of course, the alcoholic's *human* needs are as real and insistent as those of anyone else. But his need for more than human pleasure is deeper than it is in the social drinker. This need is personal. To meet it, he has to re-examine his early strivings, and bring them forward to the place where he finds himself in search of recovery. Money, power and sex are the goals of our human nature. Freedom, creation and love are the goals of our personal nature."

"If we learn how to be free, to create and to love, we don't give up the human fun, do we?" Arthurs was anxious.

"Certainly not. Actually, 'human fun' can only have genuine meaning, if we seek a higher goal than the one human desires can bring us. There is the chance that human desires may enslave us, just as alcohol does. The seeking of money, of power, or of sex-thrills can become an addiction like that of alcohol, and just as self-defeating. The prize recedes, then disappears, in the very process of wanting, even needing it, desperately. If the alcoholic sets out for these human prizes, in a recovery effort, it is not surprising to see him turn again to alcohol."

"That's strange, isn't it? Why should he, if there is anything in the view that alcohol is only a substitute for human pleasure?"

"I think I see the drift of all this," said Sully. "Alcohol attracted and held him in his search for human pleasure, yes, but in his search too for something more than those human goals. He responds to his peculiar kind of thirst. If he ever gets to understand it, he will see that his thirst is personal, not just human. Money, power and sex are simply not enough to quench that personal thirst. This is what I meant when I said that the world of my youth was rich, before I was trained to press everything into useful channels. Money and power are *useful*, nothing more. So is sex just useful when all it means is chemical relief, or a conquest to satisfy my vanity. Now then, alcohol happens to me, and I discover new riches in its early deceptions. It seems to meet the urges and the longings of my personal needs. The harsh demands of a world driven by money, power and sexual thrills are softened in drink. These human goals get less important, while alcohol grows more vital in everything I do. You know the story. At last we see that we are sick. Alcohol destroys the hope of reaching any goal, be it human or personal. To have money, power and sensual pleasure grows meaningless in addictive drinking, even if they can be had. To be free, to create, or to love, is utterly impossible in addiction. Yet these are the goals of early drinking and of sobriety."

"Thank you, gentlemen," concluded the therapist. "The goals of sobriety described by Sully make sense to us all. At our next meeting I'll do a talk on the equipment we shall need to move towards these goals. This equipment takes the form of ideals—tendencies we want to train and develop in the search for enduring sobriety."

The Sober Ideals

If the alcoholic were to settle for nothing more than the goals of money, power and sex, and abandon drinking for a time, we are certain he would soon resume his addiction to alcohol, or be in grave danger of doing so. Arthurs set forth the interesting theory that drinking was just a substitute for money, or power or sex, or all three. When I asked "Would you stop drinking, if you had these in abundance?" he replied neatly, "I wish I had the chance to find out." But there is so much evidence of alcoholism in men and women whose human needs are more than well filled, that we cannot believe the alcoholic simply to be a person whose human goals are thwarted. Now it may be true that the alcoholic, or any other addict, has much to do in reordering human appetites and their satisfaction, but we suggest that the reordering will come primarily from new insights into his personal ideals—feelings he will try to cultivate in pleasurable sobriety.

The alcoholic in his drinking days behaved in a way to earn him these labels: dependent, sensitive, idealistic, impulsive, intolerant, inclined to wishful thinking. If he seriously sets out on adventure in sobriety, he is by nature well equipped at the start. For the tendencies he shows as an active alcoholic are closely akin to those qualities of adventure which, if practised, will bring him an acceptable and rewarding sobriety. The main agency in making the essential changes from his drinking tendencies to their counterpart in the qualities of adventure will, of course, be the hope of change and a desire for it in a purposeful effort to achieve sobriety.

The six ideals which will replace his drinking tendencies are these: personable, creative, dynamic, active, singleminded, imaginative. A little thought will reveal that these qualities are similar to those of the alcoholic in the state of addiction. The difference between them is radically marked by the new purpose, the new goal, of his proposed adventure in sobriety.

Personable

This quality means what is usually understood by the word—pleasant to talk to and exchange views with, kind, considerate, humorous, friendly, entertaining. But much more is intended by the word in our searching analysis. We mean by it a kind of knowing, an attitude towards ourselves and others that plumbs below the conventional surface of life. To be personable is to cultivate the practice of personal knowing, an action involving more than the knowledge of the senses, more than what people usually mean when they say they "know". Much of what this action requires can be found in children, whose capacity to wonder, to imagine, to love is often lost in the business of growing up. In personal knowing, the adult has to regain this capacity, if he is to become personable. The alcoholic, childish by nature, has less difficulty than most in developing this capacity. He has only to become aware of his latent talent for personal knowing, strive after it, and it can be his.

It is this awareness that differentiates the man from the child and which can bring to the alcoholic the maturity he needs. Being aware of oneself and of others is neither necessary nor desirable in children. It is essential in adults, especially in those of us who tend to be neurotic, to be troubled by the problems of life. It is therefore useful to the alcoholic.

What is it to become aware of the act of personal knowing?

First of all, it is to realize that underneath the superficial facts of sense perception and of routine behaviour, underneath the world we see, there is a dynamic play of forces hidden from the eye, more important and more powerful than what we view in the world of common sense. In this world, hidden from plain view, dwell the forces which generate both good and evil. In harmony and directed by healthy purpose, these forces emerge as good. In conflict, lacking creative design, and bent towards destruction, they emerge as evil. These forces are the basic tendencies in every human being to identify and to resist, to love and to hate, to be attracted and to be repulsed. In themselves, in their primitive state, they can be called neither good nor bad, neither true nor false. "Good" and "bad" apply to systems of value consciously worked out. "True" and "false" apply to systems of science and to sentences, also consciously worked out. But the basic tendencies to identify and to resist simply *are*. They are events, dynamic, capricious, unpredictable, unless one takes measures to understand, direct, and modify them. Even the effort to know and direct them could only be partly successful. There always remain spontaneous and impulsive events in the best of well regulated lives. And it is well that this is so. Otherwise, human beings might become mechanical reasoners, unable to get into action, for action takes its source in those deep unplumbed depths of impulse, without which there can be no vitality.

All the good there is in the world, and all the evil, can be traced to the dynamic play of those forces in us all—the basic tendencies to identify and to resist. To say that "the kingdom of God is within you", and that "the things that come from within your heart defile you" no longer appears as a contradiction, when we realize that the source of good and evil is one and the same.

To identify is good when it puts us in touch with others and in tune with ourselves. It is destructive when it robs us of our own integrity, when we are so blindly drawn to some one else that we become his pawn, dependent for our very souls on his whims and desires. To identify creatively is to lose oneself in the experience at hand, but not to lose one's sense of identity. "To lose oneself" means to abandon all petty concern about our immediate human needs. It does not mean so to lose oneself as to destroy insight into one's life. Let us distinguish the tourist from the adventurer. The tourist does not easily identify with what he feels and observes. He does not easily put himself in the other's place, when he takes with him on his travels all the familiar comforts of home. The adventurer sinks himself in the new experience. He is conscious of his own goals and purposes, he is in tune with himself, but he wants to know what it is like to be in the place of those who are now foreign, but who will grow familiar as he more and more identifies with them. The tourist *observes*. The adventurer wants to *feel*, to deepen his personal knowledge of others and of himself, to change his ways, if necessary, or if desirable.

To resist is good when it fosters respect for the other as for oneself, respect for the other's integrity as for one's own. It is evil in all forms of hate, self-pity and pride, because it blocks personal knowing, and we subscribe to the faith that knowledge is good, for in knowledge there is the light we need to guide us in adventure. Personal knowing *is* adventure, an adventure of the first importance. All the other qualities we shall describe are somehow in it and flow from it. Personal knowing covers all forms of knowing because all knowledge springs from some combination of the tendencies to identify and to resist. But here the stress falls on that form of personal knowing we call empathy—a deliberate act of identifying both ourselves and others in the adventure of seeking truth, beauty and peace. In this act we learn to become aware of what we are doing, and in becoming aware we learn to direct, not others, just ourselves. We seek, then, to identify with others, to respect them, and to enjoy personal growth in the process. "Personable" is the word we chose to describe this kind of growth; it appears to be apt in avoiding the tendency to regard empathy as either too sentimental on the one hand, or too objective on the other. In empathy, actually, one corrects the tendency to be either sentimental and weak or objective and cold. Sentiment clouds knowledge just as much as the so called "impartial" observation; both are false because they are not true to the real course of identification and resistance. Sentiment puts something into our feelings which belies them. "Objective" attitudes take away something from our feelings, which is abstract, workable in certain forms of science, but false to the facts of personal knowing, if it goes no further. No one can be without feelings, and know anything significant about personal experience. Thus "personable" seems to be the word that best suits that quality of adventure which respects the impulses, feelings, and meanings of purposeful human life, and is able to identify with them.

Creative

The alcoholic, in his early drinking days, sought adventure in the gay evenings, and in the long talks and excursions he shared with fellow drinkers. Sensitive to the wear and tear of daily routine, he came to value the relaxing and liberating experience of pleasurable drinking occasions. But, ignorant of the fatal tendency in him to become alcoholic, he gradually lost the ability to use drink as a means to adventure. He became addicted, and in this unhappy servitude, his sensitivity responded now only to the fear of getting hurt. His sensitivity became negative. It led, then, to a pattern of painful imitation. He became sensitive chiefly to his sick need for alcohol, in which, monotonously, he endured the same old round of blackouts, remorse, fear, guilt and painful tapering off. This pattern, repeating itself over and over again, bore no semblance at all to those lost days of pleasure, diversion, novelty. The early adventure bogged down in a routine of addiction more distasteful than anything he ever knew in sober living.

Yet, the alcoholic is sensitive, drinking or dry. He has the temper essential to adventure if only he chooses to seek adventure in sobriety. The tendency to be sensitive is essential to art, to the creative urge that will not rest satisfied with life as it is. The imitator, skilled though he may be in the techniques of art, lacks the one essential requisite for creative work, the courage to be himself. There is a sure place for imitation in everything we do. The past furnishes us with clues and plans that we value as indispensable, and among our acquaintances we see qualities that we wish to duplicate.

The young swimmer or skater learns his skill from an exemplar or model. We follow the pattern of the best people we know if we feel it is worth while as a means to better living. But it is not enough to be attracted to the best that has been said or done, to the best we see around us. It is essential, but not enough to qualify as adventure. We need the courage to be ourselves, to express in our own way whatever we learn or imitate. To do this is to be creative, though we neither sing nor dance, paint nor play, neither visit museums nor patronize professional artists.

At first, the alcoholic believes he is trying to be himself in the release of his tensions in drink. And for a while, never more than a few years, he seems to achieve a personal freedom unknown in normal living. But repeated hang-overs reveal to him that, far from being himself when drunk, he reverts to a level of life in the dim past, he relives the processes of infancy—no control over elementary physical functions, babbling, repeating words, ill-fitting tears and laughter, even the curled-up position of the foetus in a womb. There is just another step to go, beyond this—back to nothing, death. This is the irony of addiction. It begins in the thirst for richer life, it ends abruptly in near-death. Of course, we all must die, but we die best in learning how to live according to what it is in our nature to become. Imitation at best is only second-best. Its tendency is either to be static, or to regress prematurely to decay. To imitate, as a habit, and fail to create, is to repress the natural tendency of life, which is simply growth, the expectation of change, and the hope of being ourselves.

Dynamic

The alcoholic is a perfectionist, not always, not even often, in action. But that is the way of all perfectionists—their dreams and schemes are out-size, they can rarely follow through in life what their ideas demand. The perfectionist is rigid, he winces at the prospect of any change in his plans. He tends to be static, and fails to see that there are only two paths open to him, growth or decay, of himself and anything else in the universe. He seems even to cherish perfection more than life, for clearly there is nothing perfect, nothing static in life. But the alcoholic deceives himself into the belief that to him, and for him, all things are possible, if only there were not so many stupid obstacles wilfully blocking his way. Sober, the obstacles seem insurmountable. But drunk, the path clears, and, for a brief span, for as long as he is conscious, he is king again. He is grandiose. In his reveries, in his boasts, the world becomes what he wants it to be, made to order, tailored to fit his dreams, and with none of the pedestrian effort of sober living!

Now in this tendency to be idealistic the alcoholic has the discontent essential to a vigorous adventurer, discontent with things as they are in the sure and safe world of one's familiar ground. He has only to grow convinced that perfection is possible only in logic, and that logic is not life, but only a monument to thought. If there is one feature of humanity that stands out above all others, it is that human beings make mistakes. From these, they benefit, and set out again, humbler, and yet determined to approximate their goals, if not reach them. Those of us who relish adventure will always have a trace of the grandiose spirit within us, but if we are wise we will often settle for less than, or something other than, our original dream. We will be prepared to change, and to be changed, though we will not turn back to anything less than we are. In feeling deeply the meaning of change, we will know that *to be ourselves is to become persons.* It is to see, feel and live the dynamic nature of life, ceaseless change. The only unchanging thing is change itself. Forgetting that change is not an adjective, but in the very substance of life, you may object "But you just said, simply be ourselves! Now you suggest that we change, and become persons." The paradox breaks if we can sense that being and becoming are one process, one action. We *are* ourselves in *becoming* persons. What, no final goal? No, no final goal. Becoming a person is lifetime activity. Final goals, all neat and finished, are for perfectionists, who never reach them. But needless stress and strain are averted, if we settle for the truth of dynamic living, and abandon the outrageous claims of rigid arithmetic, of headstrong conclusions, cemented in advance of experience. These are only for perfectionists who love the laws of logic more than life itself. Fleming set out on a pre-planned experiment, and along the way discovered penicillin. Cabot set out for India, sighted Newfoundland, and returned to England to die of a broken heart. Fleming is the kind of adventurer for us. He modified his plans, he changed his course, he was flexible, and in letting what he saw, speak for itself, he was drawn to it, diverted from his main course, and came out with something of inestimable value to the whole world. To the truth, wherever he found it, Fleming was loyal. In this, he was single-minded and unflinching. As the great scientist will always seek the truth, and follow the path wherever it may take him, so the alcoholic will be single-minded as to sobriety, though its freedom will open up a variety of ways in which to strengthen it. The restless, groping tendency of the alcoholic that degenerates into futile dreams we call grandiose can, instead, become *active*, practical and real, once it is seen that adventure, if not dynamic, is nothing.

Active

Common much-used words, whose meaning is seldom pondered, are active, acting, action. We shall distinguish an event from an action. The first just happens, it shows no sign of human or personal control. Rain happens, so does a disaster or accident, or certain types of sickness. The second, action, is deliberate, choiceful, conceived. He who engages in action is *active*, even if he acts on or in an event. The recovering alcoholic, consciously in pursuit of sobriety, is active, though much of his action takes place within and around the event of his addiction.

All action springs from the events of impulse. Without impulse, there could be no action. But this is not to say that impulse *is* action. For some unknown reason, human beings are both animal and potential person. To achieve the balance between these two is the greatest challenge in the adventure of personal life. In the freedom, whose source is a mystery, that man can create, he learns how to act. Now, though man cannot act without impulse, it can hardly be said that impulse alone can become action. It seems to require other persons with a conscious common goal or purpose to harness an impulse, give it form and direction, so that it is transferred into an action. But that purpose or goal, which in this adventure is sobriety, endows impulse with a new quality which makes of it an action. Thus impulse should not be contrasted with action, as though they were opposites. An action *needs* impulse for its raw material, for the very life that any real action exhibits. Impulse undirected easily becomes a compulsion.

The alcoholic has lots of impulse. He comes to the adventure of sobriety well stocked in those vital surges that the adventurer must have for vigorous actions. But wayward impulse, undirected by purpose, or too vaguely understood, easily degenerates into a compulsion. The alcoholic, or drug addict, finds himself overcome by the compulsion to indulge. He can no longer exercise his personal power because he has been too long repressed, either in childhood, or by the crippling effect of over-stern morality, in which he detects human weakness. His gods tumble, and when they do, he loses his own balance. The ability to be himself is lost in addiction, because he never had a goal, or purpose he could really call his own. But he has it now. Sobriety is a bright and sufficient goal. When he appreciates its value, he will find it strong enough to pull him out of his addiction, and to direct his strong impulsive tendencies into *actions*. But sobriety has to be *his* choice. In deciding for sobriety, even if at first it is only the honest admission that sobriety is more desirable than alcohol, he takes the first important step in the series of actions necessary to his adventure.

Single-minded

The alcoholic's tendency to grow intolerant is not hard to understand. After he has become a problem drinker, he knows it, and he knows that all his acquaintances know it. In defense, he is driven to criticism of others, and of intolerance of them. This he must do to escape the pain of guilt and self abuse. There is enough of that in his hang-overs. But intolerance, turned to positive creative use, is a quality worth cultivating; when guided by a productive purpose, it becomes "single-minded".

The alcoholic needs nothing more than the sobriety goal to put his intolerant tendency to fruitful use. For sobriety is a goal well suited to all the qualities of adventure. It is not rigid, it is not static, it is not final. Sobriety, besides abstinence from alcohol, means freedom, not abstract freedom, but the rich capacity for actions not possible in the alcoholic state. A single-minded devotion to sobriety furnishes the alcoholic with a simple easily-understood plan of life. Unlike other neurotics, whose difficulty stems chiefly from a lack of knowing exactly what is wrong, the alcoholic can range all life's problems under two heads—drinking and sobriety. He need never worry, however, about the simple nature of sobriety. Once he has tasted its joys, he will find surprise and pleasure in all the new avenues of experience that sobriety, as a positive force, opens up to him. But let him be single-minded about his goal. It is disastrous to sidetrack the alcoholic with views which tempt him to believe that "drinking is only a symptom" of anxiety, wife trouble, or bad luck. These views tempt him strongly, for he would *like* to believe, in the service of addiction, that drinking is not really the problem at all. But it *is* the problem. When we realize that the chemical known as alcohol, C2H5OH, is not the only ingredient in alcoholism, that it requires a *relation* between it and the person who drinks it, then we are on the way to an understanding of the problem drinker, and are ready at last to abandon all efforts to solve alcoholism either by prohibition or by dismissing the problem as "just a symptom". By alcoholism we mean a personal disorder whose chief expression is an intake of alcohol followed by damaging behaviour. Alcoholism is a disorder of the whole person and drinking is the central symbol of that disorder. We have explored the entire area damaged by alcohol, and in doing so we went into the deepest recesses of personal life. Drinking and thirst are still our guiding symbols, as we have often indicated. It is important to keep the symbols of drinking and of thirst well in the foreground. Thus we struck out on a study of "adventure" because it seems that the basic thirst which led the alcoholic, unawares, to alcohol, is a thirst for adventure and its gifts. Alcohol tricked and tripped him, and he was plunged headlong into addiction. The problem, then, is to help the alcoholic, *if he wants help*, back on the road to adventure, to pursue, in response to his deepest thirst, the values of life he once groped for, though he never knew just what it was he wanted in his restless search for "something more" than normal life seemed able to give him.

So we urge the alcoholic to turn his intolerance to good use in a single-minded devotion to sobriety. This is to qualify as a genuine adventurer, for in sobriety in its wide area of freedom there is a rich variety of choices to keep his life dynamic and exposed to changes which favour his personal growth. He may perhaps fear the criticism that he has become a prig, a teetotaller, a kill-joy. But this fear will fade, and he will be amused at this danger when he is able to pour a drink for a friend, without resenting that friend's ability to take it, and exult in the quiet thrill of freedom. He is free, he is rid of a tyrant. He is, indeed, a released man who is becoming a person, and in becoming a person, with all the exciting changes that this action brings, he has his goal steadily before him—single-minded he pursues sobriety, for only in sobriety can he become a person, with the promise of all the freedom and all the changes that being a person brings forth.

Imaginative

The wishful thinking of the alcoholic developed long before he became addicted, but his drinking nourished it and gave birth to a complex tissue of alibis, fabricated in the interests of his desperate need for drink. In this complex of alibis goes a lot of effort, the work of imagination. So by nature the alcoholic has all the imaginative powers required of the real adventurer. In sobriety, he has only to shift emphasis, and no one will find fault with the wishful thinking now employed in the service of sobriety.

Among the many and varied uses of imagination in support of sobriety, there is one to single out for special stress. For a long time now, the drinking habit has been fought with what is called "will power". Many sincere people have exhorted their alcoholic friends to use will power, make up their minds just to stop drinking, keep repeating this resolution, and all will be well. But all is disastrous with this method. Why? Because there is no imagination in this dull imitative negative mumbling of words coming out of the mouth, but not from the heart. Even if it does come from the heart—many alcoholics have been sincere enough in resolutions to exercise will power—they forget that the "heart" requires more than negative exercise. As a symbol of impulse, as the source of action, the "heart" pleads to do something *positive*. But a resolution, exercised by will power, is always negative, "Don't drink". But why not a resolution of "Do", a resolution of action, action that replaces drinking, crowds it out, and becomes more desirable than drinking.

Resolutions of will power are what I call imitative or copy-book morality. The drys, or social drinkers, those responsible for judgments of value in our society have rarely understood the alcoholic. So, lacking the imagination required to feel what it is like to be alcoholic, they have declared "Be like us, just don't drink. Or, if you do, drink moderately". This reveals how difficult it is to imagine and understand the feelings of those who are unlike us, for among those people are many who are kind, well meaning, and sympathetic. But they are not *empathetic*. They find it hard or impossible to know what it is like to be alcoholic, or else they care little, one way or another. Copy-book morality, all those general maxims intended for all to copy, regardless of whether or not they work for everybody, copy-book morality is lazy, unimaginative, imitative. When it is prevalent, staleness sets in, convention dominates, art suffers, because the creative element in moral living is stifled in orthodoxy. Adventure dies, or is suppressed. Creative morality arises in imaginative departures from what barely passes as good enough for some to what is best for certain persons in certain trying circumstances. The whole deception of the will-power ethic is to be found in the hidden fact that those who preach it will never need it! If they did, they would discover, as alcoholics do, that is is plainly false and phoney.

It seems to require imagination to realize that sobriety is good because it is desirable. It is not desirable because it is good. This insight is imaginative, because it takes courage to depart from what orthodox society holds dear. There is simply no genuine inducement to become sober if the alcoholic does not at least dimly suspect that sobriety is more *desirable* than drinking. Now the benefits of his imaginative powers can be called forth to entertain for a while this fancy notion that sobriety, far from being a dull affair, is an exciting experience outdoing anything he ever knew in drinking. He is offered, not just release from the misery of addiction, but a great array of new adventures made possible in this new freedom. Such positive prizes are conceivable in a lively use of the imagination. Without it, there is no prospect of anything but life without alcohol. With it, with wishful thinking now in full support of sobriety, the future opens up with great hopes and images of high adventure.

It would be simple, and perhaps easy, if all the alcoholic had to do was shift his capacity for wishful thinking from support of drinking to support of sobriety. But there is a lingering hang-over of the tendency to be easily hurt, to criticize, and to be fearfully suspicious of others. Fear needs to be transformed to wonder, and wonder to be extended to curiosity about his fear and what it means, and thence to love of others.

In this talk we have sketched an outline of the six qualities which seem to be essential to adventure, and tried to show that the tendencies of alcoholic behaviour resemble these qualities of adventure, requiring chiefly the attraction of the sobriety goal to make the transition from a life of alcoholism to one of adventurous sobriety. The whole theme assumes the right of the alcoholic to his thirst, and the right to be himself, whatever that may bring forth in his effort to be sober. But we suggest that his abnormal thirst is basically a longing for adventure, for something more than normal life appears to provide. This is the real thirst. Of course a sick thirst develops in addiction, a thirst specifically for alcohol, because, trapped, he knows of no other way out. But the sick thirst is *ersatz*, it is the thirst which students discuss when they say that alcoholic drinking is an escape, or that the alcoholic drinks to dull pain.

Such conjecture is right within its limits. But to go no further is to neglect those sessions of drinking in which, for example, people drink "just for the hell of it", or equally, just for the heaven of it. To explore what this means is to trace some of the *positive* reasons why men drink, and why, in doing so, they become alcoholic. It is in the spirit of this approach that we have stressed the alcoholic's thirst as basically a craving for adventure, for exploration of positive experiences not found in orthodox living.

Now it happens that he becomes addicted. And here is where medicine enters the picture. If it were not for addiction, if alcoholics were simply wilful and misguided, it would be a simple matter to persuade them to give up drinking and put the force of their potentially rich qualities behind sober living. But addiction is a disease entity, and medicine, or at least the moral support of medical opinion, is valuable in helping the alcoholic recover. There may have been serious physical damage inflicted by prolonged drinking. There are certainly nutritional defects to be put aright and in the early period of recovery from alcoholism, the medical doctor is a timely and increasingly necessary friend of the alcoholic. It is this crucial state of the alcoholic which has led most students to concentrate on the disease side of the problem and to infer that alcoholic drinking is the result only of neurotic traits. This is to neglect the deeper aspects of the problem, to forget that alcoholics sometimes drink for positive though vague reasons, even after addiction is well lodged. The addict who begins a binge knows if he is honest, the misery that lies ahead of him, and he may know too that he is under the sway of an irresistible compulsion. Yet, uppermost in his mind, is the dim and distant memory of the pleasure he once knew when he could say fairly honestly and truly that he drank just for the hell of it.

I suggest that these positive, but vague, reasons for drinking are in some mysterious way the desire to be in better accord with the world, and to give stronger expression to what it means to be oneself.

Thus, real thirst in the alcoholic is a longing for adventure in which these dreams may come true. It is clear to him that drinking fails to satisfy those deep urges, but the trap of addiction imprisoned him, and there seems to be no way out.

But once the alcoholic has been helped out of his trouble by medical assistance, once he sees, even dimly, that from now on much of his recovery depends on himself and others like him, the way of his adventure will take the form of making values, of trying to find himself. He will locate the fears which beset him in addiction, and revive and clarify the objects of his *real* thirst, the longing which impelled him to drink, long ago, just for the hell of it. We can say that this personal longing was the urge to be free, creative and loving. The six ideals we have set forth are the feelings the sober alcoholic will strive to cultivate in order to satisfy his personal thirst.

4.

ALLEN'S STORY—TWELVE YEARS LATER

EARLY in this book we became acquainted with Allen, a typical alcoholic, who told us about his early break from the drinking pattern. Here he tells of his discoveries after twelve years of sobriety. You will recognize that much of what he says is familiar. From him, over the years, in many talks, a lot of the material for this book was gathered.

"The best way for me to begin is to say how grateful I am. When I tend to be depressed or upset, afraid that life is not giving me what I want, all I have to do is think of my sobriety. Now sobriety is not all a bed of roses. Sobriety is life, with all the ups and downs that any fully active person goes through from day to day. But I know that the only way to face life, good or bad, is to be sober. So I am grateful because I am freed from the urge to drink.

"There are many times when I have to pinch myself to realize that I am sober. It still seems to me like a miracle. And then, quietly, I pray. I do not ask for anything. I simply say 'Thanks, God.' The only kind of asking I use in prayer is to say 'Help me endure whatever I may be called upon to endure.' Over the years, I have found this the most effective kind of prayer. I do not believe I have the right to ask for anything that God would expect me to do for myself. But I do know that without His help I could not get through a single day. It is through His help that I learn to distinguish between things I can change and things I cannot change.

"I have found out that the search for cure and recovery is

226

hopeless. Once in a while, over the years, I played with the idea that something magic in a pill or in a technique might solve the alcohol problem. Now I am convinced there is no cure and no recovery, although an alcoholic can enjoy permanent freedom from alcohol. Of course I understand what is meant when a person uses the word 'recovery' and I often use the word myself. But there is no cure and no recovery from alcoholism, just as there is no cure and no recovery for life itself! Whenever I use the word 'recovery' I mean freedom from active addiction. Life I want to enrich. I want to stay alive as long as possible. For me, sobriety is life. But— and here is a vital truth—there can be no sobriety for me of a kind that I can endure if I ever forget that I am an alcoholic. My alcoholism is the prime condition of my sobriety. So I accept it, because I need it. If I could be cured, I'd drink again. So far as I know, there is nothing from my drinking days, or from my life before I drank, that I want to duplicate.

"After twelve years' sobriety, I am no better able to take a drink than I ever was during my worst binges. I never could say, and I cannot say now 'I will never take another drink.' To say this is to believe that I have mastered my problem. I will never master my problem, I will never gain control over alcohol. And what's more, I will never master anything by myself, no matter what it is.

"Always I feel the need of help. When I seek it, and get it, I realize that I am comfortable in my sobriety only when I feel deeply that I cannot live by myself alone.

"So I can be reasonably sure that I will not drink, and that I will enjoy sobriety more and more, as long as I continue to find myself through my fellow-man.

"There is no seniority in sobriety. I do not understand the mystery that has enabled me to stay sober twelve years. I do not understand why some of my fellow alcoholics have had more trouble than I have had. They have been as sincere, as desperately needful of sobriety as I have, and they have tried hard to maintain it. For me, honestly, I must admit that it was not hard. I cannot claim any credit for living as deeply and rewardingly as I have these many years, despite setbacks and tragedies in my personal life.

"If the way had been difficult, if the urge to drink had struck me as it did many of my friends, I have no doubt that I would have slipped. The simple truth is that I lost the desire to drink in December, 1948. Then gradually there developed, more deeply as the years passed, a desire for something stronger than the desire to drink. And I knew, all along, that to enjoy this 'something more' I had to stay away from alcohol. When you desire something more than anything else in the world, the pattern of your life in other areas falls into place. But this desire has to be positive and give promise of richer life. Like many alcoholics I began my sobriety simply because I was sick and tired of the troubles of drinking. I was fear-ridden, despondent, ready and desperate to do anything to break the bonds of addiction. But such fear and distress are not enough to sustain abstinence. These negative feelings may lead you to a sort of self-righteous dryness, but they are not strong enough to maintain a comfortable sobriety.

"I was astounded and pleased to find a rich reason for being sober. When I did, I no longer had any trouble fighting alcohol. Alcoholics who have trouble staying sober are those who are unable to find anything in life more satisfying than drink. They are dry only because they are afraid to drink. I discovered that I could stay sober only if life held out for me the promise of something richer and more pleasurable than the best that alcohol could give me. I call this the rich ground of sober living. All the rest of my talk will be the effort to explain this creative and exciting reason for sobriety. Right here I want to say that I did not stop drinking to confirm a berth in heaven, to stop laughing or to dry up the world. Sobriety had to be enjoyable, and lenient or I could never have held on to it.

"I have to turn to my own experiences in order to say anything that makes sense. There is so much of the unknown, the mysterious and the unpredictable in the way of life that maintains the alcoholic's health that at best I can only offer clues, hints, invitations. Sounds like a party or adventure, doesn't it? Well, that is more or less what sobriety is, as I see it. Let's never forget that a patient seeking health is necessarily selfish. He wants to get well.

"The clue to health, when you've lost it, is found in the meaning of the symptom. And the symptom, if drinking prior to addiction can be called symptomatic, I found in my early pleasure drinking. Before I had any trouble with alcohol, I believe that I was trying through intoxication to tap the unknown world inside myself and to get in closer touch with others, more than I was trying to escape from something. I had fun and high adventure. Once in a while, on cloud thirteen, I'd be high enough to feel I had the pulse of everything. I just knew why without thinking it necessary to explain either to myself or others.

"Early drinking for me was pleasurable. Everything good is pleasurable, or at least bearable so long as it's lasting, so I see nothing wrong with the fact that I enjoyed drinking If it had continued to do for me what it used to do, I'd still be drinking. Intoxicated, I could tolerate, even indulge, the square world with it's banalities, routines, and pathetic seri ous preoccupations. What, I used to think, was there to be serious about in a meaningless world, where the weak we deluded, and even the power boys eventually became th own victims? All that made sense to me was to seize pleasures when I could.

"Intoxicated, I could tolerate the sober world, tenderly despise it, and explore the experiences of the adventurer in those precious hours of pleasure.

"What changed all this? Fear? No. Not all the vicious fear of a hang-over, the threat of loss of prestige or job, or of wife or family ever successfully turns an alcoholic onto the path of sobriety. No, it was not fear. Strangely, the fear of drinking only worsens drinking. Fear may initiate abstinence, but it never sustains sobriety. There is only one fear worse than the fear of drinking and that is the fear of sobriety. Any way you take it, fear is useless in the act of getting well. It worsens addiction because addiction itself is a pattern of fear.

"At the time I took the course which these twelve years I've tried to follow, I suspected that underneath the pleasure I had in drinking, something else was driving me. Of course, by the time I stopped drinking, I was in trouble. Hang-overs, fears, guilt, incompetence—all these proved to me that problem drinking is rough going with little left of the early pleasure of years gone by. The love for drinking came sharply under question because now this great love changed, as all blind devotions do, to a possession of me by the compulsion to drink. I first of all began to hate alcohol, that is, to hate myself, and then alternately, feel sorry for myself. Hate or resentment is love gone wrong. You are devoted to drinking, only to learn that it does you in. Surely this is love gone wrong. And surely there is resentment as a result. I next saw that I had to try to understand what I really wanted out of drinking, if I was to overcome the resentment against alcohol and against myself, and against others, the resentments which made efforts at sobriety prior to 1948 a sorry mess. I re-examined the meaning of early drinking. I long thought that it was simply the pursuit of pleasure. Unless it was something more, unless there was something more in all life itself, then there was no answer but despair or clowning. I had enough of both of these. I began to hope that there was something more in life than gloom, maudlin sentiment or fluff. So now I'm trying to understand those resentments which I call love-gone-wrong by seeking a sounder meaning of the experience of intoxication.

"If the philosophy of pleasure is sound, then addiction is its logical outcome—blind unwavering devotion to experiences which yield pleasure. If you say, ah, but one has to be moderate to be in control, then you contaminate the pleasure theme by introducing other measures whose value you imply to be higher than the state of being pleased. Also, you have only to be an addict to learn' that the zealous pursuit of pleasure leads without exception to pain and misery.

"Searching then, for more than pleasure as a reason for my drinking, I saw at last that I drank, oh yes, I drank to feel pleased, *but I wanted to feel good in order to feel free*, and to experience in such freedom the elusive something more that curiously evades us in sober life—the elusive feeling that you get once in a while in early drinking, but which moves further and further away as the problem grows.

"Now the meaning emerges more clearly. I drank for fun and I drank to be free because I could only be free if I could forget the fetters which made me less than I wanted to be. And being free has its greatest merit in being able to be interested in the things and in the people you love. Drink damages the course of love by incurring resentment. Resentments are love gone wrong. They are in the same groove as love because they betray interest, even if such interest is destructive. They go wrong in failing to yield any experience of any value to anybody. Actually they destroy both the resented and the resentor.

"So I have a new meaning for intoxication at its best. It is this; I *tried to be free to love what was love-worthy*. I had to be free to do this. And the best way I knew to be free was to be pleasantly high on alcohol. As to the meaning of life, I began to see that *the only knowledge worth having as a personal experience, must arise from the act of loving*. 'To be, to love, to know—all the same thing.' Whatever meaning there is in life must rest on my capacity to love something, somebody, somewhere. I certainly demonstrated in my own life more convincingly than all the text books I know that the philosophy of pleasure, for its own sake, is as dead as yesterday's newspapers. But this is not to say that there can be no fun, no laughter, no high times. Not at all. The paradox of all life, which screams to high heaven, is that I can be pleased, I can be at peace, I can rejoice in life only when I know deeply that at any price I must be as free as possible, provided I know that I cannot be free alone.

"So all this threw great light on those damaging resentments. It was silly to hate and fear alcohol. While I did this, I went back to it time and time again. It was equally absurd to hate or fear myself. This only led deeper into self-pity. It was again equally silly to resent others. How could I come to know them, to get their help, to earn their respect if I was blocked off in the ignorance of resentment? And finally it was real crazy to fear or hate sobriety because if I was to live there was nothing else to do but be sober. I'd have gone on drinking and be drinking still, if it were possible to gain my freedom, learn how to love and live with my fellow-man, by being an active addict. But another paradox that hit me straight and hard was that the original drinking act which helped me to feel so free and easy became a colossal taskmaster who kept driving me deeper and deeper into trouble.

"So I could not be free and I could not know love and I could not savour the meaning of life as long as I continued to drink.

"To look for substitutes, to overestimate the value of occupational therapy, is only an attempt to save face, to fear a radical change, to stay pent up within the pride of my anxious self. There could be no fooling around any more. I had to face the fact of loss of freedom—that I was powerless over alcohol. Surrender is total. It is a recognition of a power greater than your intelligence, skills, self-discipline and talents all taken together. It is a recognition of otherness. And in this recognition I began to respect, rather than resent, my addiction. I began to accept it and so I stopped fighting it. This respect for addiction, this acceptance of it, I see now to be the righting of that love gone wrong that defines hate or resentment. My devotion to alcohol became, after I was addicted, a resentment and fear of it. The form it had now to take was respect for it. And believe me, I do respect it now.

"Complete resignation to the fact of your addiction can

open up two main paths of action. When you cease to resist evil, you have a choice. Either you go on drinking still devoted to your need for alcohol and still devoted to the pleasure psychology, even though you know now that devotion to pleasure is devotion to pain. Or, you ponder the chance for recovery, knowing that you cannot expect to be comfortable without alcohol unless you do something about those other evasive facets of addiction that concern your feelings, in short, your whole way of life.

"If the decision is to go on drinking, the mind closes in, gaining a measure of peace in the conviction that 'this is it' and 'what the hell' shutting out the confusion and pain that might develop if you were to be open-minded and hope there was still a way out. If the decision is to try recovery, then a hope has to grow that recovery is really possible. Now a hope something like this began to take form after my admission of loss of freedom in 1948; perhaps there was somewhere in the vague area of otherness a power as great, even greater than, the power of addiction. The recognition of my addiction to alcohol first brought to me, with stunning clarity the fact that there *is* a world, a fascinating world, made up of more than I can ever feel, understand or know—a world of nonsense as well as of sense, a world of feeling as well as of logic, a world of others, many kinds of others, whose meaning I could never well know, but whose existence I had, at last, to acknowledge as real. While most of all this was forever barred from my knowing and my control, I could yet manage to get glimpses of it all if I tried hard enough. For the rest, there was nothing to do but respect it and to wonder about it. My hope for health was based, then, on the faith that in the no-man's land of powers and experiences I did not yet know, there was a power and experience enabling me to break from alcoholism if only I could find a clue somewhere to the path of release.

"In the ten years prior to 1948, I had tried and failed many times. The reasons for my wretched failure from 1938-48 are very clear to me now. I regarded my drink problem as most of us regard a tooth ache, stomach pain, a hole in the chesterfield, a payment on a car—a trivial annoyance that an intelligent person can manage by himself. If he can't, he ought to be ashamed of himself. Pay the dentist or doctor, bring in the upholsterers, work harder and keep your bills paid. Alright, you drink too much. Wise up, and watch yourself. Even when I knew I'd lost control over alcohol, I kept going to my books, and was often high or excited about the brilliance of an idea, a subtle explanation, or a neat theoretical game which put the whole problem where it belonged. But I continued to get drunk because I was still looking for the answer in the network of my cerebral cortex. Without realizing it I still believed in will power—the ridiculous view that you can do something you don't want to do just by thinking about it. Actually you can't even do something you very much want to do just by thinking about it. Conditioned reflexing is a modern slick form of the will power pitch. That is why the deterrent drugs won't work on the long haul any better than the old pledge. Even the great search now for the drug enabling alcs to drink socially is pathetically out of line with the facts of the problem. Let us suppose that such a drug could be found. What the researchers neglect here is that though their drug could make me a social drinker, I'd still be stuck with all the emotional garbage that defines alcoholism quite as much as the excessive drinking act itself.

"I believe that we alcs are psychologically fortunate in having such a clear graphic centre of reference in the symbol, alcohol. Our pathological drinking we learn to associate inseparably with our psychological and social quirks. Take away the physical problems of addiction and we are still left with the deeper more insidious features of addiction. These, the harder to cope with, would be left untouched in a deliverance from the physical compulsion to drink. The deep meaning of loss of freedom would be lost and I would retain most of the worst features of addiction if a well-meaning scientist could enable me to drink socially. I would not experience the adventure of otherness—I would slink back into the shell of isolated self-concern, shut in with all the old fears of self sufficiency. Eventually I would drink again, and cultivate once more a physical sensitivity to alcohol.

"Anyway, where in hell is the alc who wants to drink socially? Four simple questions I ask fellow alcs who are not sure of their condition. The first is, 'Did you ever go on a water wagon?' The second is, 'Would you like to be a social drinker?' If he answers 'yes' to both of these, I say he is alcoholic. If he answers 'yes' to the first, and 'no' to the second, he is alcoholic. If he answers 'no' to both, he may not be alcoholic. For him, a third question is in order. 'Does drinking interfere in any way with your life as you otherwise want to live it?' A fourth 'Does your life in any way interfere with your drinking as you want to drink?'

"The dawn of real insight came, not from an idea, not from a drug, not from a concern with physical health, not from the fear of drinking, but from other persons. Remember this whole story of mine is a story of personal freedom because the story of addiction is a story of hate and fear and slavery. You cannot be freed by an idea, by a programme of techniques, and obviously you cannot be freed by fear. Romantics can fall in love with love, but not with fear. And sadists and masochists can fall in love with hate and fear, but not alcoholics, not alcoholics as such.

"The act of surrender, and the hope for health came together when I experienced the marvellous feeling of being free and easy as I listened, astonished, to the stories of two fellow alcoholics. I did not yet know what lay ahead of me— more trouble with drinking was all I'd ever had to go by. I was just exhilarated by this experience. Looking back I see now that I must have been at least a little well disposed towards those two. I was receptive to the stories of their trouble. It was lucky for me that I was well disposed towards them. That's why I say tritely, but I am convinced, very truly, that good will is the solid ground of all communications, of all knowledge, of all sound recovery, of all life.

"And where did this good will come from? It came, no doubt, from the deflation of my pretensions, conceits and pride. It came from a complete resignation to the fact that I was powerless both over my drinking habits and my whole life. I was finally able to listen, to try to learn because there was, without doubt, no power of my own capable by itself of solving my problem. So now I had it. Addiction was a pattern of fear other than anything I alone could manage. And now besides that, there was a power other than myself, also more than I alone could manage, but which I had some hope of living with, as I could not live with addiction. Good will came to mean something much deeper than I had ever learned before. It comes, partly from desperation, and partly from the need to respect others. The trouble with my old idea of good will was that I thought I had to be considerate of others, not for myself, but for them alone. I know little of others' feelings. At best I know something of my own. I honestly believe, still working on the evidence of my feelings, that one of the main reasons why Jesus came out of the wilderness to mix with all sorts of people was because *there was nothing else to do*. It was, if nothing else, an act of sheer desperation. But I believe, too, that he saw, as in a divine coincidence, that this was also the best thing to do. After all, there was a choice. He did not forsake temptation because he had to resist it as the life he most wanted to live. He saw his life to be more desirable among others, than to be alone in slavery to the addictions of power, prestige and pleasure. He could only be free among others, in shared experiences of the kind that matter most. Being free is simply the ability to choose and want the soundest way. So He said 'Resist not evil', the whole catch being that we shall *want* something so much more valuable in life than resentment, that we do not waste energy in hating, fighting or fearing the things that matter least, especially when such acts do nothing at all for even the things that matter least!

"If I was to be well, I saw that I had to depend on the help of others. It was, frankly, a selfish condition. I was thinking

only of myself. But then a curious process set in. The longer
I listened, the more respectful I became of my fellow alcs.
I discovered what I could never have learned and felt out of
books. It is this: as you grow more healthily selfish, you
grow, at the same time more truly unselfish. The more
deeply I sense my own greatest needs and do something
about them, the more richly I shall serve your own greatest
needs.

"What my exemplars taught me, early in the game, was
that I was on the right track only if I put sobriety ahead of
everything else in the world. If I did this, they said, all other
experiences and values would fall easily into place. I soon
found out that sobriety meant not just abstinence from alcohol, but a way of life, a new psychology, philosophy and
religion.

"As I listened to my exemplars, and watched them in
action, I was gradually able to identify in an intelligent way,
all the tendencies in them which, because they were a mirror
for me, I could see in myself.

"Now I had a very satisfying and strengthening experience. I learnt that the great obstacle to growth is not the fact
that you are built in a certain way you can do little about.
The great obstacle is your inability to see how you *do* feel,
whatever that feeling or group of feelings may be. I have said
that the alcoholic cannot recover alone because he is powerless. He needs the help of others. The bridge between the
isolated helplessness and loneliness of the alcoholic and the
world of otherness is built on those feelings I can share in
common with others like me, in pursuit of a common goal.
And it was easy. In no other way I know of could I have felt
so relaxed and insightful as when, with lots of good humour,
I could at last see myself for what I was, an alcoholic.

"The ability to laugh at yourself, by the way, is a wonderful antidote for self-pity. It blows up prideful pretensions, and severs useless preoccupations with the wrong
methods.

"As long as I live I must try as hard as I can to understand better the feelings both of fellow alcs and of fellow non-alcoholics. I understand little of the feelings of others. But I must keep trying. It is not too hard to understand the feelings of others when they resemble your own. But always within the requirements of our growth there is the adventure ahead of becoming as familiar as we can with feelings that are foreign to us. Whatever progress we make, however, in reducing the fear of the foreign must be based on what is familiar to us. The work of wonder and imagination is important here. There will be many tries and many mistakes but we must go on trying. When understanding reaches its limits, the game is not over. We have still to learn to respect, without question, what we fail to understand.

"In the act of putting himself in the place of another the alcoholic is able to experience the next great act after his discipline of freely imitating recovered fellow alcoholics. He selects what he values most and develops his own personal style, but he never stops learning. He becomes himself in his own right.

"This is what he always longed for in his drinking days, to be himself, to become himself. He knows now that this can only come about by becoming as free as possible, as pleased as possible, in order to love what is loveworthy and maybe, but he shouldn't bargain on this, maybe be loved in return. The only way in the world to achieve such personal life is through the capacity to put yourself in the place of others, and to accept what you fail to understand in the act of respect.

"How, you may ask, can I say this? How do I get the nerve to set this belief forth when I admit that I have little or no capacity for it, excepting in small measure among fellow alcoholics? Well, it is a statement of faith; an ideal. I must hope that my belief is true, even when I fall so short of it in my efforts.

"If goodwill is not the only experience in the world which can be called good without exception, if it is not possible for me to wrench at least a little clear of my human trap, if I have to live without friends, and if fellowship is an illusion, then there is indeed nothing, and I may as well die drunk. I may not get far in the adventure of freedom and love but if I can stay sober there is still hope. Without this hope there is nothing.

"And what keeps the hope alive? It is the spectacle of recovered alcs working together in common cause with a common goal. Men and women who discover that the practice of understanding one another becomes also their goal. We learn to be free, to be pleased, to love and be loved. And this is what we wanted out of drinking, except that we got them in the wrong order. We sought pleasure to be free and easy, sentimental or aggressive, in the vain pursuit of love objects. Now we seek, first, to be free, than pleased, in order to love and be loved.

"I have made mistakes, and I will make more. I have had many laughs, many kicks, and, at times, many tears.

"I stopped drinking because I had faith in what I was trying to feel in intoxication. I believed in it. I wanted to be free and happy. I wanted to be myself. That is what I wanted when I drank—that's what I want now and always. Drink failed me (or I failed drink) but that does not blot out the deep yearning to be and become myself, wherever the mystery of sobriety may lead me. And that is the strongest most exciting reason to be sober that I yet know."

5.

FROM INSIGHT TO ACTION

"To be free, to create, to love—these are the goals, then?" Arthurs recalled the last group session.

"As I see it," said Sully, "these are the only goals to seek, if we believe we should respond to our early strivings, to the urges of our personal thirst, in the days before addiction."

"Either Sully follows me, or I follow him," the therapist observed. "Anyway, that doesn't matter. We are on the same track. It is interesting to remember that the three goals of sobriety are more attractive than the corresponding goals of active alcoholism—which were to be defensive, attention-getting and self-sufficient."

"I see that," said Alvin. "But there's more I need to see."

"You can say that again," nodded Arthurs. "There's a lot more for me to get, if I expect to make any sense out of it."

"I once mentioned the vague search for something more," said Milton. "We seem to be getting closer to it."

"So did I," added Wendell. "Always incomplete, nothing had a satisfying climax, even in alcohol."

"Let's look at the three personal goals and what they mean to us," the therapist suggested.

"I think I understand what they mean, in a way. My problem is, how do you put them into practice?" asked Sully.

"Yeah, what can we do about them?" Arthurs meant business.

"Learning how to work them is essential to understanding them. The first is, how to be free, and for us, this means concretely how to be free from alcohol. That is the first step in the recovery process."

"Now, I want to get this straight, from the start," insisted Arthurs. "You said that the three personal goals we have to seek will embrace the three human goals. So I think right off that this freedom-deal will have to embrace money. Is that what you mean?"

"Yes. I see that you intend to keep me hooked down to earth. So I'll try to keep it as clear and sensible as I can, Arthurs. But it is important to understand and to feel that words tend to become rigid, but really stand for functions, events, actions, or persons. Even when they are place-names, they represent vitality and movement. So the meaning of one symbol merges into another. I hope this grows clear as we proceed."

"I'll let you know when I fog up."

"The initial step in learning how to be free is to imitate, consciously, recovered alcoholics. This is therapy that money cannot buy. I may be able to suggest to you that it is wise to do this, but *you* have to do it. No amount of money can buy for you the desire to imitate the behaviour of well recovered alcoholics."

"But what will induce me to develop that desire?" Milton asked.

"That is the crux of all therapy—the patient's desire to get well. In our case, it begins to develop when we suspect that alcohol is not the answer to our personal thirst, and that our personal thirst is worth understanding and study."

"So we proceed first on the faith that recovered men understand their personal thirst, and are acting on its demands for satisfaction in a personal way, in the only way that suits our personal nature, without recourse to alcohol?"

"Yes, that is the ideal. Naturally, recovered alcoholics are human, and will often fall short of the ideal. That's why it is dangerous to choose just one exemplar, and slavishly imitate him in every detail. The day will come when he will let you down, not intentionally, but just because he is human like you are. He may slip, in thinking, speaking, feeling, or in a hundred different ways other than a relapse into drinking. With more than one exemplar, or model, you can find it in yourself to say 'He is not perfect, he was trying hard. What did he forget, how did that happen to him?' In this way, there are others to rely on when the going is tough, and by comparing experiences, you learn about the sort of imitation I called imposed, that is, addiction, and its danger signs."

"Well and good, but is this what is meant to be free?" asked Arthurs.

"It puts you on the way to freedom. Even only to begin to understand the compulsive nature of addiction, and consciously to keep imitating recovered alcoholics is an act, deliberate, planned, and therefore free. We can contrast it with addiction by saying that in the recovery process you begin to act; in addiction, you are *acted on*. Just the other night, a woman alcoholic, complaining of her hang-over, said to me 'I drank two bottles of beer, and they didn't do a thing for me.' As alcoholics, we expect things to be done for us, to happen to us. We are passive. In recovery, we have to learn to *act*, even if the beginning is modest, like simply trying to understand and feel, *in our own way*, the attitudes of recovered men and women who communicate to us the techniques they use in keeping sober."

"That is free imitation, then, and that is our start in learning how to be free?" Milton remarked.

"Yes, and for Arthurs' sake, I stress that it is something money cannot buy."

"Yes, but how is it a substitute for money?" asked Arthurs. "I mean, how does it bring us money? Remember, you said that the new goals embraced the human ones, and gave them their real meaning."

"Well," Sully observed, "you'll at least have the money that you might have spent on drink. And that is a substantial item. There is a statistical figure, I think, which shows that alcoholics spend half, or more than half, their means on drink."

"Sully is more practical than we thought. With the extra money you have in sobriety, you can spend it on family essentials and luxuries that you couldn't afford in your sickness. But most important of all is your new discovery that to be free from addiction is a prize you can't measure in money. If you find this out, you will understand that freedom is better than money, a more worthy goal than riches or material security."

"I want to tie in the difference between action and event with the difference between freedom and money," said Sully. "It seems to me, the way we've discussed the problem, that one pair of ideas is similar to the other, maybe mean about the same, really."

"Go right ahead."

"Yeah, let's make this clear or give it up."

"Well," Sully began, "to be free means to act. But you have to act to be free. Now, that's not my own. Read it somewhere. But now, it really means something to me. Related to us, that means we have to look at the pattern of our imposed imitations in the addictive stages of our drinking, realize that we were not free, that we could not really act in the grip of our addiction. We have then to practise consciously the imitation of recovered alcoholics. In that practice, we act more than we do in first understanding the addictive stage, and we grow more free as we continue to follow recovered alcoholics and strengthen our insight into the eventful course of addiction. All this, of course, is to take for granted that we want to be free—primarily from addiction to alcohol. That's why we are here."

"What does this drill have to do with money?" queried Arthurs.

"I'm coming to that," said Sully. "To look deeply at our addiction, our slavery to alcoholism, is an action. The addiction by itself is an event. The careful scrutiny of it, charting its course and its use as a lesson, is an action. It is an action done by you with the help of others like you. So, in the same way, money, by itself, is an event. It is nothing and can do nothing. If it is spent irresponsibly, as it is by an alcoholic, it is spent by one who is not capable of genuine action, as we now understand the word. The use of money by one whose life is obsessed with the event we call addiction follows a bookkeeping plan governed chiefly by the sick need for alcohol."

"O.K. You say that money in the hands of an alcoholic who drinks is an event, nothing more. He can't handle it." Arthurs wanted it simple.

"That's clear and to the point," Sully agreed.

"Uh-mm. Well, I could never put any aside. They say money talks, but I never had it long enough to say hello."

"To finish my point, we have to learn what addiction is, and what it is to be free from alcohol, before we can properly handle our money."

"I see all this well enough," said Milton. "But I thought we were to re-examine our early strivings, and forget our addiction."

"That's right," nodded the therapist, "I did say that. But we first want to understand why we propose to undercut addiction, before we return to consider the early days of drinking. Besides, we cannot resolve to forget our addiction, if we do not first know it for what it is."

"Why, then, do we undercut it, as you say?" asked Alvin.

"Because it is an event that happened to us, an event we cannot fight or control. And this leads us directly to the problem of the second human goal, power, and to the need to embrace it with creation. Addiction will again assert itself, if we do not learn that it is useless to fight it. Addiction never dies. And this is precisely what I mean by forgetting addiction. To forget addiction is to cease trying to fight it. Let it be. To forget it is to accept it. Did you know that forgetting is an act of memory?"

"That's something I'd have to think about," said Milton slowly. "But the main point now is what you say about not fighting, but accepting, addiction."

"It's power I want to speak of. Power is no good to the

alcoholic where he most needs it—in control over alcohol. But he has no control over alcohol. We all know that. Power restrains, inhibits, controls, and even cripples or kills when we so desire, and when it is effective. But you cannot kill addiction, you cannot reduce it, you cannot control it."

"Looks pretty grim to me." Arthurs looked the part.

"It is grim, if we cannot express energies which take priority over addiction. But I know we can. We can replace power with creation. We can learn how to create new patterns of behaviour, out of the old ones wherever possible, as, for example, we do when we re-examine our early strivings, bring them forward, and try to meet them in the light of what we are now, try to meet them without alcohol. We cannot fight addiction, but we can stop drinking."

"How, with will power?" asked Wendell, reviving old discussion.

"That will come up again, many times. Just now, I will only say that will power, without a desire for sobriety, is worse than useless, because it is a specific case of the second human goal, power, in the form of self-coercion. And this may well lead again to drink."

"You gave concrete examples of freedom. It makes it easier to understand it. Will you just do the same with creation? What is it to create, and how do we go about it with our particular alcohol problem?" Milton shared Arthurs' need for clarity.

"That's the spirit, Milton. Let's get down to instances."

"Sully is the artist, the poet. Let's turn to him for his views on creation. He did pretty well on the first personal goal."

"We were over some of the ground before," said Sully, "when we said we were creative even in imitating recovered men. You remember? Personal effort and all that."

"Well, yes. That is what I mean when I say that the words we use really stand for movement and life. It's difficult to cut up a dynamic pattern so that the pieces fit neatly, one following the other separate and distinct. One episode really flows into the other."

"So we developed the view," Sully added, "that to bring forward, through memory, our early strivings was to perform an adult act, not to return to childhood."

"Yeah, I remember. Seemed kind of vague to me." Arthurs was puzzled again.

"We mentioned imagination, too, and saw the differences between it and fantasy. Now, I want to trace the theme another way, just to exercise the imagination, and not to go over the old ground again in the same way."

"That's a good idea."

"Well, after the creative act of imitating recovered alcoholics, and after the start you get in seeing for yourself, in your own way, how they keep sober, you revive the memory of those early strivings—you know, to gain confidence, to feel better, to be a better person, to be liked and to savour the sense of wonder."

"That's all familiar," said Wendell.

"Sure it is," Sully said. "We've been over it enough. But now you get more creative. Up to now, you've been following recovered drunks, and you learn from them that it is wise to forget your addiction, and all its misery, and to think and feel, instead, about what your thirst really means. So you begin to do this *yourself*. Friends and fellow alcoholics are absolutely necessary, right through the long road of sobriety. But there are things each of us has to do for himself. To recall your strivings in your own way is to be much more creative than you have been up to this point in the recovery programme. You have had friends to help you, now it's up to you to contribute to the friendship. You begin to contribute actively to the relationship with recovered drunks, and with new drunks who cross your path. You make friends now, instead of just being carried along."

"When we started these discussions," said Alvin, "you and I felt that personal initiative was essential to knowing our problem."

"Yes, yes. And the whole answer to our problem as I see it now, is to concentrate on the meaning of our thirst, and to satisfy that thirst in a personal way. That will be to be free, to create, and to learn better to know both ourselves and others. At first it is fellow alcoholics whom we should try to know, later it will be all sorts of people with whom we shall try to be friendly, and to respect as we do ourselves."

"That means," Alvin added, "that persons can only be known in and through the act of liking or trying to like them."

"That's it. Only I'd add that we get to know ourselves in that act too. That's important—to know ourselves, if we plan to steer clear of slips, and to make sure that we get neither too disgusted, nor too concerned with ourselves."

"Now what about some concrete examples, Sully, before you fellows plunge ahead with your . . . your sense of wonder, is that it?" Arthurs interjected.

"Examples of what?"

"Creation. I have got to be shown. You see, it was something I could hang on to where you said that being rid of drink was to be free of it. Then I saw that a fellow was free to do other things he wanted to do, once he quit the booze and stopped fighting addiction with will power. They were good examples of freedom, for me. Now what about creation?"

"You remember Alvin and I wanted to tackle this whole problem in a personal way, right from the start?"

"Yeah, you got into that memory stuff, and a long song and dance about personal thirst, and strivings, and what have you."

"Well, you see, Arthurs, all that was creative, and everything you said was creative, too, because you were interested in getting some real answers in your own way to a problem that none of us ever tackled like this before."

"Uh-mm. Is that all?"

"No. This could go on indefinitely."

"Just take it the short way."

"You once said that you felt disgusted with a drunk, if you happened to be sober?"

"I did say that, yes, but I see it another way, now. I *think* I do. I'll have to find out."

"Well, when you do feel differently, if you do, that will be a creative act. When you can imagine yourself in his place, and still stay sober, that will be a creative act. Is that enough for now?"

"That'll hold it for the moment. But—ah—never mind."

"Something's puzzling you. Let's have it, Arthurs, we're all in this together."

"Well, what Wendell there said one day, and Milton too. I'm just trying to put the pieces into a kind of pattern."

"Yes?"

"Uh, you see, there's that sex problem and that feeling they spoke about, the feeling that nothing was ever quite complete. Where does this come in? And you said that love was what should embrace sex, like freedom and creation embrace money and power."

"Well, well. That's our biggest problem yet, and Arthurs is going to make sure we don't by-pass it. To be frank I must say that love is such a diffuse ideal, and yet so important, that we must approach it carefully, knowing that we can catch glimpses here and there of what it means. It means so many different things to different people. But Arthurs is right. We have to look at it as concretely as possible, as it affects us and our drinking problem."

"Wendell and I," Milton recalled, "brought up the sex problem and with it the frustrated feeling that seems to accompany most of the alcoholic's activity. We are just as interested as Arthurs in knowing how to cope, not just with women in sexual relations, but, damn it all, with everybody we have to deal with. This is a problem not just of sex—this is a problem of getting along with people."

"I am not going to try to say what love is. Instead, I am going to assume that every one of us knows more or less what it is to be in a love relationship with a thing or person. We may love a picture, or poem, an animal or flower, or some material object, or we may love persons. Because our problem concerns people, I'll restrict our discussion to love among persons. Though we all more or less know, as I say, what love is, we are sometimes in doubt. That doubt may occur for us in situations which are very important to our sobriety. Following Arthurs' insistence on examples, I'll suggest situations that have to prevail before we can say that love exists."

"This is going to cover, not just sex, but all those other experiences that for me were just as frustrating as sex. Is that the approach?" Milton asked.

"Yes. Love as it concerns us here, consists of two kinds of relations with persons. The first is the love between man and woman which embraces sex, the second is the friendship between persons, regardless of sex, which is perhaps the most pleasant feature of civilized living. But in both sorts of love, there is one essential attitude. Without it, there can be no love in the ideal form. In all loves we have to recognize and accept the other as a person in his or her own right."

"I always thought I used my wife well," said Wendell. "I really don't think I neglected her. I was decent, I am sure."

"There is something rather more to be than decent. We'll start with sex. Here we have to know what a woman needs. This is not commonly learnt in our tradition of decency. Tragically, it is perhaps our decency which keeps us and our wives from finding out what a mature sex relationship requires."

"Drink didn't help," said Wendell. "I learnt that. At first it seemed to relax me, but something else suffered in that relaxed feeling, after a time."

"We won't explore the techniques of sex any more than we did ways and means to make money, or to have power. For these, we go to legal counsel, to science, or to psychotherapy. And the third, indeed, may do us more good than tips on the stock market, or the marshalling of scientific controls."

"Will sex literature tell us anything we don't already know? What does love add to it?" Wendell asked.

"If you love your wife, besides desiring her, you do not discover anything radically new for yourself. But you do discover that what you have, and in a sense always had, is more valuable. And you work on love all your life. It does not just happen to you. So your sense of frustration, and Milton's feeling of lack in all other experiences, not only sex, will disappear in learning through love, to know and understand yourself and the other better, in day by day effort. This will be to appreciate and practise respect for the other as for yourself, as a person both like and unlike yourself. This is to act, rather than to wait on wonderful things to happen to us."

"You suggest that I regard my business deals this way too?" asked Milton.

"Yes. Money is not the only interest of your freedom, power is not the only interest of your creative talent, just as sex is not the only interest of your love."

"Milton's Paradise regained." It was Sully.

"Not before we eat the fruit of knowledge, if we're going to talk in pictures," added Alvin. "I suggested a little while ago that we'll get that knowledge of persons in and through the act of liking or trying to like them."

"And I stressed that we should get to know ourselves in the same act," said Sully.

"Let's remember how we started out," Alvin noted. "Our original thirst, its meaning, and where it leads."

"When we understand the meaning of our thirst, when we realize that it is personal, and when we meet it as persons, I suggest that we shall overcome the disturbing feeling that nothing seems to have a satisfying climax. Arthurs likes everything specific. So I'll put it this way. As we grow more *free*, more *creative*, more *loving*—notice the accent is on action—we better meet the strivings to be better, to feel better, to gain confidence, to be liked and to enjoy the sense of wonder. And this is to satisfy the deep thirst that alcohol could never quench."

"Uh, this is rather moral, isn't it," said Sully, "sort of persuading us to be do-gooders?"

"Well, in this way I think you'll *make* good. I wasn't thinking of doing good for the sake of being moral. That's rather gloomy, and tends to kill the sense of wonder. No, just think that everyone in his own way wants to be a better person, especially those of us who are disturbed or sick. Far be it from me to set up a gymnasium for the exercise of your character. I'm just groping for a way of recovery from alcoholism."

"At this stage," observed Sully, "that will be to go on and see what kind of people we've become in response to our original thirst."

"The tree of the knowledge of good and evil," suggested Alvin.

"Well, yes, in a way. To note what our behaviour tendencies are as alcoholics is to learn what is good, what is bad, with relation to our sobriety goal."

"And what, in your opinion, are those tendencies?"

"Somehow or other, in response to our personal thirst, we innocently developed attitudes which were nourished in drink, or which drink gradually developed within us. Now these attitudes or behaviour tendencies all mean essentially the same thing, just as money, power and sex are three different expressions of our humanity, and just as freedom, creation and love are three expressions of our life as persons."

"Why so many, then. Why not keep it simple, if they all mean the same thing?" asked Arthurs.

"Well, only because it is easier for me, as it is for you, to think and feel in terms of specific situations."

"What are these tendencies?"

"All together they mark our personal trouble. But that isn't descriptive enough to distinguish us alcoholics from other types of neurotics. So I break it down, only as a matter of convenience, into six traits. In any of these six, all the others can be found. But I arbitrarily chose six in the effort to locate the specific quirk which makes us alcoholics, and not some other brand of incomplete person. We tend to be dependent, sensitive and idealistic, impulsive, intolerant and wishful thinkers. The first is our main general trait, the second is the one in which we'll note our specific addiction to alcohol, the rest follow. Any one of them is an expression of the alcoholic as he is, all of him. It is not just a fraction of him. All these traits developed within us in response to our original thirst, that we have come to understand as essentially personal in nature. The traits, as we see them in the alcoholic, block personal growth. This is the irony of alcoholism. What we have become is the very opposite of what we wanted to be. And what we really want to become is outlined in my talk on the sober ideals—personable, creative, dynamic, active, single-minded and imaginative."

"I can't help thinking about addiction and the desire to drink. After all, they are our main problems, aren't they?" asked Wendell. "What in the world, I ask you, am I going to do about the consuming urge to drink, if I don't fight it?"

"Well, all along, just that has been my headache, too," said Clemens.

"Goes for all of us, doesn't it?"

"Naturally. But please don't try to fight addiction. Instead, try to keep the sobriety ideal uppermost. Failing that, try at least to desire recovery, even if there is only a spark of hope just now, and even if the desire is only half-hearted. There is an answer in the end, if you try for it."

"And what is that?" asked Clemens.

"You will lose the desire to drink."

"In our self-searching programme?" Sully asked.

"Yes, just doing what we are doing now, and propose to do."

"When we understand our tendencies as addicts and do all we can to redirect them towards sobriety—that was your talk on the sober ideals."

"We find that we create a new way of life in knowing one another in fellowship."

"Is this fellowship, rather vague to me, is it directly related to alcoholism? Is it really?" asked Wendell.

"Fellowship is a form of love more important in recovery from alcoholism than anything else I know. I say that in the downright interests of recovery from alcoholism."

"If I follow this," said Sully, "that means we have to put our highest value on the desire to be persons, each in his own right. That, for us, will be to want sobriety more than to desire money, power or sexual pleasure."

"If you can't be sober, you'll lose all of them. I see that, I wish I really felt it, all over." Arthurs sounded wistful.

"Arthurs has struck the heart of the matter," said the therapist. "It is one thing to see or understand a problem, it is another thing to put our insight into action. In my next talk, I want to set forth a programme of action, based on the experiences of men and women who have found their sobriety to be free and easy, productive and enjoyable. Before I present the chart on action, let us look at the woman alcoholic."

The Woman Alcoholic

There is troubled ground, common to all alcoholics. Let us look at it before we distinguish the problems of women from those of men.

The common ground, in review, is made up of six qualities—all are dependent, sensitive, idealistic, impulsive, intolerant, and given to wishful thinking. These are just ways of describing the alcoholic's basic pattern of feeling in order to have something concrete to work with, in an intelligent analysis. The term "immaturity" is too general and too loose to be practical. I have found that an analysis, along the lines of the six qualities mentioned, is helpful in gaining insight into the kind of person who becomes an alcoholic—man or woman.

Released from adult responsibility by alcohol, the drinker reverts to childish ways and dreams. There is a longing for the affection known in childhood or for the affection lacking in childhood. The alcoholic suffers from an imbalance of parent love. It is not a coincidence that alcoholics resemble helpless babies in very drunken or near-passout stages. Most babies get attention from some one.

But alcoholics would not differ from all sorts of other neurotics who are "dry" were it not for the second tendency, "sensitive".

Alcoholics have either a constitutional or developed body defect which reacts like gasoline to a flame. There is an explosion. So far as I know, no scientist is yet sure about the nature of this body defect. All we can do is accept it as a fact, whatever may be its exact cause. Until more is known about it, we can only describe this body defect as it appears in behaviour. And to me, it appears as a sort of explosion. The drunk, soberly composed, suddenly goes to pieces after drinking. He or she loses touch with reality, and takes off into a world of fantasy in "pieces" because there is so often little sign of coherent action or thought. The imps of the unconscious break through and destroy the civilized control of the drinker's life. "Defeat in a controlling area" is the crucial experience of the alcoholic, defeat in an area normally controlled by a healthy drinker.

It does not require precise scientific knowledge to say that no matter what the body defect is, or how it is caused, the alcoholic is sensitive in many ways other than his or her body defect. These other ways are important since they furnish clues to the alcoholic's motives for drinking.

Alert to fancied abuse, to ridicule, fearful of being less than they ought to be, they are inclined—men and women— to be grandiose, especially when drinking. The tall story, the expansive gesture, the big effort—these are seen and heard in various stages of a binge. But in the hang-over, they continue to be sensitive in a grandiose way except that, sober, they look for punishment rather than praise. Having made much of themselves, they become the more sensitive to the distress of the hang-over, and to sober living. Inflated or deflated, they mean to produce an imposing effect, either in seeking attention or supposing it to be there when, actually, most people couldn't care less. Alcoholics are not noted for balanced living. They move from the extreme of elation to that of gloom. Either way they act impulsively, when they can bring themselves to act at all. They are inclined to resent advice and authority externally imposed, especially measures to keep them from drink. Sensitive to their own defects, they become intolerant of similar faults in others, faults, very often, they are not conscious of in themselves. The sensitive nature of alcoholics is most obvious in their wishful thinking, a pattern of alibis developed over years of active addiction to protect and excuse their defects and fears. The whole issue of wishful thinking, as it grows more elaborate, appears more and more childish, not only to those who know them well, but also to people who require only a few inconsistent examples to spot the fabulous designs and alibis of addicted drinkers.

So much for the common tendencies of men and women alcoholics. Alcoholics Anonymous, stressing these common tendencies and striving to overcome or redirect them, does a remarkably fine job of recovery, whether the members be men or women. A.A. asks for honesty, humility, searching self-analysis, mutual aid and fellowship. Without these, no drinker, man or woman, can hope to achieve lasting recovery. The need to *surrender*, a process calling for humble recognition of powerlessness over alcohol and assuming that the victim is at least capable of freely choosing to surrender, brings scientific aid and genuine religious power together in one dynamic force. From there out, the help of recovered fellow alcoholics bolsters the desire for sobriety and gradually enables the members of A.A., of either sex, to do for others what has been done for them. This process, here briefly reviewed, has gained the recognition of the medical profession, of clergy and of the bulk of fair-minded citizens in society at large. It is recognized as the greatest single agency, presently known, for coping with the drink problem in its follow-up phase.

Still, members of A.A. and all others close to the drink problem, do not regard alcoholism as completely solved. The A.A. member, indeed, believes the continued open mind on the complex problems of addictive drinking is a "must" in his recovery programme. There is always another step to go. In this spirit, it is important to think about the differences, if any, between men and women alcoholics.

If some women do not respond to treatment as well as men do, if their problems are more deeply lodged than those of men, and if there is a special reason why the real problem comes to light only in an intimate interview or friendship, all of us interested in the woman alcoholic will want to know as clearly as we can what distinguishes her from the male drunk.

Dr. Giorgio Lolli makes these special points about the woman alcoholic.

1. A problem suddenly imposed from outside may shock her into heavy drinking. For example, a man generally loses his job because of drinking, a woman will drink because she has lost her job.

2. A woman whose husband's success suddenly elevates her into a new social climate becomes insecure and anxious and may resort to heavy drinking.

3. The career woman, faced with the fear of a childless life and no husband, may relieve her depression in alcohol.

4. The threat of bodily ills or disturbances such as cancer, the menopause, a hysterectomy, or removal of ovaries may induce a woman to drink heavily. (Separation from her children may so depress a woman as to cause addiction. This fact has an interesting symbolic relation to the threat of bodily ills: personal identity is threatened.)

5. Men are more likely than women to blame themselves

and feel guilt during hang-overs. Women, thinks Lolli, are inclined to blame the drink for their misfortune and misery and to minimize their personal responsibilities.

There is much value in these observations based, as they are, on clinical experience. Still, I believe, also on the strength of evidence, there are other important points, which, though perhaps implicit in the above five, need to be made clearer in any analysis or treatment of the woman alcoholic.

A man's world, outside the circle of his family and friends, is often competitive. A woman, today, freer than she ever was, also may develop a competitive spirit as she becomes more and more active in the world of struggle and gain. But this spirit of drive and push is developed at the expense of something peculiarly feminine—the role of supporter to her husband or loved one. Competing with her husband instead of supporting or loving him, regretting that he does not measure up to the ideal of her father, she forsakes her role as woman and lover, and unwittingly begins to think like a man, one man in competition with another—her husband.

All this is not to say the trite and obvious, "A woman's place is in the home". But it is to say that a woman is happiest as a *partner*, not as a competitor. Partners are not slaves, neither are they masters. A partner is ideally thought to be someone who has what the other partner has not. Similarly, the other partner has something which the first partner needs.

Central in a woman's life is the need to be loved, to be wanted, and in return to feel that she is needed rather than tolerated or pampered. This basic need is more important than the drive to be competitive, on the same basis, with her husband, or with other men.

The hard-boiled attitude of many women alcoholics is a cover-up for an intense feeling of guilt and shame created by early teachings about sex, and by a strong father need which somehow failed to be satisfactorily met. Even in the strictest homes, boys are indulged compared with the taboos and fears hammered into the heads of otherwise healthy young women. Dad, to the young daughter, becomes a paragon of virtue and the standard of manhood. If she is thwarted in her need for father's affection by a possessive mother, she will go through life vaguely seeking her lost male ideal. On the other hand, if she is completely indulged by a father who grants all her wishes, she is likely to compare her husband with her incomparable dad. Of course the comparison will limp—the husband never makes the grade. Then a curious change takes place, though the woman will not be aware of it. She *becomes* her father; psychologically she abandons hope of finding her greatest feminine need, so she plays the role of a man competing with this fellow, commonly recognized as her husband. But once bring her deepest need to the fore, stir in her the need to be loved and wanted, and she will respond, as all women will, to her true nature.

The woman alcoholic displays an I-don't-care attitude because she is fearful of society. Her training has made her that way. Actually, such an attitude does protect her to some extent. She feels that nobody would be more tolerant or kind if she did tell the truth about her feelings. It would only make her more vulnerable to jibes and curiosity. The woman alcoholic whose excesses follow illicit intercourse appears to be completely relieved when she learns she is neither pregnant nor diseased. On the surface, it looks as though she is rather hard-boiled, concerned only about the inconvenience of an unwanted child or the worry of venereal infection. When these fears are dispelled, she goes merrily on her way—so it seems. But probing deeper, you will learn that a feeling of guilt underlies her "sin" and the suspicion that she is "dirty". This goes back to her childhood, to the fears instilled in her about the good life, and she turns to alcohol for comfort. This is one good reason why women alcoholics are often so much harder to treat than men. Men are less inhibited about sex than women who, under pressure of social stigma, have to conceal the sources of their trouble and are compelled to put on a hard-boiled air to cover up their real feelings—feelings of guilt, shame.

But the woman alcoholic may be helped well along the road to recovery if she accepts the fact that the perfect man is a myth, and if she recognizes her true role as a woman supporting a man, and giving him evidence of it. Her greatest need is to be needed—not just for sex, but in every way that she as wife and mother can fill the role of partner. There will then be no frantic need for vicarious sex relations, competitions for honour and prestige, and best of all there will be no occasion for that excessive guilt and anxiety which lead to the bottle.

All alcoholics—men or women—appear to be sensitive. The all-important task for each problem drinker is to learn as honestly as one can just what forms this sensitivity takes. Common forms are noted in the tendency to be childish, grandiose, impulsive, over-idealistic. No matter how much the tendencies of one alcoholic may differ from those of another, the *body sensitivity* is present by the time the drinker seeks help. It is the real danger signal. By it, the alcoholic knows that he or she must either stop drinking completely, or go on to disastrous trouble. So far, nothing is known to science that can cure the body defect except to stop drinking. Abstinence is within reach by knowing the forms which the general trouble, *sensitivity*, takes in day by day behaviour. The drinker, if he or she is honest, best knows what these are, aided by a friendly recovered alcoholic. And if the alcoholic, seeking recovery, comes to believe that these forms of sensitivity are harmful, and if steps are taken to alter their course, the body sensitivity will lose its most insistent feature—the craving for drink.

By all odds the most important initial step for the alcoholic to take, man or woman, is to say "Yes, I am alcoholic, because drinking interferes with my life. I need help."

We know that women problem drinkers share basic tendencies and hopes in common with male alcoholics. But in the conversation which follows, they explore their difficulties in the light of their special problems—personal and social.

A woman's personal life is more complex than that of a man. Her husband, children and friends expect her to be the moral model of the family. Her social life, whether married or single, is more demanding than that of a man, since society forbids to her what it often accepts, without question or criticism, from a man.

Though her feelings are just as strong as, if not stronger than, male feelings, she must control her behaviour more carefully than a man.

And yet the trend in North America has been to place women on the same social basis as men. The ensuing competition is often in conflict with the role of women as mothers, wives, lovers.

Even so, with understanding and diligence, the woman alcoholic can learn to be comfortably free from her drinking problem. She can, if she wishes, achieve this freedom as effectively as a male alcoholic.

The conversation of Margaret, Jane and Lucille is drawn from the experience of patients who provided much of what has been said in the foregoing statement; they confirm more or less what Dr. Lolli had previously reported in his studies of the woman alcoholic. Other personal observations reveal that women alcoholics have problems of feeling usually more concealed and more difficult to unearth than those of men. But good communication shows how effectively such problems can be brought to light and managed.

"We all know that our problems are similar to those of men alcoholics," said Lucille, "we're here to discuss what we can add, or modify, as women problem drinkers."

"We have much in common," Margaret noted.

"Their theory of thirst applies to us," Jane agreed. "Everyone wants to be liked, to be a better person, and so on. All that applies to us as well as to men."

"Certainly we are just as sensitive as men," said Margaret. "Perhaps more so. Then there are the forms this sensitivity takes—grandiose, impulsive, over-idealistic. And the basic pattern—being dependent. This is our pattern too."

"Yes, but there's definitely something more," said Lucille.

"A therapist helped me become aware of my problem in three or four stages," Jane began. "First of all, a long forgotten experience was unearthed. It took some time because the experience was distasteful and concerned my father. Something he did upset me, when I was about five years old. I can't be sure whether it was intentional or not. I like to think he meant well, that he meant no harm."

"It could be an experience with a man other than your father," Lucille added. "I can recall an occasion with my uncle similar to the shock you mention."

"Well, anyway," continued Jane, "my therapist pointed out that the shock of that experience with my father set up a dislike of physical contact with men. At the same time, I had a strong urge to be liked and wanted by men. It looks as though I both liked and disliked my father, sort of torn between feelings of warmth and the experience of distaste. He was happy-go-lucky, not much good according to social and professional standards, and my mother began to take over as head of the house. She wore herself out trying to make the most of her family—perhaps to make up for her growing indifference to my father. Her persistent efforts were annoying but she had her way. My brother got through university and I went to the best schools. I remember having to take piano lessons with some one to supervise the practising hours. I hated it. But mother insisted. She tried so hard to be helpful, saying that such discipline was for our own good, and I'm sure she meant it. But, without her quite realizing it, she was really satisfying her own thwarted desires through me and my brother. Before I married, mother had become like a girl friend, and less like a mother. But she was like a girl friend in an over-devoted way, sort of like a servant. The early discipline was relaxed, and she now bent over backwards to satisfy my every little whim. But what was strange, until I realized what had been going on, was that mother was never really affectionate. I cannot ever remember kissing her."

"Is there still that 'girl friend' feeling between you and your mother?" Lucille asked.

"No. Frankly, I grow bored with her efforts now to oblige me, and to share all the little intimacies we used to discuss. I'd do anything in the world to help her and make life easier for her. But I love her now because I feel sorry for her, sorry for her because she seems to have missed something important in her own life. I don't need mother as I used to. I don't lean or depend upon her now. But I did just that for so long that it was hard to cultivate the right relationship with my husband. You see, before I stopped drinking, I felt the urge to control my husband rather than really love him, to control him and live through him, as mother had controlled and lived through me."

"Well, how did you solve this problem?" asked Margaret.

"When I learnt through bitter experience that men want love and not bossing, I saw that it was no use to go on trying to run my husband's life. Besides I was very unhappy. I was torn between the old tendency to lean on my mother and the tendency to find my own identity through bossing my husband. In this conflict, I could see, after a while, that there was no filling of my real need, a genuine love relationship. I felt uneasy among women. In their company I felt different, slightly on edge all the time. I was far more comfortable with men who I thought could sense my troubles. I enjoyed the company of men as long as I felt they did not desire physical contact with me. Well, anyway, about the time I realized the meaning of my mother's thwarted life, I began to see the meaning of my own. She tried to live through me, possessing me. I naturally tended to lean on her. But, groping to find myself, I tried to control my husband's life. I saw that I could live tolerably well without my mother, but I grew very lonely, and at last I realized that I wanted desperately to be loved—not possessed, not to control. So after I stopped drinking, I developed a new attitude towards my husband.

When I did, I gave in to him on many issues. And he responded warmly to this change of heart. It isn't all it should be—not yet. But I've found the right approach, I'm sure of that. I think I'm beginning to learn what love means."

"Jane's story," observed Margaret, "shows that we women have to work on our problems often in a different emotional setting from that of men. I am reminded of some good practical clues I picked up in an article by Dr. Georgio Lolli. My therapist suggested I read it."

"What are they?"

"Well, as I recall the article, there are five main situations that bring on alcoholic drinking among women. The sudden loss of something important may do it. A man generally loses his job because of drinking, but a woman will drink because she has lost her job. If your husband is successful, and suddenly you find yourself in a new social climate, you become insecure and may resort to heavy drinking. If you are a career woman, faced with the fear of a childless life and no husband, you may grow depressed and turn to alcohol for relief. The threat of bodily ills, like cancer, or any of those operations on women, or perhaps the menopause may upset us enough to become addicted. Separation from our children may also depress us and induce us to drink. He says too, that we do not, as a rule, feel guilt or blame ourselves to the same extent that men do, in the hang-over. We are more inclined to make drink the cause of our misfortune and to minimize our personal blame."

"Never knew many men anxious to take their share of blame," said Lucille. "They're about as good at the alibi as any woman I know."

"My story is different in some ways from Jane's, and similar to it, as well," said Margaret. "Jane's father put her off— mine was a model of everything a man should be. Anyway, here's the gist of the problem I had with my husband, Ron. Ron's life, outside his family and friends, is competitive. I grew competitive too. I developed this attitude because I went to work, wanted more things for the house, and wanted to show Ron that I could help to keep our show going the way we wanted to. But after a while, something happened. I got good raises, and my salary was soon nearly as much as Ron's. Then *we* were competing, Ron and I. I began to think of my father, how much he had done for me, and how little Ron measured up to him. I was competing with my husband, I was losing hold of him as the man I loved. I was thinking and feeling like a man, one man in competition with another."

"I know the drift," said Lucille cynically. " 'A woman's place is in the home.' I can't swallow it, not all of it."

"I appreciate our freedom as much as you do, Lucille," said Margaret. "A woman, today, is freer than she ever was, and of course we don't want to lose what we've gained. But we need to be careful about this danger of competing. What's the good of being free, if there's no one to love? I mean, a woman is happiest as a partner, not as a competitor. Partners are not slaves, neither are they masters. A partner is someone who has what the other partner has not. They share."

"Men need to know that as much as we do—that sharing you speak of," said Lucille defensively.

"The most important thing to me," said Jane, "is to be loved, to be wanted, and to feel that I am needed, not tolerated or pampered. This is far more important to me now than the desire to compete with my husband, or other men."

"I'm not so sure about the straight feminine line," Lucille retorted. "I know you think I'm rather hard-boiled. Well, I'll tell you why. That attitude is a cover-up for an intense feeling of guilt and shame created by early teachings about sex. My parents were strict about morals. But my brothers got off light compared with the taboos and fears that were impressed upon me. Like Margaret, I thought my dad was just about perfect, a paragon of virtue, an example of what men should be. Mother was possessive, and rather resented my affection for dad. But that didn't keep him from showering me with favours and trying to satisfy my many whims. Anyway, to cut it short, I became disillusioned about men after I left home, because none of them could measure up to my father. That's how I see it now, though I didn't realize it at the time. Then I came to see, after some sessions with an analyst, that I sort of became my father; I gave up hope of filling my deepest feminine need. So, in many ways, I played the role of a man, competing as Margaret says, with my husband. I see that much of Margaret's view. What I can't take is something deeper than that."

"But," said Jane, "once you bring your deepest urge to the fore, and see that you want to be loved and wanted, you'll respond, I'm sure, as we all do, to our true nature. The don't-care attitude, the hard-boiled line, will disappear."

"It isn't that easy, Jane," replied Lucille. "I, like many others, display an I-don't-care attitude because I'm afraid of society, of other people. A long training has made me that way. It isn't just turned off like a tap. And anyway, that attitude does protect me to some extent. I suspect that nobody would be more tolerant or kind if I told them the truth about my feelings. It would only make me more vulnerable to jibes and curious enquiries. I have talked with girls who started drinking heavily after their affairs with men, worried about pregnancy or disease. They appeared completely relieved to learn they were neither pregnant or diseased. On the surface, such girls look hard-boiled, concerned only about the prospect of an unwanted child, or some sort of infection. When you see their fears vanish, and they go merrily on their way, you sort of think, well, they're just tough, hard-boiled. But probing deeper, you'll find a feeling of guilt underneath the shell, and a suspicion that they are dirty. This goes back to childhood, to fears instilled in them about being good and decent. So they're glad to turn to drink for comfort. Now we are not all subject to misgivings about sex relations. But women generally are more inhibited about sex, and more concerned about the proper way to behave, than men are. This makes it harder for us to respond to treatment than men alcoholics. Just think of the social stigma we have to watch for! So we tend to hide the sources of our trouble. With me, it takes the form of a hard-boiled attitude. It covers up that guilt and shame, from away back."

"But now listen," countered Jane. "We can get well along to recovery if we accept the fact that the perfect man is a myth, and we see our true role as women supporting our husbands, and giving them some evidence of it, like staying sober, and doing something about the condition of the house, let alone the children. Our greatest need is to be needed— not just for sex, but in every way that we can be partners as wives and mothers. To realize this is to see that there is no need for illicit sex relations, nor for competing prestige. Best of all, there will be no occasion for that dreadful guilt and anxiety which lead to the bottle."

"That's all very well," said Lucille, "and I see nothing wrong with it, if it works for you. But what if you find it hard, perhaps impossible, to make those changes? What if you find it just too much to be an ideal wife and mother? After all, I'm an alcoholic, and so are you. It isn't easy to make a quick turnabout."

"Yes. That's fair enough," said Margaret. "Jane and I may find the ideal of being a loving wife and mother more appealing than you do. Is that it?" Margaret was probing tactfully into Lucille's love problems.

"Exactly," agreed Lucille. "I'm no doll, no housekeeper. I have no children."

"Well, it isn't as easy as you think, for Margaret and me, to make the changes we agree on," said Jane. "It's just that we agree on what we have to do, if we want to stay sober."

"I don't think we should let personal differences separate us so much that we forget our common problem, alcoholism," said Margaret. "If Jane and I have something in our recovery plan, it should follow for you too, Lucille, only you express yourself in your own way, to suit your own particular case."

"I often hear the men say that their sobriety comes ahead

of everything else, even their wives and families," said Lucille wonderingly.

"It's the same for us, then. Whatever you find to do that best keeps you sober is the best thing to do for your husband, or for anyone else."

"Well, this is beginning to make better sense to me," Lucille conceded.

"Going to work was not good in my case," Margaret said. "It may be just what you need. Your husband is far easier going than mine. It will give you something to do, some purpose. You used to be a nurse. Why not try it again? Just think what you could do for other women alcoholics. You don't want to replace your husband's love and respect. But if a woman has no children, she sort of needs to find some."

"The way it works out, Lucille, you have about the same needs as we have, only you satisfy them a little differently."

"Well, you girls seem to want to put me to work. Isn't there some other way out for me?"

"That was just an example," said Margaret. "The main point is to develop some meaning for your life. You could do anything, for that matter, that interests you most."

"The men made a lot of 'creative effort' and 'love' in their discussions," Jane observed. "If it's important for them, it is more so for us. By nature, we are indispensable in the creation of life, and we do this through love."

"I have no children." Lucille appeared evasive.

"For heaven's sake, Lucille, that doesn't matter. So you have no children. But you're a woman, and you have all the instincts and tendencies we have." Margaret was again searching. She was not sure about Lucille.

"The day soon comes, anyway, when your children go. You can't hang on to them forever," Jane said stoically.

"But you still love them," said Margaret. "They're yours, and you'd do anything in the world for them, even when they're on their own."

"So, if I find a substitute for children in persons I can help,

I shouldn't try to be possessive, but encourage them to grow in their own right." Lucille was trying hard to find a clue.

"Now we're coming together on this," said Jane. "Love is more than sex, as the men kept saying. It is an activity that means a growing respect for others as for ourselves. We are women, and the art of love really comes to us more naturally than it does to men. The poor souls! They did such a lot of talking about what we know by instinct."

"If you give in a little more, Lucille, to what you really are, you will not find this so hard to understand." Margaret was kind.

"Yes, but you must admit that what I said about childhood fears and taboos complicates our life." Lucille could not let her defences go.

"Of course it does," agreed Jane, "and it makes us think and feel too much like men. Fear ridden and suspicious—it takes us some time to adjust to our real role as women. With too much to fear, we set out to control situations around us, just as men do in the struggle to live. But it is more or less natural to men, their lives are necessarily struggle and gain in order to keep alive. Even the men have to see beyond struggle and mastery to what they call fellowship, if they expect to stay sober."

"What then," asked Lucille, "for goodness sake, makes it harder for women alcoholics than for men if we come more naturally by creative and loving efforts?"

"The answer to that is in your own story," Margaret replied. "A woman alcoholic has more to unravel than a man, and a rougher time with social attitudes."

"A man's growing up, what they called 'becoming a person', is a growth that moves step by step from lower to higher," observed Jane. "He is a child before he is a boy, a boy before he is a master, a master before he is a person who can be free, who can create, who can love. That seems to be the way their discussions developed. But a woman? She has mature instincts at sixteen or thereabouts. And all along the way, she is taught to be afraid of everything that her natural urges impel her to do. She is instilled with the same caution, the same need to control the outer world, as her brother."

"Are you saying a young girl should let go, just when she feels it? That's radical, to say the least."

"No, Lucille, I'm not saying that," Jane replied. "I'm no expert. I don't know what changes should be made in youth education. Here we are, three women alcoholics. We're just trying to understand how we became what we are."

"I think a lot can be done to improve the training of our children for the problems ahead of them," said Margaret. "And it looks as though some improvements are being made. But, as Jane says, we are alcoholics. The fact is that we failed to make the difficult and abrupt adjustments that the majority of women managed to make better than we did, at least so far as drinking is concerned."

"Well, anyway," added Jane, "we sort of developed a masculine psychology, responding to control and wanting to control, like men have to do sometime in their lives. Maybe the father image has something to do with it, too. Both of you seem to think so. I'm not as well read as you are, on Freud and Jung and the others. All I know is that a girl has more to 'unravel', as Margaret says, than a man. We have to learn to become women all over again, and into the bargain there is all the criticism a woman is likely to get, that a man usually escapes. A woman is taught and conditioned to be more sensitive to social prejudice than men are. So that, for me, is enough to explain why the way to recovery is harder for us than for men."

"It's too bad that more women won't go to A.A.," observed Lucille.

"Especially in small communities," added Margaret.

"You have the reason," said Jane. "In big cities, she is less afraid of gossip, more at home with other women whom she meets there. In the small district, she hesitates because of social opinion and the fact that so few women will be there."

"But if only that fear could be broken down," said Lucille

earnestly, "getting rid of social concern would be a substantial part of her treatment, it would be the best way to strengthen her native feminine traits."

"After all, everyone we know is aware that we have a drinking problem," said Margaret.

"That's the insane part of it all," said Jane. "Women know this, and yet they hesitate to go to A.A. because it might be known! The stupidity of this attitude can only be explained by the stupidity of our social fear."

"Of course that applies to men alcoholics, too," Margaret added.

"And something more," said Lucille. "The resistance to A.A. is just the awful difficulty of admitting 'I am an alcoholic'."

"Well!" observed Jane, "you seem to be solving your own problem pretty well, Lucille."

"I suspected the right solution all along," Lucille confessed, "but I like to keep probing. I'm afraid of easy solutions. The real clue is in A.A.'s 12th step. There I can have children, watch them grow, and see them strike out on their own. And I find that fellowship there too that the men were talking about."

"That sure is no pat answer. There's a lot of effort there," said Margaret.

"Yes, I know," said Lucille pensively. "I resisted both of your solutions. It all seemed a little too clear, too straightforward. You see, women are not simply women, and men not simply men, with differences that completely separate us. We have within us, as the men said, the urge to be persons. Men, if they are nothing more, are fighters, destroyers. Women, if they are nothing more, are child bearers and house servants. This isn't good enough. As persons, men can be tender and yet manly in the best sense of the word, and as persons, women can be resolute, expressive, and yet be feminine. In the qualities we tend to share, men and women can cultivate one another in fellowship. This does not mean that men will surrender their manliness, nor women their feminine nature. Somehow we need to come together more often, to know ourselves better and to explore the meaning of our lives."

"You have a deeper view than I first suspected, Lucille," said Margaret.

"Thank you, but I have that eternal misgiving."

"What can that be?"

"To put into practice, with all the faith it needs, the ideas I've just expressed."

"When you marry young, you and your husband are both struggling to get ahead in the world—he in the business world and you as wife, mother and a useful person in the community." The other girls could see that Margaret was off on one of her real excursions. "As the years pass, he becomes more successful in business—his field of operations, so to speak, broaden, become more interesting and challenging. He faces these challenges, meets them successfully, and goes on to fresh horizons. You, as a wife and mother, also meet your challenges, do a good job raising your children, meet your ever increasing social and community activities with pleasure and success, and are considered an excellent mother, housekeeper, and hostess *but* there is the feeling it is not enough! There are not enough challenges, no far horizons to conquer, no great future unrolling before you. Then you begin to feel frustrated, to feel, well, where do I go from here? Then a feeling of resentment grows, *not* against your husband and his success, but against the fact that you are a woman and your field of endeavour seems so limited! It is all very well to say, 'Go out and do things to help other people.' It is quite possible you have been doing that all your life, it's part of your very nature to do things for others. You just couldn't live without doing them. Well, then, where do you turn this driving force instead of getting so frustrated and tense that finally you resort to drinking.

"Don't forget, too, that this has to be something that

comes from deep inside, so that the feeling of growing and broadening and 'near horizons' can be yours as well as your husband's."

"What is it you are seeking? It isn't success, you *are* a success, at least in the broad meaning of the word. It is, I think, to learn, somehow, to be satisfied with yourself, as you really are, and not try to be six different people with all their successes, but just yourself. In other words, don't strive so hard for the 'far horizon', but just enjoy the one you can really see."

The Sobriety Programme

Before we begin our study of the creative sobriety programme, it is important that we notice a distinct change in the order of our approach to life as sober persons.

When we drank, our pleasure came first, misery and pain followed. Now, in sobriety, we have a few difficulties at the start, and work towards pleasure as our reward.

Addiction is a process of illusory freedom and fun gradually growing into a pattern of pain and imprisonment. Sobriety, on the other hand, is an act of discipline and learning which leads to progressive improvement, day by day. We are eventually rewarded by an enjoyable and pleasurable life. The time it takes to reach relaxed and enjoyable sobriety depends on how deeply we want it. If we set out on our new programme grudgingly, half-heartedly, it will be difficult, long and drawn out, and possibly a failure. If we embark on it with all our effort and desire, it can be easy and adventurous.

I suggest that a simple and clear way to regard the whole problem is to say to yourself "I want sobriety for the same reason that I drank in the first place." This is the same as saying "I want the same care-free, easy going experience in sobriety that I got out of drinking at its best."

But now we note, from our long, expensive experience as

problem drinkers, that an *intelligent* pursuit of pleasure is very different from a haphazard approach to it. To be easy and care-free without damaging our health and without hurting others is a far more intelligent action than getting drunk, and a far more effective way to be happy. We learn that we cannot be really happy by chance. We cannot be happy unless we are *free* to be happy.

So the difference between pleasure in drinking and pleasure in sobriety is the difference between chance which leads to addiction and action which is disciplined. Thus our programme of sobriety will be a programme of *disciplined* pleasure. In disciplined pleasure, there is initial adjustment to a programme with an intelligent plan and a rewarding goal. At the very beginning, therefore, we must expect to initiate practices and attitudes and to remove obstacles to the interesting programme ahead. In the discipline of pleasure, we learn how to be free. And, of course, the whole object of our recovery is to learn how to be contentedly free of alcohol.

Initial Sobriety

Regains physical health, restores memory and mental functions.
Practice of self-honesty.
Pre-occupied with sobriety.
Growing open-minded.
Removal of needless guilt.
Freely discusses alcohol and its problems.
Mild depression, anxiety disappears, mental functions more alert.

Learning Sobriety

Loss of freedom acknowledged, and accepted.
Alibis replaced by sound reasons for sobriety.
Social pressures disappear, threats replaced by encouragement.

Grandiose behaviour replaced by give and take of real personal relations.
Aggressive behaviour replaced by willingness to learn.
Persistent remorse disappears, peace initiated.
Abstinence graduates into sobriety.
Change of pattern of thinking.
Regains friends.
Job improves.
Sobriety-centred behaviour.
Regains outside interests.
Acceptance of friends.
Sense of humour replaces self-pity.
Acceptance of environment.
Regains family faith.
Acceptance of the personal qualities of others, replaces resentment of them.
Protection of family interests.
Proper nutrition.
Learning to cope with mild "dips", depressed or anxious states.
Improvement of sex relations.
Better understanding of wife.
Learning to enjoy a good breakfast.

Accepting Sobriety

Loss of desire to drink becomes lasting.
Improved ethical perception.
Improved thinking.
Improved feeling.
Keeps company with persons one can respect or help.
"Dips" become few and far between, easy to manage.

Creative Sobriety

Loss of desire to drink becomes permanent.
Fear, anxieties, depressions are understood and overcome in interpersonal relations.
Appreciates deeply freedom from alcohol.
Explores new freedom to use it in other activities without fear.
Single-minded sobriety—defines assurance there is no compromise with sobriety.
Genuine religious desires centred on new way of life.

Alibi system replaced by deepening quality of intelligent
  sobriety.
Appreciates need for help, both for sobriety and as a guard
  against drinking in daily effort.

Pleasurable Sobriety

Self-unity, at peace with oneself.
Socializes easily, at one with the world.
No hang-overs.
Rewards clearly exceed tough times.
Feels well, enjoys sobriety.
Anxiety, shyness, etc., disappear in genuine interpersonal
  relations.

There are seven steps in *Initial Sobriety*, the first phase of
the creative recovery programme. These are:

1. For step one you have the advice of the medical doctors
and nursing staff regarding protein, vitamin and mineral supplement, proper diet, relaxation and exercise. A great deal
of any disturbance you've had in memory functions and
body stresses will be removed by the scientific counsel
designed to restore to you optimum physical health.

2. It is often difficult to think and feel clearly about yourself in the practice of self-honesty until you have worked
well on step one. When the body functions well, the mind
will clear. After all, our mental and emotional functions
cannot probe to the depths of self-honesty if we are tired,
irritable, poorly nourished, and restless. Self-honesty will
largely mean the scrutiny of old alibis, in the effort to remove them. This is not done all at once. It requires practice
—the putting of thought in between impulse and action.

3. Just as drinking was deep in the centre of our thoughts
and desires when we were practising problem drinkers, so
now, we must deliberately put sobriety in the centre of our
life in the recovery programme. By sobriety, we mean
simply the all-consuming desire for the richness and abundance of life. (Please do not confuse sobriety with fear of
drinking.)

4. Growing open-minded covers a limitless area. At first, we can settle for this objective; learning to accept fellow alcoholics without disgust or resentment. In this way, we learn to accept ourselves.

5. We remove needless guilt when we learn not to be ashamed of the fact that we have undergone a sickness.

6. It is healthy to discuss alcohol and its problems as freely as we might discuss polio, cancer or heart trouble.

7. Physical and mental functions are knit together. As we grow healthier in sobriety, we can be certain that our depressed or anxious states will pass and be less severe. The more we learn about ourselves, the less will emotional "jackpots" disturb us. This faith must sustain us in the initial sobriety.

There are twenty-three steps in *Learning Sobriety*, the second phase of the creative recovery programme.

1. Loss of freedom acknowledged, and accepted. All the knowledge in the world about alcoholism will not necessarily equip us for sobriety. Knowledge can be very helpful. We believe in it in our clinical work. But, without the deep feelingful admission that we have lost all control over the use of alcohol and addicting drugs, we cannot learn sobriety. This admission it is well to accept whole-heartedly.

2. Every time we are tempted to invent an alibi for drinking it is well to try to match it with a reason to stay sober.

3. You are encouraged to improve the skills of sobriety as you notice the lessening of social pressures formerly due to your drinking. Fear of the law, of business associates, of disapproval of family and friends will disappear as your sobriety grows longer and sounder.

4. Grandiose behaviour is like a balloon. Sooner or later it collapses. We were often the victims of such behaviour in our drinking days. As we check our actions with friends and associates, our behaviour begins to show the rewarding effects of realness and truth. These effects can only emerge in

the give-and-take of honest communication of our problems and plans with people we learn to trust and respect.

5. Aggressive behaviour easily becomes an obsession to have it all your own way. Allowing others to assert their opinion, and respecting them, is the only way we can ever learn anything about personal problems. To learn is to grow, and to grow is to become yourself. Having things our own way is the surest road to isolation and fixation. It is strange, but true, that the best guarantee I have of being myself is to let you help me.

6. The rewards of sobriety become clear as we lose that former persistent cloud of remorse. For the first time in years we begin to enjoy a quiet feeling simply known as peace. It is not spectacular or exciting, but it is very worthwhile— just to be at peace with yourself.

7. Abstinence graduates into sobriety as we learn not to fear alcohol, not to be ashamed of our problem, and as we come to see that sobriety is not penalizing, but rewarding. There is something to learn anew, something to *gain* in the sober life. Easter is a clue to the truth that our greatest burden can be borne lightly within sight of new free life tomorrow.

8. We learn to change the pattern of our thinking. This consists in dwelling on the present and future, and discarding regrets about what "might have been". The past is valuable for its lessons, but it is the present and future which bring new life and new hope.

9. We gradually regain our old friends on a new sound basis which restores our self-respect and brings pleasure in genuine fellowship.

10. Our job improves with our new thinking, a pattern of thinking devoid of fear and strengthened by easy communication with our friends and associates.

11. Our behaviour grows sobriety-centred. In the care of every act we perform there is our growing awareness that

sobriety is the necessary condition of business, pleasure, love and faith.

12. We deliberately cultivate favourite interests, long forgotten or neglected, interests of a personal sort other than our business or vocation.

13. After regaining our friends, it is important to learn how to *accept them*, without criticism and without feeling easily hurt by tendencies of theirs which are simply different from our own.

14. It is deeply valuable to cultivate a sense of humour to replace any of the old tendency to self pity. A sense of humour is the achievement of wise people—especially the ability to accept yourself and to laugh at yourself.

15. We gradually extend the acceptance of ourselves and of our friends to the acceptance of the whole environment in which we live. Here a good slogan is "Live and let live".

16. Deliberately, we restore to ourselves the faith of our family. We repair the weakened confidence they had in us by daily evidence of increasing trust in one another. There is no longer anything to hide.

17. We have learnt to regain and accept our friends. Now we extend this attitude to *all* our associates, replacing our resentment of anything foreign or threatening by accepting the personal qualities of others in the same way we accept the weather.

18. Formerly in addiction we grew obsessed by "protection of our supply". Now this emotional energy is transferred to protection of our family interests. The family now becomes our primary concern.

19. We are learning to discipline ourselves in the use of a well balanced diet. Proper nutrition is the basis of healthy sobriety.

20. Proper nutrition and plenty of rest enable us to cope with mild "dips", depressed or anxious states. We are learning the lessons of endurance, and patience, knowing that "dips" grow less serious and shorter, as our sobriety lengthens.

21. Sex relations are known to improve notably, as sobriety becomes stronger. We come to regard sex as a factor in richer and more mature love relationship with one's partner.

22. With a sounder attitude towards wife or husband, we gain a better understanding of our partner, based on a sharing philosophy, not on a possessive one.

23. "Learning to enjoy a good breakfast" illustrates improvement in total personal growth. It shows that we have rested well, can take the time to relax and enjoy the first most important food of the day. It also sets the mood for a day of good humour, and gives pause for gratitude.

In *Accepting Sobriety*, there is a total of six steps. Here they are:

1. You know you are well launched into acceptance of your sobriety when loss of desire to drink extends from day to day, week to week, month to month. Loss of desire to drink begins to be known when our need to drink disappears. But we have to be vigilant in the practice of learning sobriety to be sure we no longer need to drink.

2. Improved ethical perception will be noticed when you find yourself growing more sensitive to fair play, the welfare of others, and better performance of your own duties and activities. Accepting sobriety includes the awareness of our notorious tendency to be sensitive—but now we accept this sensitivity, determined to make it positive, and not negative (as, for example, in the old form of getting hurt).

3. We know we are accepting sobriety as our thinking grows more clear, more considerate of all those with whom we associate.

4. Also, even more important than thinking, our feelings are sounder. Replacing the old wishful thinking—a kind of thinking based on alibis—we now base our thinking on feelings shared with others, also seeking or favouring sobriety.

5. Our sobriety grows more acceptable as we find ourselves seeking the company of persons we can respect, help,

and from whom, in turn, we regain the self-respect and enjoyment we so much need.

6. The early "dips" following initial sobriety lessen in frequency and duration. At first, these were something of a problem—we were depressed, or anxious, or even elated. They once might have been the cause of a relapse. Now, however, we have learnt that they pass, they cannot last. Maturely, we learn to accept them, as we come to appreciate the great value of endurance. After all, *every* human being has to endure the occasional discomfort or tension, even tragedy. There are times in the lives of all of us when there is no way out of despair or grief. It is to be endured. Certainly alcohol or drugs will be of no avail. We accept our sobriety when we hear "the still, sad music of humanity" as well as the richness and variety of life in all its joy, seeing both for what they are, deeply and clearly.

In *Creative Sobriety*, there are eight experiences that we should strive to feel and know. These are:

1. Loss of desire to drink becomes permanent. We should realize that this admirable state of feeling has to be practised and worked over daily. Freedom doesn't keep.

2. Our old fears and depressed states are more and more overcome in the strengthening and practice of our interpersonal relations.

3. We really come to appreciate our freedom from alcohol, as contrasted with the resentment of our early abstinence.

4. We begin to extend our new freedom positively in other areas than our main problem, and this we do without fear.

5. We develop a strong single-minded sobriety in the sense that there can be no compromise at all with drinking.

6. The vague fearful religious needs of late state addiction are replaced by genuine religious desires which together centre on our new way of life, a life of freedom—free from alcohol, free from fear, and free to love and enjoy life.

7. There is intelligent effort to clear away all traces of the old alibi structure. This is replaced by deeper and stronger reasons for our new way of life as exemplified in attitudes at work, at home, and among our friends.

8. We are constantly aware of the need to help and be helped. This need we recognize both in the interests of our sobriety and as a guard against drinking.

The rewards of sober living we can classify in six main experiences.

1. We achieve self-unity, and in this unity we find peace. Self-unity means that the old fearful conflict is gone—the conflict between the urge to drink and the urge to abstain. The conflict disappears as we succeed in bringing our purposes into harmony with our impulses. Loss of the desire to drink replaces the old urge to indulge, and a genuine desire for sobriety grows strong from those impulses which no longer serve the urge to drink. In our self-unity we therefore bring our impulses and feelings into the service of an enduring love of sobriety.

2. We mix more easily with others now. With our new confidence and peace, and freedom from fear, we find ourselves able to get along much better with our fellow-man. This ability, in turn, strengthens our self-unity, and deepens our sense of peace.

3. There are no hang-overs. This in itself is a prize reward of sobriety. There may indeed be a few ups and downs. But these we learn to manage, to accept, and to modify, because we have learned to discipline our feelings.

4. We have the evidence, at last, that the rewards of sober living exceed our frustrations and tough periods. This evidence comes in many forms in daily life—in business, at home, and among our friends.

5. We come to see sobriety as an experience of value for its own sake. We see it now as a way of life. Without thinking of any rewards at all, sobriety is good because we feel well, and enjoy feeling well.

6. If, however, we must think in terms of the "pay-off" of sobriety, we have only to give evidence to the fact that our anxiety, shyness and all other forms of fear have disappeared. If they have not completely disappeared, we know that we can cope with them now in the faith and practice of interpersonal relations—finding ourselves through others.

6.

THE PRACTICE OF FREEDOM

THE more complex the man, the more complex his practice of freedom in acts of sobriety. It is well to come to the truth in the open-minded manner of children. But many of us have grown over-defensive, more concerned with protection than growth in finding our way through life.

Here we meet two new characters, Buxton and Ward, who illustrate that sincere new insight is often hard to achieve, even after a long sober period. There are not only the techniques of a sober programme to learn and to put into action; there is also the deepening of a whole new way of life.

The sobriety programme of action is a reliable guide, with its five phases of fifty steps. But we shall see that the ability to follow it is found in the way each man deepens his personal desire for sobriety. In this act, he practises his freedom. And this he will do all his life. He keeps his freedom, and gains more, by learning to use creatively the same feelings which, not understood, can lead him again to drink!

Buxton is a man who, in previous sessions, had shown much trouble in accepting the trend of the discussion. Suddenly, he gave himself to the theme, as in these opening remarks.

"First of all we want sobriety. But there is something more. Sobriety is what makes everything possible that we value most. Sobriety is life. How is that? Sobriety is life. Yes! Without it, we are headed for death. As drinking men we are afraid of life, so we seek slow death in drink. Fear has to be conquered, so we need help. We need our fellow alcoholics to give us the courage to be ourselves, to get honest with ourselves and then, only then, are we really free. Now, then, where do we go? Oh, yes, we see personal freedom as the goal of sobriety, freedom not only from drink, but freedom to do ever so many things that our old slavery kept us from doing."

"You're doing pretty well, Buxton. Is that the end?" asked Arthurs.

"No. I can only be free because other people make it possible. I am free because of you and the others here. So are you. This is personal. But it is religious too."

"Why?" probed Arthurs.

"Because this freedom we give one another is what keeps us sober. Without sobriety we are lost. With it, and only with it, can we hope to make the best of ourselves. Anything so important and all-embracing must be religious."

"Umm. Sobriety, personal freedom, fellowship. God. Is that the sequence?" Arthurs looked doubtful.

"The sobriety programme is all one piece," said Buxton. "One phase involves the other. I see now that the personal life is the religious life. God is both inside and beyond. I can only know Him as I experience Him. Yet, He is beyond me because I need you to have that experience. And I think it must be the same for you. I somehow can't believe that you or someone else has a special access to God not possible to me. He is beyond you as He is beyond me. Yet He is available to us both if we help one another, if we recognize our mutual limitations and encourage each other to make the most of himself and to be himself."

"Come now, Buxton, old sock, haven't you made a real quick turnabout? Now mind you, I follow, all right, but . . . but it's a little too neat. It's what I'd expect to read in a slick know-how book. Coming from you, after all your doubts, it's a shocker, isn't it?"

"Y-e-s. You're right, Arthurs. It is too neat, I'm afraid, but

I think I see. The outline is clear in my thinking. How far this takes hold in living remains to be seen."

"Take hold in living?" queried Ward. "What about the problem of being what we are? How, I ask, can we *really* change, how can we be other persons? Even when I create and grow, I remain what I am, don't I? For example, you say the alcoholic is inclined to be impulsive. When he is trying to be sober, what will replace his impulsive urge to drink? What can he turn to, if he is naturally impulsive, drunk or sober? How can I be sure I shan't turn to drink, but to something less harmful, when I *know*, if your analysis is sound, that I am impulsive by nature and likely to do what I shouldn't do? How can I be reasonable and impulsive at the same time? Surely I have to be one or the other. Buxton's turnabout, as Arthurs said, is rather too neat."

"This is deeply important," observed the therapist. "Your idea that we have to become other persons—and this is impossible, except in sickness—follows an historic error in all our thinking about human problems. It is a sort of double rut."

"Well, I have a point then. All of us have to proceed in our thinking as we've been taught."

"I think your argument is very challenging, Ward. If there is no error, no double rut, as I call it, in our past habits of dealing with problems, your questions are difficult, perhaps impossible, to answer satisfactorily."

"How did this error get started, and what accounts for its persistence?"

"It started in the interests of natural science. Researchers found they could make great progress in their control over nature if they kept human feeling out of their calculations."

"I remember once a friend of mine dropped a pint of whiskey on the pavement," said Arthurs. "As he watched it trickle away, he turned to me and said, 'You can't beat the law of gravity.' To this I replied with real unscientific feeling, 'No, but it's a damn shame, and a hell of a waste'."

"Well, the method of natural science is to keep feelings like yours out of the picture, Arthurs."

"It works, does it not?" asked Ward. "Now who would be so absurd as to say that science has not brought us real progress and power?"

"Surely no one. Science has given us control over nature, and has increased our power over everything but ourselves."

"What about medicine? Just think of penicillin, and now the polio vaccine."

"All right, Ward. But what about alcoholism?"

"Perhaps one day we shall have the drug that will put an end to alcoholism."

"Will you, then, become another person? You said, or inferred, that one could not be two persons at one time, excluding the disorder known as schizophrenia. Even in schizophrenia, one does not readily become two persons, as we have developed the meaning of person, but rather simply a very confused human being."

"What do you mean by the failure of science?" asked Ward.

"Science does not fail in its proper area. It just fails when it tries to do too much. This problem can be traced to the error of trying to apply the methods of natural science to personal problems."

"Ah, yes," nodded Arthurs. "The law of gravity does damn little about my sorrow over the loss of a pint of whiskey. That's clear."

"You have to keep your human feelings out of a problem that by its very nature is personal through and through, if you are scientific about it."

"What has this got to do with my question about being impulsive?" asked Ward.

"Just this. Many people tend to assume that reason and impulse are two forces in conflict. That is what your questions implied, Ward, and you put those questions just as many intelligent people would put them who have been trained to believe that scientific thinking is the only correct kind of thinking."

"Well, aren't reason and impulse separate and distinct?"

"In scientific work, it is often convenient to proceed as though they were. But in dealing with personal problems, I think it is a great error to do so."

"Will you please go into that?" requested Arthurs. "I want to tie in this verbal deal, if I can, with that lost pint of whiskey."

"We should not suppose that becoming more reasonable will make us less impulsive, or less emotional. If I become more reasonable, in the sense that I act or do something, I must at the same time become more impulsive. If my reasonableness carried me into activity, even productive thinking, for it is an activity, I am *moved* surely to do so, and the more I reason, the more I am moved, or impelled to do so. So, you see, I do not grow less impulsive as I grow more reasonable."

"All this sounds tricky to me. What are we missing?" asked Ward. "If this is going to make sense, you'll have to strengthen your argument."

"I don't wonder that you say that. There are three hundred years of thinking to challenge. Tradition is not easily changed."

"Take it the other way for a while," suggested Arthurs. "Do we become less reasonable as we grow more impulsive? Ward thinks we do."

"In any practical sense of the term reasonable, I enrich it as I show drive, sincerity, spontaneity. I enrich it, I don't impoverish it. The confusion about reason—impulse arises from the neglect of personal growth, an act that cannot be mechanically broken up into two abstractions, opposed to one another."

"Come, now. Surely there is a commonsense meaning which makes it intelligent to say that one man is impulsive, contrasted with another who is reasonable."

"Of course. Only I think we need to be careful about what we mean, when it concerns the important problem of sobriety."

"What's the difference between the impulsive guy and the reasonable one?" asked Arthurs.

"The man commonly called impulsive is a man without clear goals. He dissipates his life, because he is less free, less creative, even less able to love than the reasonable man. The reasonable man conserves and enriches himself, and may even generate fresh impulses for new actions. I should insist that it is a mistake to contrast these two types by the labels 'impulsive' and 'reasonable' if you mean that the reasonable man is not rich in impulsive resources."

"Yes, but what about the impulsive guy?"

"I was waiting for that, Arthurs. You cannot say that an impulsive man is as reasonable as the reasonable man is impulsive because of that act—personal growth—which is so much neglected in our thinking about these problems. The impulsive man grows, he creates, he learns to love. And these he does by learning what it is to be free. In this creative process, he becomes more reasonable, in the practical sense of the word. Perhaps 'more wise' would be a better way of putting it."

'To go back to my question," said Ward. "You suggest that if I believe in growth, I shall see how it is possible for an alcoholic to become reasonable and yet retain his identity as being impulsive."

"Yes, and what goes with that is most important. You need to have faith in personal growth and this is to believe that you can change yourself, though you remain the same person."

"More or less biological, isn't it?" asked Ward.

"Organic growth is, but not personal growing. Personal growth implies action and freedom. These are not part of science."

"Why aren't they?"

"Because science studies *reaction*. Anything which acts,

a person, for example, is free. And science seeks to determine, not to liberate. When he excludes his own human feelings from his study of persons, the scientist fails to enlighten us on the actions which bring sobriety to an alcoholic. But it would be unfair to project blame onto science for something it cannot do. In my talk today I want to describe resistance in its three main currents of human feeling; these we are wise to accept, though we shall want to change or modify them. But we cannot ignore them. In their healthy form, they are downright human, and pave the way to personal life. If we just observed them, and did not admit we felt them, we would regard them as only reactions. We have to admit we feel them in order to know them, and to make them become actions with a goal. If it is possible to change a reaction to an action, then it is exciting to know we can make use of obstacles."

Making Use of Resistance

Resistance is to be found not only in the physical factors of addiction, but also in the stubborn persistent traces of pleasurable sensation lodged deep in the memory and in the dark recesses of your feelings.

Resistance to recovery, to influences of a beneficial nature —in the treatment of alcoholism and of addictions in general, not to mention many other disorders—is a common and persistent challenge to all therapists and patients who experience it. Resistance is by far the biggest problem in the treatment of addictions. What is most elusive and difficult about resistance is that it is largely unconscious or unintentional. Most therapists and patients mean well. It is the unknown or uncontrolled forces in people which put obstacles in a well meant path to their goals.

RESISTANCE INDEX

Personal Thirst—to feel better, to get on better with others, to sense adventure.

The Pleasure Principle—to dominate, to be taken care of, to gain release and fun in drinking. The human will prevails.

The Tenderness Taboo—a social clamp on give and take of personal affection.

First Phase of Resistances

A. Projection of Blame $\begin{cases} \text{dependent} \\ \text{sensitive} \end{cases}$

B. Over-idealization $\begin{cases} \text{idealistic} \\ \text{impulsive} \end{cases}$

C. Fear of the Foreign $\begin{cases} \text{intolerant} \\ \text{wishful thinking} \end{cases}$

Personal Thirst plus *Pleasure Principle* plus *Tenderness Taboo* plus *Resistances A, B, C.*
↓
Transitional Imitation (Drinking begins)
↓
Conscious Imitation (Drinking becomes a problem)
↓
Imposed Imitation (Loss of freedom, addiction)
↓
Later Phases of the Resistances

A. Projection of Blame $\begin{cases} \text{childish—anxious} \\ \text{persecuted—paranoid} \end{cases}$

B. Over-idealization $\begin{cases}\text{grandiose—elated}\\\text{compulsive—obsessive}\end{cases}$

C. Fear of the Foreign $\begin{cases}\text{hostile—depressed}\\\text{fantastic thinking—}\\\qquad\text{defective thinking}\end{cases}$

(Various physical disorders often accompany the later phases of the resistances.)

EMPATHY INDEX

Personal Thirst—understood, accepted and cultivated.

The Freedom Principle—to be free, to be creative, and to sense adventure in love. The goodwill prevails.

The Tenderness Taboo, and *Resistances A, B, C* understood. Accepting oneself as discovered in the Resistance Index, in discussion, and by reflection in others.

Genuine Resistance—after resistances A, B, C and the tenderness taboo are understood to be fights against the self, genuine resistance is experienced in *respect* for both alcoholism and sobriety.

Personal Thirst plus *understanding of tenderness taboo and of resistances A, B, C* plus *genuine resistance.*
↓
Transitional Imitation (Spontaneous putting of oneself in the place of recovered alcoholics)
↓
Conscious Imitation (Goals and disciplines of recovered alcoholics studied and practised. Genuine resistance to alcoholism sustained throughout life.)
↓

Free Imitation (The life of sobriety becomes attractive in free imitation of what he admires most in recovered alcoholics)

↓

Becoming oneself—quenching personal thirst—in one's own way in the practice of empathy. Genuine resistance to sobriety becomes devotion to sobriety. Acceptance of principle "It is better to be free than pleased."

↓

The Personal Ideals (Chapter 3)

↓

Follow-up in A.A., out-patient clinics, and in friendships—gradual growth, extending personal ideals into all areas of one's life. The gifts of adventure. Freedom in fellowship.

The resistance index is a clue to the problem drinking pattern. The potential problem drinker begins with personal thirst and the pleasure principle which early governs it. Please note that the pleasure principle reveals three outlets —the urge to dominate, to be taken care of, and to seek release and fun. The conflict between the first and second produces the third in initial drinking, after the tenderness taboo has done its job. He then experiences the first phase of the unconscious resistances, illustrated in the "drinking" tendencies which correspond to them. They are, of course, unconscious resistances because the prospective drinker does not yet realize that his fight against freedom, years later, will be traced to them. If he is aware of them at all, he but dimly recognizes that they are self-defences, protection against the threats of a difficult world.

Personal thirst, the pleasure principle, the tenderness taboo and the three unconscious resistances in their early phase together lead to *transitional imitation* when he tries drinking because others seem to enjoy it. This trial is haphazard, experimental and adventurous. The next stage is *conscious imitation.* He finds the attractions to which many people are drawn—money, power and sex—less than sufficient for his personal needs. He seeks the added zest of intoxication, consciously and deliberately. He discovers value in drinking, and grows more and more dependent on it for solution of his problems and for his deepest enjoyments. He begins to *need* alcohol.

The problem drinker settles into a need for alcohol with occasional ability to make choices. But at last, in addiction, he experiences *loss of freedom.* While he may seem able, very often, to "take a few" and quit, he is never sure when he will drink more than he originally intended. The deepening of unconscious resistance makes control virtually impossible when the corresponding drinking tendencies overpower his conscious decision not to get drunk.

Well into addiction, the drinker will continue drinking, after he has started, for very sound physiological reasons, and then he clearly demonstrates loss of freedom due to chemical needs of the body.

But we want also to stress the experiences of loss of freedom in the problem drinker *even before he takes a drink,* often if he has been dry for some time. No feeling in human behaviour is born immaculately. Every experience we have comes partly from an experience preceding it. Thus there are important feelings, prior to the actual evidence of loss of control in problem drinking, that contribute to what we understand when we say we have lost control over drinking. It is these feelings we should know in order to accept and then modify them where we can, if our sobriety is to last. Simply to stop drinking is not to cope with the unconscious feelings which may well lead to drinking again.

Loss of freedom soon reveals a pattern of *imposed imitation.* By this is meant the repeating of behaviour imposed upon the drinker by his deepening unconscious feelings (resistances). *Addiction* is one type of imposed imitation. Situations around the drinker, and the deep resistances within him, trigger off excessive drinking. These situations and feelings he learns to rationalize, to make appear reasonable, to himself as well as to others, as *alibis* for drinking. He does not know the meaning of those situations and feelings, but he is urged to give them the semblance of sense and reason. In this process the feelings that we have called resistances A, B and C are more and more deepened, and more vividly illustrate loss of freedom. The resistances run deeper, evidenced in the worsening of the drinking tendencies, as shown on the index.

Alcoholics are not always aware of what makes them fabricate their alibis for drinking. Far from it. Actually, most problem drinkers appear to be completely unaware of the resistances to sobriety illustrated in the "drinking" tendencies—the traits from which the alibis arise. If problem drinkers *were* aware of these resistances, their problem would be simply an exercise in elementary logic. They would have only to learn that they should not drink, and that fact would bring the problem to an end. It is because resistance is chiefly unconscious that makes addiction a problem deeper than their intelligence can handle.

Of course, problem drinkers can count on a great reduction of their trouble from the day they stop drinking, and that is a substantial practical gain. But we must go further, if sobriety is to last. We must try *deliberately* to identify ourselves with the resistance-experience, each in his own way, if we are to reduce the real obstacles to creative sobriety. The three resistances though deeply lodged and often unconscious can be made familiar to us all, with a little study.

The Shifting of Blame

A repression shared by oneself and others is projected outside oneself. The potential problem drinker unconsciously projects his undesirable traits onto others. Without knowing it, he locates the source of his difficulties and aversions in others. In self defence, he blames others for trouble whose source is in himself. For example, he attributes *his* inability to break the "tenderness taboo" to the failure of others to appreciate and love him. There is a part-truth here, because people other than potential problem drinkers suffer from the effects of the tenderness taboo, and find it as difficult as he does to break through it. But for many people the human goals of aggression seem to replace their need for affection, and for still others the need for tenderness does not appear to be as urgent as it is for those who easily become alcoholic.

The feelings repressed by the tenderness taboo show up in drinking situations in sentiment and romance. The effort to break the tenderness taboo is a leading causal condition of alcoholism.

Such a resistance is, therefore, also a fight against sobriety, until the drinker can be convinced he is capable of giving and receiving affection without fear, and without the support of alcohol. Resistance to sobriety caused by the tenderness taboo is shown in the drinking tendencies, "dependent and sensitive". In these tendencies we detect the self-defensive resistance—projection of blame. The drinker, even before drinking becomes a problem, is more dependent on repressed needs for affection than he realizes. There are four outlets, mature give and take of unashamed personal affection, being taken care of, the urge to dominate, and, in his case, drinking. The weight upon him of the tenderness taboo blocks off the first; his consequent sense of shame tends to reject the second though he may want, more than anything else in the world, to be taken care of. The third and fourth are more or less socially acceptable. The potential problem drinker easily shifts from failure to have it his own way and to relate well to others, to dependence on alcohol. Drinking releases the repressed needs.

He feels better, he relaxes, he gets on better with others, and he finds adventure in the timeless carefree state of intoxication. This experience, though short-lived in terms of calendar time, remains indefinitely as a memory image of pleasure, not to be measured by the dull units of time used in the competitive world of clock watchers. Such memory images of pleasure have a logic of their own, difficult to penetrate by the logic of common sense and science. They contribute more to the fight against sobriety than any other cause. The drinker, though he goes on to experience loss of freedom and misery in addiction, never forgets that alcohol solved his problems in the early stages of his drinking, and gave him much pleasure. Vaguely but deeply he treasures this experience as he grows more dependent on alcohol, a dependence in which pleasure of the sort he once knew dwindles, until it becomes no more than a memory. As he grows more dependent on alcohol, he grows more dependent on others; it was just this deep need to "be taken care of" that led him, at first, to the comforts and hazards of drink! But alcohol he never blames for his troubles. He tends to defend himself by blaming and disliking the people on whom he has grown more and more dependent.

But he is incapable of composed feelings in any sober effort to wrench clear of dependence on those against whom he rebels. His conflict is this: he cannot get along with those on whom he depends because he resents the need to depend on them. But, equally, he cannot get along without them, as long as he drinks. Dependence on other people and dependence on alcohol are psychologically of the same order. But it would be wrong to suppose that to stop drinking requires withdrawal from others. He needs other people and will always need them. His problem is to learn how to relate to others, to need them, indeed, and be unafraid of needing them, but without leaning on them. The healthy form of projection is simply the ability to attribute to others what really belongs to them—their right to be themselves.

A "disorder of the social disposition" results from the tenderness taboo in sensitive people. (This is the view of Dr. Ian Suttie.) When they drink, they find that mild intoxication alleviates this disorder, in the early stages of drinking. But, in the long run, drink worsens what at first it helped. For example, the drinker was companionable and forgot his sober shyness when, in the early years, a few drinks took the uncomfortable edge off his dependence and sensitivity. But, in addiction, after he has gone the whole course, drink, far from easing those traits, makes them worse. The traits, "dependent" and "sensitive", become "childish" and "persecuted" and finally "anxious" and "paranoid". The last two are clearly signs of problem behaviour. They appear well into the third or last phase of the resistance we call projection of blame.

Over-Idealization

This human tendency, in its early mild form, can be observed in most young people. There is the lad who idealizes his girl friend, the local hockey star, an older school chum, and he seeks to impress them. There is the young girl who makes a hero of her school teacher, camp leader, older brother and she wants desperately to please them. Both boy and girl may also idealize their parents, and set up goals for themselves difficult or impossible to achieve. Perfectionist and rigid moods can be observed if such idealism persists unchecked against real life. There is nothing wrong in attention-getting and in dreaming in its healthy form—the downright personal need to be accepted and recognized.

But when youngsters are of the sensitive sort to indulge deeply in their dreams and ideals, and find drinking pleasurable, it is not long before their sentimental and romantic excursions lose all footing in real life. What was, at first, a quite common and natural idealism becomes, after loss of freedom, grandiose and expansive behaviour. During sober periods, they may build up a feeling of expectancy in otherwise good health that is best described as "feeling so well they can't stand it". Former impulsive tendencies become compulsive. Such drinkers may, after a bout has been started, go on drinking, not because they prefer it, but because they must.

Over-idealization in its distressing form refers chiefly to the resentment and self-pity which spring from the collapse of ideals wrongly imputed to others and to oneself. It functions as a fight against freedom both before and after plans for sobriety. Before the decision to get well, it simply builds up in addiction; intoxication more and more appeals to him as the only experience in which his fantasies can be indulged. After the decision to recover, resistance B can be observed in short-term abstinences during which the abstainer had idealized still far too much in himself and in others, and has expected too much of sobriety, in too short a time. He seeks attention through extravagant claims, well-intended, but unrealistic. When these excessive ideals collapse, a "slip" may occur. In this stage his rigid idealism is fused with the confirmed physical factors of his addiction. The retreat into himself deepens his dependence on a change of body chemistry in order to escape the pain of coping with the collapse of ideals. The traits "idealistic" and "impulsive" of the early phase of over-idealization become more unmanageable in the traits "grandiose" and "compulsive" and finally out of hand in the traits "elated" and "obsessive".

Fear of the Foreign

Early indications of this experience are seen in most human beings. The self-sufficient person, if you observe him well, always reveals a fear of anything foreign. Many of us are at ease and self-sufficient in familiar situations, and cautious in unknown or foreign predicaments. Self-sufficiency, fear of foreign, in its mild and modifiable form is seen in persons whose lives, for one reason or another, usually beyond their control, have been formed in prejudice, indulgence, intolerance, excessive or defective moral standards, stiff competitive settings, clear cut divisions of class, creed or culture. When such persons like to drink, and relish alcohol as a solvent of the problems occasioned by the limits of self-sufficiency, drinking will eventually worsen such problems, though at first it provided relief and pleasure.

Anything foreign to the problem drinkers' chief needs is not well tolerated. The prospect of sobriety, though *logically* clear to him, is deeply resisted because the threat of life without alcohol is greater than the familiar fear of death from drinking. At least he knows now what drinking involves, with all its troubles. But sobriety is so foreign and frightening to him that he can conceive the most fanciful alibis to justify continued drinking. Self-sufficiency is a fear of the unknown, a form of ignorance deepened by the isolating effect of his acute periods of sickness in addiction—lone drinking. This "unknown" appears in the form of persons and situations which may intimate to him some knowledge he cannot bear to experience. It ruffles his efforts to be complacent. It makes him intolerant and resentful of such persons and situations —even the prospect of their "shadow" in his path. Then a tragic paradox emerges. He begins to experience, in his alcoholism, the nameless fears and loss of support he dreaded so much in the prospect of sobriety! It is these which lead to the breakdown of his alibi structure, after his self pity is vaguely felt to be a last desperate inadequate stand, and after his depressed states grow intolerable. The traits "intolerant" and "wishful thinking" of the first phase of fear of the foreign become "hostile" and "fantastic thinking" and finally in the last phase, "depressed" and "defective thinking". Clear physical impairment of the brain cells, reversible or permanent, coincides with the incoherent and inconsistent behaviour to be observed in the late stage denoted by "defective thinking".

The Practice of Freedom

You gain practice in the use of your freedom when you understand and feel the three self-resistances to have been strong forces in the advance of addiction. To a great extent, they are brought out of the uncontrolled area of unconscious life when you see them for what they are, named, understood and consciously felt. Then you make use of them in finding ways and means to cope with them. There is always a residue of these resistances which remains impulsive and unconscious. That is why sobriety is a life time's job. There is always something to remind us that our freedom has to be active. You take a long step in the right direction when you understand the play of resistance in your own life. It is wise to realize that the tendencies to shift blame, to overidealize, and to fear the foreign are always there inviting the actions of our freedom. If we understand them, we accept them as enduring human tendencies, essential to the play of freedom. Without them, there would be nothing to try to be free from! (The empathy index is a clue to the sobriety pattern.)

Now what have we to understand about resistance besides the three main types which, in addiction, operate unconsciously? Well, there is what we can call *genuine* resistance, which will be any reasonable objection to recovery after the three unconscious resistances have been well understood and their errors as far as possible, removed. Genuine resistance to recovery will be, equally, respect for recovery. A sound and reasonable argument against recovery will, by implication, require also a sound and reasonable argument for recovery. Otherwise, the argument could not be sound and reasonable. But, because this is largely a logical, or academic operation, it does not yet identify the whole person with the *life* of recovery, or of resumed drinking. It is an intellectual operation.

The fairness of the argument, though still only an intellectual operation, can also be expressed in another form. *Genuine resistance to recovery will involve genuine resistance to alcoholism.* Respect for recovery requires respect for the meaning of alcoholism. It will be *respect* for the needs of an alcoholic who is still sick, still unaware of the unconscious nature of the drinking tendencies, yet groping for the same goal as the sober man! It will be equally a respect for the recovered man intelligently seeking what he tried, but failed, to find through the pleasure principle of drink. (At every turn, throughout therapy, the therapist deliberately identifies with patients' resistance, thus helping them to become aware both of the value and of the distress of their drinking experiences. This approach works well because interference with pleasure, either as memory, or as present and prospective experiences, is much more disturbing than interference with pain. For example, the patient usually cooperates with the medical doctor in removal of the distress of acute alcoholism and the hang-over. On the other hand, he often resists stubbornly the effort of the therapist, if the therapist threatens to rob him of his pleasure experiences by talking them down during the course of therapy, in the period following recovery from physical distress. The problem, in long term sobriety, is gradually to divert the patient from his absorption with the pleasure principle to a scrutiny of the higher principle of freedom. The patient, not quite realizing it, is tactfully drawn to a level beyond pain and pleasure, and pulled out of his absorption with pleasure when he is able, in group therapy, to look at the resistance index and see himself within it, as if he were another person. Such an operation detaches him from his drinking pattern, at least enough to enable him *deliberately* to identify with it. The suspension of thought between his detachment and his deliberate identification also breeds the prospect that from his detachment he could equally identify himself with the *opposite* of what he recognizes in his drinking pattern. Thus, if only in thought, he can resist drinking as well as resist recovery, at this stage.)

At the stage of genuine resistance, *action* in favour either of drinking or of sobriety is suspended, because resistance to the one is equally possible with resistance to the other. A sound argument for drinking calls, by implication, for a sound argument for sobriety. By this time, alibis are purged equally from both arguments, as far as possible in the human situation. Detachment is sought. It would be unfair to consider sound arguments for one activity, and then to disallow this soundness to the other activity.

The person with a drinking problem is now in a state of conflict. The two experiences—addiction and sobriety—are so opposed to one another that an action in favour of one or the other is inevitable. The effort to have it both ways always ends in a distressing catastrophe.

We at last reach a place where the argument for addiction defeats itself purely for physical reasons, if for no other. Addiction involves the impairment or destruction of the *means* to adequate judgment and productive imagination. It is well known that alcohol impairs the brain cells, the most vital instrument of sound argument and action. Thus addiction, *as a way of life*, has to be discarded. As a disorder, however, it is not so easy to dismiss.

Addiction is an overall compulsion which has lost its original value in pre-addictive drinking to give pleasure, but which continues senselessly to control the drinker's life from a source deeper and stronger than conscious control. It involves a deepening dependence on certain substances in order to provide chemical changes, at first required for the experience of pleasure, but now unconsciously required for sedation (escape from a hostile world). This chemical dependence is subtly interfused with a deepening psychological dependence on the three types of resistances. These resistances, under the pleasure principle and the tenderness taboo, constitute the main obstacle to recovery from alcoholism, or from any of the addictions.

The main key to recovery is this: make use of the resistances, of the pleasure principle, and of the tenderness taboo. When you understand them, you begin to make use of them. They cease to be obstacles.

You proceed from argument to action. Genuine resistance —a respect for arguments pro and con, though a step in the right direction, must go a step further to the experience of empathy where the problem will be solved. It is not enough to see both sides of the problem objectively. It is not enough to stop at the scientific level, where genuine resistance—a reasonable assessment of both arguments—takes place. One must go into action beyond an intelligent understanding of both sides of the problem. We have seen why addiction collapses as a way of life. It is an invasion of the centres which make a way of life possible. This is not an argument, it is a fact. Thus, if one is really seeking a way of life, and that person is a problem drinker, there is only one course now to take. It is time now for action. The problem drinker, in acting, will freely imitate the recovered alcoholics whose way of life appears attractive to him. He thus takes the decisive step from genuine resistance to recovery—the period of suspended action—to genuine deliberate identification with the *life* of recovery. He moves from respect to love. He grows devoted to sobriety. It becomes his way of life. This act still leaves a genuine resistance to alcoholism, meaning that he wants no longer to drink, but that he continues to understand and respect the needs of an active alcoholic, a person still sick and still unaware of what makes him drink. In this act of understanding, the recovered man "joins" the patient's resistance, strengthening his own insight and, at the same time, throwing light, for the sick man, on the nature of obstacles to recovery.

Empathy, in recovery from alcoholism, is personal action involving the conscious free imitation of recovered drinkers and leading to a creative effort in the way the recovering man works it out in his own way. In helping others less insightful than himself, he shows a capacity to put himself in the addicts' place, without himself having to drink. This is respect for the other fellow, and for himself.

The wrench from the pleasure principle to a desire for the freedom principle has to come without shock or force. Exhortations to be "good", sensible and normal are of little avail. Interference with pleasure memory has to be an interference made by the patient himself. The therapist assists him in this task chiefly by showing him that he understands and appreciates why drinking has been a valuable experience. The patient, when he becomes aware of this experience and its meaning is then ready to think about the prospects of freedom, and its advantages. He next realizes that the freedom goal has incentives and drives behind it very different from either the prospect of pleasure or the fear of pain.

We can exercise our capacity for detachment and deliberate identification by studying the two indexes, and their accompanying explanations, to see and to feel where this pattern applies to our past and present behaviour.

So persistent is the old underlying urge to drink that recourse to the alibi is evident in any stage of psychotherapy, even during the serious business of discussing a new way of life, when the patient seems well on the way to enduring sobriety.

Now the great trouble with alibis is that they are largely unconscious or impulsive. Their sound counterparts are *reason* and *imagination*. It is with our reason (or reasons) and our imagination (an intelligent technique) that we can throw light on our alibis. Alibis are excuses to make suspect behaviour *appear* reasonable, when in fact it is not. For example, problem drinking is defended by alibis stemming from unconscious resistance to recovery, sobriety by reasons arising from imagination (in a good recovery programme). Perhaps, for some time after the patient has stopped drinking, the foundations of his alibi structure will remain, unconsciously and deeply rooted in unknown feelings. This is one of the reasons why we stress our follow-up programme, and urge you to accept sobriety as a long haul project, for possible resistance to recovery has always to be faced.

We can transform alibis by changing our values, and thus solve the problems created by resistance. To change our values we have to abandon all hope that drinking can ever solve our problems or bring us lasting rewards, and we have to have faith in the basic principle that *we can change our human nature* after we know our limits. Positively, we shall try to see in sobriety *a gain*, not a deprivation. As long as we suspect that drinking still has attractions, that we might be able to drink again, we shall have trouble and we shall resist the radical demands of sobriety.

With a sincere conviction that our values must change because we can change, we solve the problems of resistance through knowledge gained in the talks, a change of attitude and inner feeling in the group therapy, cooperation with the clinic's medical programme, and genuine self-searching in the interviews. If possible, join an Alcoholics Anonymous group, it can fill all these needs of your follow-up programme, if you are well disposed towards it.

A patient, ideally, stops drinking for himself, not just for the sake of his job, or prestige—not even for the sake of his family or friends. Any one of these reasons, or all of them, can serve as good ground for seeking recovery, and we welcome a patient's desire for sobriety, *on any ground*, because we believe in sobriety for problem drinkers. But we hope, as it continues, that each patient will come to regard sobriety as desirable primarily for himself, as a great gain in personal growth. The other reasons for sobriety will easily fall into place.

We have seen that alcoholism, or any of the addictions, invades all areas of human life. To chart your way to recovery, long after the clinic course is finished, we need some guide, some view about human nature embracive and sound enough to avoid every kind of pitfall, and to promote every kind of new creative experience. This view will embrace physical, mental, social and personal activity. To neglect any one of these might be to neglect just those experiences which, unknown, might lead to a relapse. Obviously such a view will be ideal, but it is better to have an ideal to work towards, if it keeps us sober, than to settle for goals less than good enough to insure sobriety.

This view, though ideal, and one we often fail to reach, is yet practical. It has emerged after much experience with alcoholic patients. It is not just theory or speculation, because patients who are well recovered will tell you, in a thousand different ways, that these personal ideals enable them to maintain sobriety and to enjoy it. The resistance index coupled with the personal goals and ideals (Chapter 3) helps you to understand how resistance can become an aid to freedom.

Few people can live up to these goals and ideals, but the great merit of it is that just trying is all one can be well expected to do. The mystery of it is that there are few defined goals except to live as well as possible. The reaching of goals is less important than striving towards them, in deeply felt actions, as outlined in the empathy index.

Ward resumed the discussion after the therapist's talk.

"Well, science is useful, anyway. There is surely a lot we want to know about reactions, if we expect to understand our alcohol problem."

"I agree. But I suggest it's also important to know action and its meaning. To do that is to go beyond science, as understood today."

"So you think," Ward observed, "that the making use of resistance, the task of changing ourselves is a question that goes beyond science?"

"Yes. It is not that science is at fault. It is only that we should know its limits."

"You can't beat the law of gravity," said Arthurs stoically.

"No one wants to. But no one should apply the law of gravity where it does not fit."

"Like trying to recover the broken pint." Arthurs was wistful.

"Yes, or like trying to recover from alcoholism."

"If science is the only approach to the problem of resistance, there is no answer?" asked Ward.

"That's right. Science offers no help on the belief in personal freedom, in the faith that we can change our behaviour. In regarding my behaviour as determined, science makes it hard to understand how I can learn to use resistance constructively."

"So my questions in the last session were enquiries of a scientific kind?" asked Ward.

"Yes, I think so. It seemed to me that you simply did what so many intelligent people are in the habit of doing. You applied science, you undertook a scientific task. There's nothing wrong with undertaking scientific tasks. But that is not to seek recovery from alcoholism, a personal effort."

"Of course, scientific work is surely personal effort, but its goal differs from the goal sought in sobriety," Ward observed.

"All right. You might say that scientific work is a personal effort, with a human goal, power and control over something outside of you as a person. Whereas, sobriety is a personal effort with a personal goal—to be free, to create, and to love —all these are actions."

"The goals are actions?"

"Yes, as distinguished from theoretical knowledge which is the goal of science. You remember Farr? He was here with us for a while."

"Bright guy," observed Arthurs.

"The poor chap simply couldn't stay sober," said Buxton.

"He could discuss the problems of drink more knowledgably than anyone I ever met."

"Yes, and he'd be drunk an hour after the session closed," Buxton added.

"Farr seemed to me to be a living example of what happens when you follow the rule of science that personal feelings have to be excluded from facts and analyses."

"He certainly never allowed his knowledge to interfere with his desire to drink."

"Wait now. What about that other fellow?" asked Ward. He was the same as Farr."

"You mean Granby."

"Yes, he knew more about good and evil, temptation, free

will and what not, than ever I thought there was to know
in religion."

"And he, too, never allowed his fancy knowledge to curb
his thirst," said Arthurs.

"It doesn't matter what your particular line is—science
itself, morals, religion, law or medicine. Both Farr and
Granby are typical of men of their time. They more or less
think in scientific terms, without realizing it, whether the
problem is plumbing, biology, religion or alcohol."

"Are you saying," asked Ward, "that the knowledge of
Farr and Granby was theoretical and failed to become active
because their personal feelings were not in it?"

"Not exactly, they projected blame for their alcoholism
onto science. Because science provides no cure, they said,
there is no hope. Their feelings were in it because projection
of blame is a feeling. The whole point here is that in their
effort to be objective and strictly scientific, they could not
see their own unconscious resistance."

"Didn't you say, once, that science is imitative?"

"Yes. Science imitates, and imitation is good as far as it
goes. Farr and Granby had much to offer. It's only a pity
they did not stay long enough to see what could be offered
to them. They gave us imitations of someone else, but little
of themselves. Their scientific knowledge was excellent,
their classifications impressive. But none of us got to know
them."

"That sounds strange—science is imitation. Really now,
what about new science?" asked Ward.

"New science is art. Einstein was an artist. Those who
follow him imitate."

"Well, we do this all the time, every day, in ordinary
human behaviour," said Ward.

"Yes, I know. And it saves a lot of time, doesn't it? Not
having to face strange situations in new ways makes life
easier. We are creatures of habit, all of us."

"Yes, that's what I mean."

"But besides that, we are persons or try to be. And to be

a person is to create. More than anything else, the alcoholic must try to be a person. That is the real meaning of sobriety."

"The drive behind science," Ward continued, "is a desire to know, which extends beyond yourself, to what already is there, waiting to be understood. It's a desire to know by control, by exercising power over things outside you, outside your feelings. I'm just trying to see better what you mean by imitation, what you mean when you say that science is imitation."

"Yes, you sort of copy what you see, you copy according to the principles laid down by the particular science you follow. What you see and know has to correspond with what you *should* see, with your personal feelings out of it. Science is naturally afraid of the danger of reporting what is *not* there. And it has very definite ideas about what "there" means. All we have to do is to think of the mice, and exotic animals that many of us have seen, to realize that something very important is left out of their calculations."

"You mean our sick fantasies. No one in his right senses would think of calling them scientific facts."

"Of course not. But they are real, and you know it. They are real, because you feel them, even if you realize they are not "there". Even science concedes that they are factual in the sense that we inwardly experience such fantasies. But science tends to discourage their full title to reality. There is more to being real than just being out "there". It is this that many of us tend to forget."

"Like the little man who wasn't there, but wouldn't go away," Arthurs added.

"On another occasion, I tried to point out that fantasies are aimless, and happen to us, whereas symbols and images that we consciously evoke are acts of our imagination. There is much in our imagination that science fails to deal with, because it is left out for the same reason that fantasies are excluded."

"They don't correspond, is that it?"

"Whatever fails to correspond to standards laid down, is left out of the scientific picture. That is why I say the tendency of science is to be imitative, rather than creative as we are when we call up images. Science imitates or follows what has gone before. By contrast, creative effort yields something new, something that was not previously seen. You are creative, for example, when you come to understand the three resistances to recovery, and make use of them in your sobriety."

"Surely a scientist, doing science, can sometimes act and choose just as anyone does who is doing creative work?"

"I agree. That only shows the scientist is far less scientific than he supposes himself to be. But it is still true that the objects and goals of scientific search are mainly sought to the exclusion of personal feeling and freedom."

"This is a long way from Ward's questions. They still puzzle me," said Buxton.

"Well, briefly there are no satisfactory answers to Ward's questions, if we cannot believe that we can learn to be free from alcoholism. And to learn to be free from alcoholism is to change our behaviour. To recover from alcoholism, to learn sobriety is an effort different from a scientific task."

"But there's nothing wrong with science," said Ward.

"Of course not. Scientific effort may well help us to understand much about alcoholism as a reaction. As a tool, it is valuable. But as a final answer, it fails. It can tell us nothing about sobriety—an action. Science is only fitted, by its own premises, to study *reactions*."

"And the reason again, why does it fail?" asked Buxton.

"As scientific thinking is most at home studying reactions, it tends to exclude just that which enables us to act, to make changes, and to choose goals. We cannot make changes, for example, in the tendencies to project blame, to overidealize, or to be fearful until we first accept them and realize that whatever we do, we have to take them into account in dealing with our personal problems."

"But we do not discard science. We use it as means to our

goal. Why, then, were my questions wrongly put?" asked Ward.

"Because your questions concerned the problem of action, of choice, of value. And these are personal questions which, in my opinion, can only be expressed and answered in a personal way."

"I see this better than I did before," said Buxton. "It explains my own resistance, and it also points to the dangers of just adopting another's view in an imitative way, without really feeling it."

"Your struggle," said Arthurs, "was honest enough. But you broke through too sudden like. After that, you lined up quick with the therapist. Some of us thought this was just too easy, after all your trouble."

"There is a long way yet to go," said Buxton.

"Let's hope so. Everyone wants to live as long as possible."

"This, then, is a lifetime's job—this sobriety?" Arthurs was all thought.

"Yes. If we can see that the desire to be a better person was just the desire that led us into addiction, that addiction brought us the opposite of what we wanted, we have ahead of us a lifetime's job, not a problem that can be settled in these discussions. To be a better person is not a scientific task."

"But scientific tasks can serve the alcoholic's personal goals?" said Ward.

"Yes. Scientific effort, one expression of the human desire for power and control, can help him to understand alcoholism as an event which happened to him. But he has to realize that he must create and gain freedom in fellowship as his highest goal. You see, we have no control over alcohol, so how can we expect to recover, if we rely solely on instruments of control, like science? Our whole problem is that we have lost control over alcohol. So we must seek a higher goal than control, or the hope of control. We must seek to be better persons in a way that does not tempt us to repeat the errors of trying to control drinking. We need help. We get this help from others like us, in fellowship."

"So, if I am really seeking sobriety," said Ward, "rather than the hope of control in science, I will not neglect those feelings that I can never control. In trying to become a better person, I can identify those feelings of mine in other people, and together we can make use of them in sobriety. That was your theme in the talk 'Making Use of Resistance'."

"Your theme has a guiding reason behind it," observed Buxton.

"Yes, I admit that," said the therapist.

"Your reason is in the desire for sobriety, and in putting that over to us," said Ward.

"Yes, both the reason and the desire, I hope."

"They shouldn't be separated any more than impulse and reason, should they?" Ward recalled the previous session.

"You are quite right, Ward. The reason is in the desire, and the desire is in the reason. But the guiding reason, I suggest, has to be more than just a desire to be sober, though the reason beyond is simply more of the same thing as sobriety."

"I'm still wondering," said Ward, "about the proper role of science."

"Just to wonder about life and nature. Isn't that enough to explain science?" asked Arthurs. "You birds sure make it hard for yourselves."

"But that goes for poetry too," said the therapist. "It is not enough to distinguish science by itself. Science seems to be distinguished by its efforts to control, to regulate, and to limit, and to exercise power over the controlled objects. That's why I say the desire for power and control is back of science."

"All right. Now, why should we want to be sober?" demanded Ward. "If there's a reason behind everything, even science, there must be a reason why we should want to be sober, there must be something to induce the desire for sobriety."

"Time and again, in different ways, I've said that the goal beyond sobriety, and the desire behind it—they are the same thing—is the desire to be a better person, that's all. To make the most of myself is what it means to be sober."

"This main goal," observed Arthurs, "it's not crying over spilt whiskey and its not blaming science for it—this being a person is, after all, a pretty common hope, isn't it? Nothing real special about it, is there?"

"We human beings only make it hard for ourselves by letting the instruments of living become our goals. If we could have used drink to serve personal purposes, we might have had no problem. But it changed from an instrument to an all-consuming need."

"You said that the reason for sobriety, and what it means to be sober, came to the same thing—the desire to be a better person. Well, the reason for drinking, when drinking seemed to serve the same desire, was the same too." Buxton pursued the theme all the way.

"The only trouble was that drinking did the opposite for us when we became addicted. Still, when we started, drinking was a response to the thirst to be a better person. We never drank with the intention of harming ourselves. But we didn't realize clearly enough that drinking was a response to personal thirst. If we realize that now, the way is clear."

"I was puzzled for a long time about the elusive desire for sobriety," said Buxton. "Now I see that the desire for sobriety is the same deep desire as the one that led me to drink. This makes it much clearer to me why sobriety is worth striving for. My quick turnabout, that came under the criticism of Ward and Arthurs, was more imitative than it was personal. I have more to work on now."

"I didn't mean to be critical, Bux. It was kind of sudden, your change of heart, that's all."

"That stirs up a lot—Buxton saying that the meaning of the desire to drink is the same as the meaning of the desire to be sober." Ward was impressed.

"Yes, yes, sure," agreed Arthurs. "Unless Buxton is right, I may as well go for another pint, if I lose the one I have."

"In sobriety I search for what I failed to find in drink,"

mused Ward. "There is essentially the same thirst in both."

"That's better." Arthurs was relieved.

"Learning, in fellowship, to be a better person is the goal of sobriety. It seems to be the best response as adults that we can make to the personal thirst that got side-tracked in alcoholism."

"Along the way, science might prove very helpful. Medication, and all that, and understanding alcoholism as a reaction."

"No one can object to that. I was strong on that track in the first session. But personal thirst is never quenched. When we abandon alcohol, and finish the treatment of an institution, we still have a life time of thirst in action ahead of us."

"We'll need a clinic in the outside world," said Ward.

"We have to train ourselves in sobriety all the time, the way it's working out," Arthurs suggested.

"Each of us will have to work out a follow-up plan for himself. Each of us will make his own decisions."

"Before we finish today," said Buxton, "I have a question to ask. How do I close the distance between me and sobriety? I am on the fence if I respect equally my alcoholism and my prospective sobriety."

"Ah!" sighed Arthurs. "There you go again, digging away at this intellectual stuff. Damn it all, I either want to be sober or drink. Isn't that it? Why beat around the bush with the psycho deal?"

"If you're clear, Arthurs, that's just great. I'm happy for you. But I have to see it my way."

"Okay, Bux, no offence. Shoot. Pick it up for yourself. Once in a while it's real crazy, this out-of-orbit jazz."

"Let's go ahead," urged Ward. "What you said about 'respect' makes a sound case for the scientific approach. I can be scientific. I like that."

"The great merit of learning to respect alcoholism and sobriety is that in this act you can be as scientific as you want to be. Doing science is an act of respect, though not the only one. Sympathy and rejoicing are also acts of respect. All three—science, sympathy, and rejoicing imply distance from that which you are scientific about, in sympathy with, or rejoicing over. So all three are detached from their objects of interest. They are forms of understanding from the outside. For example. when I respect sobriety, I am at a distance from it in gaining knowledge about it. I come closer and abandon my urge to control sobriety when I sympathize with it as a way of life, and when I rejoice that some alcoholics can be happy as sober people. I may do all this, and yet not be sober myself."

"This is what puzzles me," said Buxton. "Where do we go from there?"

"Get with it!" Arthurs cried. "Do it, feel it, get the taste of it!"

"The hot taste of life," murmured Buxton.

"The step to take, after you respect sobriety, is to fall in love with it. When you do that, you put sobriety into action."

"What nonsense is this?"

"It is nonsense, Ward," agreed the therapist, "because it is beyond common sense. You were devoted utterly to alcohol, to the way of life that you and alcohol developed together. A tragic love affair, and nonsense into the bargain. Sobriety, too, is a love affair and nonsense. But it's wise nonsense."

"Anyway," said Buxton, "I've found my way out of the maze. Respect for sobriety is not enough. Knowledge, sympathy, and rejoicing are necessary, but just not enough. I have to go into action. I have to devote myself to sobriety. I have *to be* sober. Sobriety is not something I own or have or that I can buy or master. Get with it, as Arthurs said."

Ward was puzzled. "Wise nonsense. Now what am I going to make of that?"

"Go after what you wanted when you drank for the hell of it, but do it wisely now."

7.

ALCOHOLICS ANONYMOUS —
A CLINICAL VIEW

ALLEN and Ward helped us to see the fallacy of theoretical knowledge when it is not tested or illustrated in action. For example, in their experience, they see now that "knowing better" does not guarantee "doing better". On the contrary, the more they knew, the less they *really* knew, before they found sobriety. We are grateful to them for their tireless and rewarding search. Here is the fallacy of separating knowledge from action. The error is to suppose that a principle which works in theory should also work in solving personal problems. This is just a warning that we are in for trouble if we suppose that logical methods, sound and fruitful within science, should also necessarily be sound and fruitful in solving the biggest problems in human behaviour.

Alcoholics Anonymous teaches you, more than any other source you can think of, that intellectual mastery is not equal to the really crucial problem facing an alcoholic, or anyone, I believe, suffering from a personal disorder. Let me illustrate. On more than one occasion during your drinking days, well-meaning friends would say "Really, haven't you had enough?" By "enough", they meant the two or three drinks that a social drinker would take, and then dutifully go home for dinner, the reality picture kept beautifully intact. You see, your sober reasonable friends were simply following a logic of quantity, which is the method of science. They were suggesting that the problem was a problem of the stuff called alcohol. Simply understand that more than a few

drinks bring changes that we the reasonable people disap-
prove of. "Watch how much you drink", or more strongly,
"Don't drink at all" was the only kind of advice you were
able to get. The logic of measure, a logic of quantity, has very
little to do with the real problem. It is a fact, of course, that
alcoholics should not drink, if they wish to live. But the
reason is not to be found in the evils of the chemical
C_2H_5OH. We have to appeal to what I call "personal" knowing in order to convince your well-meaning quantifying
friends that what is reasonable to a social drinker is unreasonable to a problem drinker. Once you get the drift of
personal knowing, you can understand, you and your sober
friends together, that it is *not* reasonable for a problem
drinker, under the sway of his compulsion, to stop at two
or three drinks. It would be nothing short of magic to expect
a problem drinker to be free of his compulsion, without any
insight, and to stop at the third drink, when every fibre of
his being called out for more. In Allen's final binge, his wife
one day appealed to one of their best friends. She reported
that he wanted to stop, but could not. What could he do?
"Nothing," he sadly decided, "nothing, because I cannot
make sense of your report that he wants desperately to quit
and yet cannot do so." Allen appreciated this honesty. And
then he began to reflect on this strange contradiction. He
knew better. He knew he should stop drinking if he wanted
to live. And yet he could not let a day pass without forty
ounces of whiskey and a dozen pints of Bass' Ale. At that
time, during that binge, he was completely baffled by the
fact that he knew as well as anyone that he should not drink
—and the fact was supported by a great deal of reading on
the problem, a great deal of knowledge *about* alcoholism.
This did not seem to matter. But dimly he began to suspect
there was help somewhere. He could not believe that there
was no choice but to drink himself to death. Vaguely he
sensed that, if there was any hope, he had to find it somewhere outside himself.

The trouble with his theoretical knowledge about alcoholism at that time was that he regarded it as a problem to be mastered by the intellect, by the logic of science. His personal feelings about the problem were untouched by his knowledge. Personal feelings. Personal desires. What about them? Logical games provided fun, a thrill of mastery. But what did they do for his greatest needs? With great dismay, he had to admit—nothing. Nothing, unless he could somehow bring his deepest needs into some sort of harmony with his knowledge. Because of this experience, it was easy for him to understand a couple of men whom he met four years later—one, a professor, the other, a lawyer—two men who could hold forth brilliantly on the pitfalls of alcoholism, citing the soundest authorities in science and psychology—two men who invariably tied one on within hours of their brilliant analysis of the problem in group therapy. These men were well posted on the tricks and techniques of argument, and like himself were the victims of the separation of knowledge from personal action. They had a keen sense for intellectual games, but no thought at all for the knowledge of feeling, as applied to themselves. It is this knowledge of feeling that I call personal knowing.

As I develop my theme, I notice a danger—it is the danger that you might suppose me to be opposed to science. I hasten to correct that tendency. Later, I shall explain why I regard science as essential in gaining freedom from alcoholism—essential but not sufficient. Just here I want to stress the all-important experience that comes with what I call personal knowing. Will power and the intellect fall short of explaining these three basic questions: "Why should I stop drinking?" "Why did I drink in the first place?" and "How should I seek and maintain sobriety?" It is curious that the will power magic and work of the intellect are cut from the same cloth. But the fabric of will power is weak, while the fabric of the intellect can be sound if properly used in science. Still, they are cut from the same cloth—a determination to achieve their ends by the control of nature—will power by stifling and containing, the intellect by destroying freedom by analysis, by the removal of mystery, and by the neglect of feeling.

The sense of mastery is evident in the will-power alcoholic. His attitude is something like this, as you recall it in your will-power water-wagon days. "By God, I'll show them. I can do this on my own steam. How can anybody be so weak as to turn to others for help. I can do this alone." And what is back of the will-power alcoholic? It is usually the spectacle of a man who does not really want to stop drinking. It is usually a man trying to be sober under pressure of family, of friends, of employer or, worst of all, of a fear-ridden conscience. There is no deep personal response to the question "Why should I stop drinking?" and "How should I seek sobriety?" Equally, the patient who seeks to recover through scientific techniques alone is one who also ignores those questions. He relies on the scientist's mastery of nature to answer questions which simply are not scientific questions, but personal ones; not questions concerned to destroy freedom, but to make freedom real. The alcoholic, sober by will power or by the prescriptive fatherly sternness of a scientific technique—"don't drink, or else"—"do this, or else" and "don't do that"—either will-power or conditioned reflex—you will notice such an alcoholic is sober under strain. What is the strain? It is the strain of imprisonment. He is sober by force, but deep down there is the urge to be free. Mistakenly, he supposes that to be free is to be free to drink. And yet through will power or outside control he has submitted to a dry regime. He is imprisoned by the superstition of will power or the chaining of his reflexes to a sobriety on the surface. But down deep, his personal feelings contradict and hate these chained reflexes. His deep feeling is a feeling for freedom, for release. On the surface, in his outward behaviour, he is in chains; to drink again is to get out of the cage. What kind of sobriety is that? Is it any better than being good and drunk? Allen told you that in his last binge he sensed that he was imprisoned—a prisoner of his own making. And yet, if he had submitted to will power, or to a conditioned reflex treatment, he would have been equally imprisoned. What about this? Well just this. Submitting to sobriety is not a satisfactory or enduring response to the urges of these deep personal feelings. Somehow or other, if he was to be a sober man he had to find a way to be honest with his deepest feelings, his greatest needs. And the sum of his deepest feelings and greatest needs was the basic urge to be free. Free to drink? No, that was and is and always will be impossible. No one is ever free to do the impossible. Free *for* what, then, and free *to* what? Well, if he was not free to drink, maybe he could be free to be sober. This, at last, is what is meant by personal knowing, the logic of feelings. It is an experience that has to be known personally. It has to be felt. It cannot be understood unless it is felt. Scientific knowledge can point to it. But only personal logic can actually know what it is to want to be free. And you have to be imprisoned, know that you are imprisoned, before you can want desperately to be free. So the personal act of recovery from any personal disorder is an act that can only be known by those who are conscious of defect, conscious of slavery, conscious of having had to behave compulsively in spite of great efforts to the contrary.

The Miracle of Alcoholics Anonymous

You go to Alcoholics Anonymous, conscious of slavery to alcohol, but wanting very much to overcome it. Allen came to Alcoholics Anonymous after he had seen two sponsors whose stories astonished him. It was hard to believe that these two people had once been very sick, as he was at that time, hard to believe that they were now sober. It was even more astonishing to see that they were pleased with their sobriety. Most astonishing of all was the delight Allen knew in finding his own sobriety easy. He had guessed it would be difficult. What else could he expect, after years of struggle? The usual did not happen. The experience was new, contrary to expectations and prediction based on past experience. All this astonishment I call the experience of a miracle—the miracle of Alcoholics Anonymous. So Allen's first greatest discovery in Alcoholics Anonymous, after his sobriety, was finding the difference between magic and miracle.

Magic, referred to yourself, is the expectation that something spectacular will happen to you, something not requiring your own effort. There was the woman alcoholic who said to me one day, "You know I had four bottles of beer just a few hours ago and they didn't do a thing for me." She expected, after the minimal effort required to swallow the contents of four bottles of beer, that something would happen to her. What I want to stress here, is that she expected something to happen to her. This passive reliance on outside substances—alcohol, drugs, pills—is a modern form of the ancient magic sought in alchemy. Of course that woman had no right to expect that four bottles of beer would do anything for her. But she was deceived, as thousands are, into hoping that the old lost lift and glow could be hers again as it was when she started drinking. Treacherously, her memory plays tricks on her, popping up with the recall of early pleasure, and submerging the memory of misery that always goes with hang-overs after the drinker has become addicted.

The practising alcoholic is always looking for magic—he keeps hoping that "just one more" will bring again the pleasant lift of the good old days—a revival of the sense of adventure and release he used to know, way back in the days when he drank just for the hell of it.

And magic is sought, too, by the alcoholic who resolves to be sober through will power, through pills, or injections. It is a hope that his alcoholism can be cured without going to the source of it, without exercising any personal effort. If you think that will power is personal effort, let me hasten to say that will power is *human* effort. Personal effort always requires more than one person. Personal effort is interpersonal effort. Human effort cannot solve personal problems.

To suppose it can is either to be deceived or to believe in magic.

Briefly, magic is happening without rhyme, reason or cause. A miracle, on the other hand, is not just a happening. A miracle is an astonishing action. It is unusual but it is not unreasonable. It only appears to be unreasonable to those for whom "reason" has a narrow dogmatic meaning. Human beings, for example, who are not also persons, are inclined to regard miracles as the invention of the superstitious. Events or actions which do not respond to familiar habits of study are thought to be either unknowable or impossible. But if we appreciate the mystery of what it is to be a person, miracles need not be regarded as fictitious. They will be astonishing, unusual, but they are not without reason. Miracles are not unreasonable. They are paradoxical only because they are not in accord with familiar human habits of knowing.

Here are some features of the Alcoholics Anonymous programme that are foreign to familiar habits of knowing; they are astonishing, paradoxical, and not at all what you expect in a twentieth-century enterprise. Though they appear to be just the opposite of what should work, according to accepted standards, they are, actually, the conditions that account largely for the wide prevalence of Alcoholics Anonymous therapy.

Usually a therapy or theory is expected to undergo a controlled test or study in order to validate it, to assess it, and declare it to be sound. Now the first new feature of Alcoholics Anonymous is the strange but true discovery that it is your constancy as patients that keeps Alcoholics Anonymous alive and flourishing. There is no problem of scientific assessment in Alcoholics Anonymous therapy because it is essentially an act of growth, a programme of creative action. Many say that if it worked according to a set pattern, there would be no Alcoholics Anonymous! It would disappear, its entire meaning would be lost if a student could say that Alcoholics Anonymous was sound, and if he had to back his observations with scientific precision. There could be a scientific study of Alcoholics Anonymous, just as there is a psychology of religion, but it would be just as wrong to say that Alcoholics Anonymous is a science as it is to say that religion is only psychology. Controlled studies of therapy usually allow a period of from two to five years or more before any decision is reached as to their soundness. What about Alcoholics Anonymous? Well, you know, they say that a man sober ten years is just one drink away from a drunk, they say there is no seniority in Alcoholics Anonymous for the very good reason that no one is ever safe, though well meaning observers may try to assure you that you are well recovered if you have been sober five years.

So it is your inability to declare you are cured that keeps the fellowship alive! This lack of certainty is not only in the constant exposure to a possible slip in drinking, it is also in your constant exposure to slips in thinking and feeling. The programme is daily—there are no graduation certificates— no assurance from students that Alcoholics Anonymous is scientifically sound. This discovery was important to Allen. It came when he gave up worrying whether a twelfth step call would be successful or not. He stopped worrying whether his effort was a success or a failure when he realized that Alcoholics Anonymous is not to be understood primarily by the effect of the actions of any of its members. The twelfth step of Alcoholics Anonymous is an action of value to the man who performs it. It is an art, without plan, and without thought of its outcome. You do it in the faith that it is worthwhile. It keeps you sober, it clears the lines of communication with your fellowman—that fellow without whom you cannot stay sober. How it turns out you cannot well know. If it turns out well, you are pleased. But how can you claim a success for yourself when, for all you know, there are a thousand influences at work in the problem? And if your effort does not bring in a recruit for therapy, is this a failure? No, your friend may have to work through a lot of resistance before he is ready for Alcoholics Anonymous. And your effort, though it may have looked like a failure, was very likely an important step towards his ultimate recovery. You do what you can, and let it go at that. You don't lose any sleep over it. Above all, you cannot force the issue. If he wants to drink, that's his affair. If he wants to stop and can use your help, you'll do what you can, if you want to.

This casual procedure, without plan, relying on the unique situation to suggest what you'll say or do is hardly the sort of behaviour which lends itself to a controlled study. This then is the first astonishing feature of Alcoholics Anonymous therapy. Of course this is nothing against scientific assessment, and it is nothing against Alcoholics Anonymous, simply because Alcoholics Anonymous is not a science, though it may and does draw on science for many of its instruments in its programme of action.

The second feature of Alcoholics Anonymous which is astonishing is the stress in our time on personal effort when experts are the fad. It is foreign to familiar habits of thinking to call alcoholism a sickness in one breath, and in the next to stress the importance of personal effort. And I must say now, if it is not already clear, that personal effort is free effort, it concerns values and choices. And personal effort means to work in concert with other persons. You cannot be personal by yourself. Now to say that I need someone else in order to be personal is to say that I recognize a power greater than myself. Later, I want to say rather more about what it means to be a person. Here it is enough to point out that right at the beginning of your programme, you hint at the greater power in the second step, and in the third step it is suggested clearly that you decide to turn your will and your lives over to the care of God as you understand Him. You start out with the recognition that alcoholism is a disease, a sickness, and then right away you encounter the need to turn to God in handling this sickness. Actually, it is intimated that your sickness has been to a large extent a failure to know God in action. Strange "sickness", isn't it, as people generally understand the word?—So the second astonishing feature of Alcoholics Anonymous therapy is that this sickness is not only a physical and psychological illness but also a spiritual defect. Alcoholism—a sickness with a difference.

The third feature of novelty is that in the very act of banding together and declaring yourselves to be powerless over alcohol and your lives unmanageable—in this very act of surrender, you begin to gain strength. This is astonishing to the twentieth century mind, but it works and that is what counts. In the three features of Alcoholics Anonymous therapy I have just outlined, and in many others as well, you experience the astonishment which enables you to call Alcoholics Anonymous a miracle. But the miracle is not unreasonable, as I'll try to show.

Let's look again at those three questions,

 (1) Why stop drinking?

 (2) Why did you drink in the first place?

 (3) How should you seek and maintain sobriety?

The first question is, or should be, the easiest of the three to answer. If it is possible to stop, you should try to do so, otherwise you die. But you want to live. The question "Why stop drinking?" arises well along in your drinking experience, at a time when you are truly sick. This question is what induces you to take the first step of the Alcoholics Anonymous programme, that is the first step after you have expressed the desire to stop drinking. In the first step of the programme you declare you are powerless over alcohol and your life unmanageable. You do this because you are tired of being sick and miserable, and give up all hope of being able to run your life, by yourself. You want to be free of your misery. Having made this surrender, this admission of utter failure to control your behaviour alone, the only reasonable next step is to look for help outside yourself.

Now, if you have any doubt about the need to make this surrender, you have only to look around at those friends and acquaintances who have tried to control their drinking, men, and women, who are problem drinkers. What do you see? You see most of the causes of slips or relapses in failure to take the first step, whether they are Alcoholics Anonymous members or not. The first step of the Alcoholics Anonymous programme is the atom bomb of the therapy. You learn that you will have trouble if you ever forget the tremendous power of the first step. The act of surrender—a deliberate act —paves the way to enduring freedom. Resistance to recovery is evident in all the trouble expressed in what we call *conflict*. Painfully dry, resentful of those who are drinking, resentful of those who are pleasantly sober, hanging on to abstinence grimly, this is a fighting effort revealing that sobriety is stifling, the opposite of what it should be.

The slip or relapse shows failure to take the first step— unconditional surrender. Instead of surrender, there is only submission. And submission arises from fear. Wherever we see submission, we see a grudging truce, and conflict and strain will prevail. It betrays the hidden hope that the alcoholic can drink again, as he once did, pleasantly. He does not feel the need to change his attitude towards life. He believes that the pleasant glow of drinking at its best cannot be known in sobriety. He regards sobriety as the *opposite* of the pleasant glow of early drinking. He cannot imagine that sobriety, if given a chance, will produce a "glow" comparable and superior to the glow of drinking. So he is tense and unhappy as an abstinent man. He secretly longs for a safe alibi to resume drinking, the kind of drinking that he can really no longer experience—the drinking of the good old days, gone forever.

Nothing shows up the nature of human delusion like the alcoholic's vain hope that he can learn to drink in a controlled way. At a meeting recently I asked a group this question. Supposing a magic pill were to be announced. This pill would ensure the drinker that it would enable him to take not more than four two-ounce drinks over an eight hour period, without any of the ill effects of alcoholism. How long, I asked, would the drinker use such a pill? One humorous and honest member of the group answered promptly, "just eight hours." And that in a nut shell, or in a pill, is the answer to that vain delusion. Drinking in a controlled way is simply not your wish because you drank in order to loosen control! You have really no desire to drink, without that definite change in feeling to which you became addicted. And that always means getting drunk.

What the alcoholic really feels when he expresses the wish to drink moderately is to drink again as he once could —and that was plenty, and it was alcoholic, though it was in that period previous to his crucial misery and worst trouble.

So the first necessary step of the alcoholic is the first step of the Alcoholics Anonymous programme, that is, the first step after feeling at least a glimmer of desire to stop drinking. This step is indicated clearly for strict medical reasons, if for no other at this stage.

In the period just before or during the time you admit you are powerless over alcohol, and your lives unmanageable, the science of medicine is your great ally. There are, first of all, the ill effects of drinking on your physical health. These must be put aright, if you are to become receptive to Alcoholics Anonymous therapy and active enough to do your share in the programme.

There are always nutritional defects to be corrected by proper diet and rest, and cellular functions to be improved by medically supervised doses of vitamins, protein, salt, glucose, and the like. There may be serious damage inflicted during your excesses—damage requiring careful medical attention for some time.

Throughout your sobriety, as long as you live, you are wise to respond intelligently to danger signs that medical men can point out for you, and to care for your health in strengthening your sobriety. You learn, for example, about cross-tolerance, you are told that it is disastrous to shift your dependence from alcohol to sedatives. Sedatives and tranquillizers can be as addicting as alcohol and worse, far worse.

Through medicine, you can shorten the difficult period of

initial recovery, with the help of skilled doctors who know the physical damage inflicted by alcoholism and how to treat it. Your debt to science is great. Many Alcoholics Anonymous members tell me they must never suppose that they can get along as a closed exclusive society, independent of the help easily available in medicine and in psychology.

So one very real and practical expression of the progress made in the first and second steps of the programme is the turning to a power greater than yourselves in the form of drastic medical aid. In the first step, you make clear you are powerless, each by himself. The only possible next move is to turn to a belief in a power greater than yourselves. But besides medicine, besides similar types of aid, the important *personal* action here is the growth of hope and of faith. It is in the nature of a miracle, in twentieth century thinking, to witness a man, abject in a state of surrender, finding, in the depths of his despair and weakness, the ground of his freedom. The miracle grows clearer as we see him, at last, making the effort to reach out beyond himself for help. He joins hands, heart and aim with others like him, and then the miracle becomes action. The miracle and the paradox is this: he finds himself *in others*, after he has admitted that by himself, he is powerless. By himself, he is *not* himself. He finds himself in and with others because it is only in this way that he can *be* and become himself.

So to the question "Why stop drinking?" The Alcoholics Anonymous initiate can say "Because there is nothing for me but death if I go on drinking. Though I am hopeless by myself, there is the prospect of recovery in working with others like myself. I want to be free. I stop drinking for the same reason I started drinking. But in sobriety there is real hope I can find what I failed to find in drink."

The miracle taking shape in moving from the first to the second step is astonishing. From an utterly powerless condition, the alcoholic finds strength in breaking through the confines of his own weakness simply by the growth of a belief from the soil of his utter incapacity to do anything for himself. It is a declaration of the failure of human will to solve the most crucial problems of life.

And yet, miracle that it is, it is not unreasonable. For, if it is true that by yourself you are powerless, it only reasonably follows that in order to be free, you must look to a power greater than yourself.

As to more about this power, we have to move on to the third step—"Made a decision to turn our will and our lives over to the care of God as we understood Him." The interpretation of the greater power in the second step was wide open. It could, if you chose, have been a medical doctor, a friend, a clergyman, or engine—anyone or anything at all. Now, it says "God". Still, it is God as you understand Him. So your belief may continue to be very flexible and very personal. Yet, it is God, without doubt.

Here I have to become more personal. How did you come to know God as you understand Him? You go back to the days before you drank, and also, to the early pleasant days of drinking when you drank for the hell of it, before you became definitely addicted to alcohol. In doing this, you get an answer to the question "Why did I drink in the first place?" When you decided to turn your will and your life over to the care of God as you understand Him, you began to relate this decision to the deepest most sincere desires of your life *before you became sick.* But to create this relation, to bring your desires into accord with God, you had first to follow through the admission of surrender in the first step, and the faith of the second step. So when you gave up trying to run your own life by yourself, you gave up belief in your human will, your pride, your will power delusions, and your faith in intellectual mastery, the worship of logical games as ends in themselves. (This is daily effort, by the way. Their struggle for expression has to be diverted daily, hourly, and on the spot. It isn't always easy.) Now, in this daily surrender of human will and its allies, the miracle continues to work. The experience of new life is astonishing. The adventure is full of surprise and wonder. Here is the real mystery of your thirst. When your human will ceases to be defensive and aggressive, it serves a higher feeling, commonly known as good will. But let me make clear that I do not believe good will to be simply another form of human will. Good will is higher than and different from human will, though the higher can turn the lower to good advantage and make use of it. Good will makes us free. Human will alone keeps us tied to addictions or obsessions. Good will is free will. Human will is restricting, determining, enslaving. Good will is of God. Human will is also of God, but only if it serves good will. Human will, without the grace of good will, is opposed to God. And human will is what governs the life of an active addict. In that period of your life you tried to get along without God, even if you thought you were religious.

Now I want to suggest the relation between God as understood now and God as understood in youth before you became alcoholic, including the early days of what is called drinking "just for the hell of it". And in this relation I want to suggest you get the clue to the question "Why did I drink in the first place?"

God, in one's youth, was the source surely of any person's meaning in the universe, the source of his proper relation with all else around him, and the source of any worthwhile adventure and mystery, not to be found in the accustomed daily round. In God was to be found the meaning of life, and of death.

Disillusioned by clues available in sober living, you were delighted from the first with the experience of intoxication. And what can you say now of the reason for early drinking, in the pleasant good old days? As you see it now, looking into the past, then bringing the past forward to the present, you drank in response to personal thirst. It happened to be alcohol, it might have been marijuana, 222's, carbromal, a tranquillizer or some offspring of mother opium. It was alcohol. It seemed to quench your personal thirst. And what was the nature of this thirst? You didn't know then, but you may know now. If you had known then, the story might well have been different. You only know that being aware *now* of the meaning of that personal thirst enables you wonderfully to support and continue sobriety as you experience it in Alcoholics Anonymous. All of you have suggested this theme in our talks.

And what was your personal thirst? Just this: to feel better, to get along better with others and to be in a genial harmony with everything in your life, and to savour a sense of adventure and mystery, not to be found in the usual sober life. But this, you may agree, is just what you had hoped of God. So drinking for the hell of it turns out to mean drinking for the Heaven of it! Pleasure drinking was a blind plunge for Paradise.

The radical difference between drinking as a way to Paradise and the genuine way to that ideal is this: as drinking continues, your reliance on alcohol grows into a sick need. Before you know the difference, in expensive experience, between hell and heaven, you likewise are unaware of the difference between human and personal. To be personal means to be free, to be creative, and to love. To be human means to be restricted, to imitate, and to conquer. The way to heaven is learning how to be personal. The way to hell is to remain human, to stay fixed at a level of growth short of what it is to be yourself. To depend on alcohol to quench personal thirst is to expect a boy to do a man's job. This is soon seen in addiction where, after all the rosy promises than drink held out to quench your thirst, you find it does just the opposite of what you originally wanted most. In addiction, you feel miserable, not better. You get along with no one, including yourself. And as for that sense of adventure and mystery, there is only a glassy stare at the ceiling and the infernal hours, ages long, in your hang-overs.

There is only one way to quench personal thirst—and that is to try to be personal. And there is only one way to find God —and that is to try to be personal. So it is that I interpret the spiritual meaning of Alcoholics Anonymous—a much debated and controversial subject in Alcoholics Anonymous circles—but much less debated than it was fifteen years ago. It is much less debated for the very practical reason that over these years you have learnt that those of us without God, without religious feeling of any sort, have not been able to stay sober.

So, in a practical sense, the spiritual is the personal. But to say this, is not to say that God or a spiritual experience is simply the highest in human achievement. No, the personal life is a life above our human desires. Were it not so, alcoholics could not remain sober. I believe it is your faith in the greater power that accounts for the soundness and continuing vitality of Alcoholics Anonymous personal therapy. The main outlines of the answer to your third question are already clear.

"How shall I maintain sobriety?"

From the third step, in my view the heart of the whole programme, you move on to the fourth, to the taking of an inventory, a moral inventory. The word "moral" indicates that you are to exercise your new-found freedom—you are to make values, to form ideals geared to the standards of your sobriety as developed in the preceding three steps. And then on to the other steps, traditions and legacy, deepening your sense of personal dignity in recognition of the rights and needs of other persons. To be personal is to be interpersonal. You need to cultivate, with the help of others, the ability to feel and understand life as they do. To begin with, this is not hard. After all, in your alcoholism, you have common ground from the very start. From there you go on to compare notes in other areas, and to respect differences where you find them, as well as to gain strength in other similarities. In this way, you grow personal, and in this way you find God, as each of you understands Him. This is not possible in drinking because the main concern of your drinking, pleasant or distressing, was a *passive* reliance on alcohol, an expectation of magic, a hope that something glorious would *happen* to you.

In sobriety there is action. And sobriety in Alcoholics

Anonymous is action that is miraculous. It is miraculous because it is wonderful beyond any dream or hope that you thought possible. It is recovery through personal thirst.

Let me illustrate briefly what it is to become personal. First of all, you are free from alcohol. And the first requisite of healthy personal growth is to be free. But this is only the basis of your freedom. After release from addiction to alcohol through the support of fellow Alcoholics Anonymous, you are free to find yourself in communication from week to week, day by day in your Alcoholics Anonymous group. You are free to express your opinions because it is the whole group who give you this freedom.

Whenever you set forth your story, you gain exercise in the discipline of freedom, so essential to personal life, and so essential to sobriety, for sobriety is life. What you say matters much less than that you are accepted. The others allow you to say what you like. Second, since you are freed from the vicious imitative pattern of addiction, you can begin to create new ways of living. It is good that Alcoholics Anonymous does not subscribe to any set pattern, chiefly because personal therapy encourages you to be yourselves. And to be personal is a creative act. To explore your lives, to seek deeper meanings of life than you ever did before, to break the fixed habits of behaviour, repetitive and viciously imitative, as in addiction—to do all this, and to find new interests or reconstruct old ones—this is truly to be creative, this is to become yourselves.

And finally, to learn that in sharing your insights with one another, to respect your fellows as well as yourselves, is not only to develop a sound therapy for alcoholism. It is also to love in the best sense of the word, when to love means to foster the freedom, the artistry and the personal dignity of each of you through your fellows. To love is to furnish the basis of all personal knowing, all communication enabling people to get well. Feeling is more dynamic, more meaningful in your therapy than information. That is why the entire programme from the fourth step to the twelfth, then through the traditions and legacy, is a programme of the discipline of feeling. A programme of action? Yes, of course, but feeling is the ground of action. The crux of the whole problem is just here. Your feelings before and during your addiction were unknown and undisciplined. That is why I call your behaviour in the old days, eventful. An event is something that happens to you. Not knowing what was happening to you, you looked to magic to improve you—magic in the form of alcohol, will power, or bits of information. Undisciplined feelings are events. Addiction is an event. Only action can cope with events. And personal life, personal growth is *action.*

Learning to love is learning to discipline your feelings by knowing them. It is to break clear from the restraints of human will, and to cherish the experience of good will. In good will you are free, and you can create, and you can love. If good will does not mean action, it is nothing. I discard the view that good will is simply an attitude of sentiment and nothing else. Ideally there can be no consideration higher than good will and the activity it generates in personal growth. There can be no human value higher than this personal value. That, in my opinion, is the meaning of Alcoholics Anonymous anonymity.

Walter Winchell once said that Alcoholics Anonymous is about as anonymous as the Brooklyn Dodgers. By this he meant that by name, by the tag of identification, that the movement has, it is indeed well known over the world. In this sense, Alcoholics Anonymous is at least as well known as the Brooklyn Dodgers. You certainly may withhold your last name and expect this will be honoured among those to whom you say you are alcoholic. If you prize your anonymity because of embarrassment to others, this is a wise gesture of respect. If you absorb the teaching of Alcoholics Anonymous rightly, you will not be ashamed that you are alcoholic. You will not be proud of the fact, but you see no more need to conceal it, as a blow to your will power, that you should conceal any other unfortunate sickness. But you conceal your last name as a member of A.A. because it is the symbol of your life in the human scene.

As I understand it, your anonymity is the foundation of your personal therapy, because *anonymity deeply means a release from the priority of human desires.* Not money, nor power, nor prestige governs either your sobriety or your Alcoholics Anonymous activity. But it is altogether commendable to strive for *personal* distinction as Alcoholics Anonymous members among alcoholics and before the general public. But such personal recognition does not require the use of last names. Everyone needs more than anything else in the world, to achieve a clear sense of personal identity —both as therapy and as a way of life. But personal distinction or personal identity is a very different goal from obsession with human prestige and human power—as a result of which someone else is always bound to suffer. Personal identity is the highest goal one can seek. When you say that anonymity should always remind you to place principles above personalities, this could mean that the principles of personal growth in freedom, creative effort, and fellowship are principles of action that are far more important than the *human* welfare of any individual member whose tendencies could get him into trouble if he went his way alone. The whole idea of this personal growth, as suggested in the programme of recovery, is based on belief in a power greater than any human agency—individual, group, gadget, medicine, or psychology. You call it God. There seems to be no better word. This power is illustrated in the practice of your belief that life is worth living as suggested in the programme of action which brings freedom in personal growth.

To sum up. I have tried to show the difference between magic and miracle, between event and action, between being human and being personal, and the importance of these distinctions in Alcoholics Anonymous therapy, from a therapeutic point of view.

Magic is an event, unaccounted for, an unreal event. A real event is something that happens. Addiction is an event.

Magic is the expectation that will power will make you sober. Being human is to live according to human desires, driven by human will, restricted, imitative, and out to conquer. It is human, and vain, to expect to cope with a personal disorder through human effort.

A miracle is an astonishing action, emerging from the concerted effort of God and person. An action is a deed done deliberately, imaginatively and with purpose. Alcoholics Anonymous is a miracle, and the work of Alcoholics Anonymous members seeking sobriety and maintaining it, is action. Being personal is to try to be free, to be creative, and to love.

The answer, then, to the first question "Why stop drinking?" is to be free. To the second question "Why did I drink in the first place?" is to be creative. To the third question "How can I maintain sobriety?" is to learn to love. Note that in the answers to these questions you have both means and end. In the first question you get your initial taste of freedom in the fact that you even ask the question! To ask the question "Why stop drinking?" is to reveal a suspension of thought in which alternate answers may be weighed. To admit powerlessness over alcohol is to achieve a freer capacity of judgment than you had ever before known. So actually you are to some extent free when you put the question, a question calling into doubt your most precious human indulgence. Thus even to put the question "Why stop drinking?" is to use as a technique what the answer furnishes as a goal—freedom, personal freedom.

In the second question, too, in seeking to answer it you *use* the answer! You are creative when you examine your lives and evoke meaning from past experience. "Why did I drink in the first place?" requires that you recall imaginatively what you were seeking many years ago. This recall you bring forward and relate to your ideals now. Personal meanings are always creative acts. So you are creative in the very act of discovering that it is the destiny of human beings to become persons, it is our destiny to create the sort of life that makes us personal. In Alcoholics Anonymous, the personal story is stressed because, I think, of the great importance of this creative effort, so necessary to your therapy, the need to cultivate the ability to express *yourselves*, and to communicate with others, on your own grounds, in your own way.

And again in the third question, "How shall I maintain sobriety?" You get much of the answer simply in asking it. You maintain sobriety in learning what it means to love. You can only well put the question among persons of good will. In waiting for the answer, you get your first exercise in the active use of an open-minded attitude. You need to be well disposed towards teachers and exemplars or there will be no answer. You learn to love as you learn to respect the views of others. And in this way you make the most of yourself to achieve the self regard you need to love others well and intelligently.

So you maintain your sobriety in the Alcoholics Anonymous programme because it is the best discipline in freedom, in creative effort, and in love that you can find anywhere. Only in a discipline that makes you free, enables you to be creative and to love, can you expect pleasurable and enduring sobriety. On sheer faith through the evidence alone of the sobriety of others, you gave Alcoholics Anonymous a try. It worked. You were astonished. Being sober was easier than you thought. You actually enjoyed it! This new found freedom was the source of tremendous support and pleasure in many areas during the early period. You had the answer to the question "Why stop drinking?"

Then after a while in Alcoholics Anonymous, you began to sense the need to go further and deeper. Freedom doesn't keep. You have to exercise your freedom if you want to preserve and enhance it.

You explore the programme, trying to remember that, above all, it is a programme of action. You go back to study your personal urges—"What did I want of life in those early buoyant years when the world looked like my oyster? Why did I drink in the first place?" And then you saw what your drinking thinking kept you from seeing for so long. Your personal thirst was vaguely crying for the effort to be yourself, to put forth the effort to find your place among fellow men, to sense the mystery and adventure that awaits any person who feels its lure. But for this you had to be a person —you had to act. You could not sit passively, ingest alcohol, and wait for this mystery and adventure to *happen* to you.

Mystery, adventure and miracles come of creative acts. You have to be creative. Now you had the answer to the second question "Why did I drink in the first place?" You drank in response to personal thirst, not knowing that alcohol for you was the opposite of what this personal thirst was craving—that drinking, in addiction, was the very opposite of what you most longed for.

In recent years up to the present, you delve further into the crucial question "How can I maintain my sobriety?" The conviction has grown that it is in Alcoholics Anonymous, nowhere else, for the long haul. Why? Because you know of no other group in the world without an angle, a human angle. And human angles destroy alcoholics, either through drink, or by obsession with human desires. Human angles also inhibit and block personal growth. If Alcoholics Anonymous ever develops an angle, that may be the beginning of the end of the greatest therapeutic agency the world has yet known. This marks the need for the greatest diligence, those who are fortunate enough to be members of Alcoholics Anonymous today—to make sure that no vested interest, no exclusive views of theology, of science or religious doctrine ever holds sway over Alcoholics Anonymous, to make sure that there is no exclusive screening of members, that no alcoholics who suffer be barred from Alcoholics Anonymous therapy.

But a purpose is not an angle, when it is a purpose above human defects. And the only purpose of Alcoholics Anonymous is to stop drinking, and to achieve sobriety. This, you find, is to try to become a person. I honestly do not know of any therapy in which this ideal is more clear than in Alcoholics Anonymous. To strive for the good will, a definite notch above all our human desires, the good will in which your therapy and your anonymity flourish, is to sense all the mystery and adventure there is time for. And it is to learn how to love as only persons can.

To you, then, the Alcoholics Anonymous programme is not a denial of personal thirst. On the contrary, it is a quenching of it. It is the programme of action enabling you to be or to become personal. To do this is to make what contact you can with the power greater than ourselves, the source of your freedom, your art of living, and your love. As to death, it is the final event. It couldn't matter less in a programme of action, except that you will want to put it off as long as possible while sobriety is as pleasurable as it is.

It is better to be free than happy, because you can only really know how to be happy if you are first free. But to be free you must have to act. And Alcoholics Anonymous is a programme of action, or it is nothing.

8.

THE GIFTS OF ADVENTURE

THIRST takes the problem drinker on his two-way journey, the one inward to himself, the other outward to persons, places and things, and then home again. Both quests are vital. To neglect one at the expense of the other is to court a half-truth, a half-solution that may well end in disaster.

Personal thirst struggles to satisfy itself. If we fail to yield to its tendency, the dynamic activity through self to others, back to self and again outward, ceaselessly tracing the movement of a ring, we live as though lost, and our personal thirst goes unquenched only to be lured into the trap of an addiction, or an obsession.

The inward search alone may be seen in the alcoholic who stays sober painfully in pious efforts of will powered stress. Ultimately, he breaks because he cannot, by himself, stand the strain any longer. He gets drunk, in rebellion against his limping conscience, a power unequal to the burden of his silent guilt. Alone too long, he is crippled by his self-righteous ideals.

Action among others, with no thought or feeling for inward turmoil, may be seen in the alcoholic who stays sober uneasily on the quicksand of his unstudied impulses. He skirts the error of the first fellow who puts all his faith in will power and shuns the help of others. But, over-zealous about the success of those who are sober, he identifies with them blindly, takes no thought of his own identity, makes gods of his models, and when they tumble—for tumble they will, in one way or another—he also falls. He feels deflated, saddened by the collapse of his gods. Before long, he is drunk. A perfectionist, his dismay grows with increasing evidence of human weakness in his models.

The lone alcoholic has had too much of himself and too little of others. The social alcoholic has had too much of others and too little of himself. Neither of them qualifies as an adventurer. The first stays too near home. The second wanders too far from home, he forgets where it is. The first fails to respond to the main lure of adventure, to fare forth into strange places. The second gets lost, and unlike a real adventurer, knows not how to take bearings and begin again.

There are three gifts the adventurer is glad to accept, for they bring him not only practical gain but deep pleasure of a lasting kind. Still, the gifts themselves are more important than the uses made of them. They are the gift of grace, the gift of peace and the practice of empathy for its own sake.

Grace

Both the inward search and the outward foray are needed to give meaning to each other, to bring adventure in sobriety to the alcoholic. It is together that these two features of adventure yield what the alcoholic longs for, and must have, above all. That is *loss of the desire to drink*. This is the first great gift that comes to the alcoholic in recognition of his efforts, and the first real sign that he is finding adventure in sobriety. Grace, too, it could be called. As an abstract word, it is hard to understand. We speak of the grace of God, but with how much meaning? Only when we feel specific situations, does its meaning emerge with life. We know what grace is when we appreciate a swimmer's form, or a skater's style. In the same way, we can, if we wish, appreciate the grace of an alcoholic who has lost the desire to drink. It is a gift, because it comes to him through others, as much as from himself. He has made, and continues to make, the essential personal effort. Without that, there could be no gift, for no gift at all deserves the name, if it is not graciously and actively received. So we can say that loss of the desire to drink is a gift of grace.

Loss of the desire to drink is felt when the alcoholic sees, in his own way, that to be obsessed by human goals is no substitute for alcohol.

For obsession with human goals—money, power, sex— generates those feelings of resentment and self-pity, false pride and sick fear, which make the alcoholic over tense and strained. These tense feelings are certain to invade and grip him, if, in his sober efforts, he fails to sense the value of personal goals, and fails to pursue them.

Loss of the desire to drink, a gift of grace, comes when the alcoholic sees the futility of those over tense feelings and the principle of action within them, and relaxes in a new desire, the desire to abandon all hope of recovery through pursuit of human goals alone. In this relaxation he loses the desire to drink, and begins gracefully and easily to receive the creative rewards of sobriety—the gifts of adventure itself.

So this first gift, important though it is, because it is not final and has to be received daily in continuous adventure, is not all that rewards the sober alcoholic.

A new world is opened up to him in the knowledge he absorbs daily in the sobriety adventure. Within sobriety, heaped into the area made vacant by loss of the desire to drink, the marvellous absence of the old painful craving, are the gifts of adventure itself. In the last three chapters, adventure has been studied chiefly as a means, a technique.

But once it is well sensed that change is in the very essence of life, it becomes easy to see that means and end, or technique and goal, are interchangeable. The qualities of real adventure bring sobriety, and sobriety becomes its own reward when the adventure that strengthens it becomes worthwhile in itself. If the means to an end are a drudge, the value of that end is questionable. So we stake our claims on adventure itself, believing that, given a chance, the lure of adventure will yield priceless gifts in a new way of life.

Once more we need to stress the difference between event and action, between event and adventure, for adventure is action. An event is something over which we have no control. It happens, as a rainstorm does, or as an addiction befalls its unfortunate victim. An adventure is an action, whose results we cannot foresee, but on which we embark deliberately in the faith that it is good. Within it are stirring incidents full of surprise and born of wonder. But an adventure, as distinct from an event, is an action guided by the overall purpose of the courage to be oneself in a daring enterprise, in which one is free to engage. In adventure, then, there is courage, readiness, deliberate engagement; yet none of these obstructs the wonder, surprise, hazard or pleasure of the stirring incidents which occur *within* the adventure.

The ideal aim, in the sobriety adventure, is to make sober living an action as natural and spontaneous as addiction was an event. Just as a practising alcoholic will drink anything available, if he needs a drink, so the well-recovered man has no choice but to stay sober. Within sobriety, there is ample room for the exercise of freedom in a thousand different ways, and the peace he has earned by the conviction now that there can be no choice between drinking and being sober, will reveal the motions of grace. He will act as naturally by the ideals of sober behaviour as he once easily gave himself to the event of addiction. In ideal recovery, in a genuine adventure in sobriety, he knows that controlled drinking and being sober are not two actions between which a choice can be made, because no problem drinker can choose to do the impossible. To drink is to die, even if physically he should linger for years. The ideally free man can do nothing but pursue sobriety. He can do nothing else. He will pursue it as the bee goes to the honey, as naturally, as gracefully, as serenely.

Let us observe some of the characters we have met in this book, and let them speak from their experiences.

Peace

"The alcoholic wants the same wonderful feeling of peace that we get in sobriety," said Sully. "But he just does not know how to go about it. The mean, short-lived peace of a pass-out is preceded and followed by hell, confusion, pain and misery. And he can't even enjoy the brief span of a drugged peace because he is not conscious. At best it is the kind of peace that is death, if he's lucky enough not to have nightmares in his sleep."

Arthurs did not get it all, but some of it came through. As Sully went on, it became clearer.

"In spite of all this," he said, "the alcoholic longs for peace. It is this longing that the practising alcoholic and the recovered person share. You see, the genuine peace of sobriety is what the alcoholic really wants, once he realizes that it can be lively and enduring. Nothing endures when you're drinking, nothing."

"We need not be afraid of people. Why should we? Others, like us, have their troubles too. Actually, your sense of peace is deepened and strengthened by having a rich assortment of friends. I visit the jail where I was once an overnight guest, and get a real thrill if a contact there works out well. I was protected so much as a boy that it is a wonderful experience to move around freely in the world, without fear, to like people for what they are, and to do for them what they will let you do. You can't help anyone, if he does not want to be helped."

And Arthurs then felt that he still had much to do. He knew that he had a way with people, but that he would never rest until he had done all he could to learn what his friends were helping him to understand. Arthurs is completely himself, and has nothing to hide, only more to find. Natural, spontaneous, he gives and gets pleasure in being himself. His wisdom, which earns the respect of all who know him, springs from the events and actions of real life. He is not perplexed by the knowledge of books and abstract thought.

What are the gifts of adventure in the creative sobriety of Arthurs? They centre round the deep pleasure radiated to others from the man himself, in being himself. The courage, the humour, the comfort, the open hand of fellowship, the amazing ability to enter into the thoughts and feelings of those around him, to give himself without stint, and above all, to be himself—these gifts make up the pleasure that Arthurs gives to others.

Arthurs does not have Ward's problem—a complex struggle to be himself. But from Ward, and others like him, Arthurs can learn that fellow problem drinkers have to grow in their own way, though they may be slow in gaining strength to stand on their own feet. But he knew, as well as Ward did, that being sober was downright practical. His income soared, life was better at home, and he was able to provide better for himself and the family. Arthurs has the gift of grace—loss of the desire to drink. The old craving has gone, and in its place, he savours the pleasure of knowing, liking and helping fellow alcoholics and having their affection in return. And he has begun to appreciate that gift his friend Sully talks about—peace. He is well on the way, for the gift of peace is impossible without the gift of grace. And Arthurs enjoys being sober, he takes deep pleasure in the great variety of actions that sobriety now releases him to do. This pleasure consolidates the gift of grace. The more he enjoys his sobriety, the more certain he becomes that he has lost the desire to drink, the more pleased to feel that he really wants to be sober. Why should he ever imagine in his wildest dreams that a drink could do anything for him now? What more could a man want?

He thought often of Sully and his deep feelings about the prize of peace. He wished he could share his serenity, and his fine thoughts. And Milton too, had something he longed to share. Arthurs was a sensible man, he did not want to be other than he was, but he wondered often about the real goal of sobriety. They talked much of peace. Did they really feel it in themselves, Sully and Milton?

Milton once said, "There are three objectives in a problem drinker's life—surrender, change of attitude towards self and others, and a contented sobriety." He knew the words. But what did they mean?

Arthurs was sure he knew what surrender was—he was through with alcohol; it was not a truce, not a patched-up deal, it was all over. No choice now. He just never thought of taking a drink. As long as he had his friends to keep the fact of surrender central in his thoughts, he was safe. And he knew, too, that his surrender to a sober life had to be renewed every day.

And there was no doubt about his change of attitude. He well understood that the way he lived, and felt, searching in himself and in others for the richer life of fellowship, was an attitude he never suspected was possible in his drinking days.

And he also knew much about contented sobriety. Arthurs could say he was happy now, as happy as any man is entitled to be. When, ever, in his drinking days, did he have such friends, friends he had longed to have all his life? And when, ever, did he have so many pleasant hours day after day, made all the better for his belief that this pleasure had a good and valuable place in the meaning of life for him now?

There was something in the "peace" Sully talked about that led him further. "What a wonderful discovery," he said, "genuine peace, the peace of sobriety." The word "endure" kept ringing in his ears. "Nothing endures when you're drinking, nothing." This he understood better when he explained that peace must last, or it is nothing, it has to last from day to day. Arthurs had to relate everything he heard to a personal experience. When he drank, the bottle was full, half full, then empty and he too was full, half full, and then empty. But now, that is all over. It could not last, if he still had a glimmer of desire to go on living. Then he met Sully, Milton, and many others who helped him to become sober. He had it! The bottle was full, half full, then empty, but nothing like the emptiness in himself. Now, it's different. "Sober, I give something away," he pondered, "and it gets bigger, the more I give. I help a fellow, for his sake, and I feel the peace Sully talks about. And there's never too much of this, it just goes on and on. It lasts. The more you give, the more you get. But it's strange, what you feel is not a greedy feeling. It's nice, but it is not selfish like I used to be. It's . . . it's . . . well, it's just peaceful, I guess."

He recalled the words of Milton. "We want contented sobriety, yes, but we need to know that it's better to be free than happy." So you don't have peace just being happy. Was that the trouble with the boys who complained of being jittery and shaky when they stopped drinking? They were trying to do it all at once, hoping the world would fall in their lap just because they were sober. They were sorry for themselves because they couldn't be happy all at once. They expected sobriety to give them what they once got from alcohol, a feeling of pleasure. But the real prize of sobriety is being free. And a man might have to work long and hard being free before he could expect to be happy. It was like this with Wendell, a fellow alcoholic he had long respected. He had a chronic tremor of the hands, a tremor that persisted for five years of sobriety. He still had it, but he never complained. To watch him drinking coffee might lead a stranger to believe that Wendell had just come off a binge. And Clemens, he recalled, was living with chronic pain in his stomach, and lost his only son only two years ago. Yet neither Wendell nor Clemens would think of drinking as a way out of pain or sorrow.

Arthurs learns from Wendell and Clemens that to know peace is to accept the tragic side of life along with its joy, to accept sorrow for what it is without flinching. He knows himself what it is to have suffered, and from this he can build the hope and courage to do what he can, within his limits. He can do this, because he already did it when, powerless over alcohol, he found sobriety among others like him.

Being free of alcoholism, *at any cost*, is a prize far greater, more precious, than any pleasant feeling or happy time that drinking, at its best, could ever yield.

This belief, worked out in Arthur's own way, brought him peace. It is an acceptance of sober living, an unconditional surrender to life, whether tragic or joyful. And on this ultimate ground, sobriety ceases to be a strain. Being sober is a strain only as long as the alcoholic suspects that he may be able to drink on certain occasions, or as long as he supposes he can still choose between drinking and not drinking. Arthurs became ready for the great gift of peace when he felt deeply within that "There is no choice now."

What led Arthurs to his belief "There is no choice now"? How is this in accord with Milton's words "It's better to be free than happy"? If it is better to be free than happy, what of the terrific final character of the words "no choice now"? Where there is no choice, there is no freedom.

There is no problem here if we recall the distinction between event and *action*. We cannot choose, in the midst of the greatest freedom, between an event and an action. An alcoholic cannot choose to drink in a controlled pattern. It is just impossible. We can only reasonably speak of choice when it is possible to put the alternatives into action. But you cannot put an event into action. If you do, it *becomes* an action. But drinking for an alcoholic is an event that cannot be put into action, because an action is a deliberate planned type of behaviour. If an alcoholic drinks, and does so deliberately, he will sooner or later be seized and overcome by the event of compulsive drinking—addiction. And within addiction, there is no action, there is no deliberate making of choices. Both the addict's drinking behaviour and his apparent sober stretches are dictated by the crippling need for alcohol, by the event of addiction.

Arthurs, through his natural intelligence and the lessons of example, saw that there was no choice, when his insight grasped the whole problem of alcoholism. As long as he hesitated between the desire to drink and the desire to be sober

—the pattern of his behaviour years ago—he never escaped the dangers and troubles of addiction. To choose, to deliberate between the two, was to put them on the same level.

No one, except a madman, deliberates between driving over a cliff and staying safely on the highway. To be hurtled through the air to his death is an *event* which befalls the tragic victim who drives over the cliff. To drive safely on the highway is an *action*, because in acting one is an agent of his own behaviour. Events may befall him, but he exercises all the controls within himself by wanting to live. The man who *acts* will have richer life than he who leaves everything to chance.

So in desiring a drink, in yielding to it, the problem drinker is plunged into the event of addiction, over which he has no control at all. But in desiring to be sober, he is led to an *action*, for sober living is action.

The problem drinker, then, cannot regard the desire to drink on the same level with the desire to be sober. The alcoholic's desire to drink is an impulsive trend towards the *event* of death; the desire to be sober is a deliberate desire for the *action* of life. After a problem drinker understands his original personal thirst, and knows that drinking cannot quench it, there is no choice between wanting to drink and wanting to be sober. The way now for an alcoholic is clear. Either he wants to be sober, or he dies. So he wants to be sober. When this logic runs deep in his feelings and in his way of life, he receives the gift of peace. The gift of grace must precede the gift of peace. With the first, the alcoholic loses the desire to drink. With the second, he is prepared for any experience life may offer.

Arthurs had pondered the word "endure" in Sully's view of peace, and learned its meaning in the life of two of his friends. Peace has that enduring quality that all human beings strive for, but alcoholics seem to need it more desperately than do most people. It has that quality of permanence which sustains and nourishes any experience at all, tragic as well as joyful, dutiful as well as carefree; love in giving and receiving, love in respecting the distance between oneself and another. Peace endures, it lasts, it suffers, it enjoys. It is an art of suffering as well as an art of creating, and because it is, the tragedies of life do not destroy or embitter, but chasten and bring light. It is through the gift of peace that the alcoholic's adventure in sobriety brings him enduring value, lasting life. Within it there is no room for boredom, fear, the miseries of addiction, or death. It does not come at once. It is gradually earned. It is the lasting gift of rich adventure, and with it the problem drinker can forever relish the actions of his life, past, present and to come.

But grace and peace in personal life are not without their price. The ideal adventurer in sobriety strengthens his courage in resisting the obsessions of money, power and sex and all the feelings that accompany them—fear, hate, arrogance, vanity. He strives to be himself, to become himself, to be honest with himself. This he does with the courage and the imagination to put himself in the other fellow's place in order to understand the other, and to do for the other as he has been done by. To become himself, a person in his own right, strong enough to stay sober, he will use empathy to guard against the obsessions of money, power and sex. Because he is human, he will want money, power and sex like any other human being. But he learns that it is more important to be free than to have money, to create than to wield power, and to love than to possess or be loved. The fact is that unless he is free, unless he can create, unless he can love, he will make no productive use of money, or power or sex.

There is no place, in the ideal sobriety adventure, for fighting addiction. To fight addiction is the same useless process as the vain attempt to choose between drinking and not drinking. The uninformed alcoholic fights addiction in two ways: (a) by desiring to drink, and (b) by using will power to stay sober. In both, there is submission, but no surrender; the desire to drink still competes with the desire to be sober. In desiring a drink, the drinker is still deluded by the hope that he can handle alcohol. In using will power, he is afraid, he is controlled by censors outside himself, and this fear can lead straight to the bottle. He rebels against himself, he is in conflict. And in this conflict, by chance, he may not drink for a time. But at last, worn out by the struggle, he will have a relapse.

The genuine adventurer in sobriety does not fight addiction. He uses it. There are two main uses of addiction, the recall of its misery, and the present meaning of the pleasant drinking occasions long ago. The misery is his assurance that drinking no longer serves any purpose in his life. The pleasant occasions, forever lost to him now, yet reveal to him the meaning of his original personal thirst. He drank at first to feel better, to be in harmony with people, and to savour adventure and mystery not found in the routine of human desires.

Empathy

Throughout this book, the technique of empathy in adventure, in the self search and in the search of others, was studied as a means to sobriety. Here we shall look at it as a goal in itself, the third great gift of adventure. It is a value in its own right, yielding truth, beauty and goodness—all that any person can ever hope to strive for beyond the pull of human desires. To be able to practise empathy is to know what it is to be honest with yourself and others, to learn the truth, to feel the beauty of life in its harmonies of joy and sorrow, and to become a better person in the search for more than the life of human desires can yield.

Though empathy is useful in gaining sobriety, it has even greater value in its own right.

If you are well, see and feel clearly, and you are not distracted by anxiety, by the pressure or prejudice of human needs, you have the first requisite enabling you to know a person. You appreciate this person as an identity against the background of everything else as "the other". He is *one* person, an identity in his own right, not to be explained away by his sex drives, his desires for power, or his social background. He has an identity of his own. Satisfied that he is *one* person, you now begin to know that he is one *person*. You explore his capacity for freedom, you are interested in the unique pattern of his acts and feelings, and you feel his love in the way he respects you for what you are.

But it is hard to see him in this way if you do not have *your* sense of identity, *your* feeling that you, too, are a person like him, though different, clearly, in the unique pattern that makes you what you are, as his unique pattern makes him what he is. The more confused you are by fear, by class, by prejudice, by sick need, or by human desire, the less able you are to see this person in his own right, and the more likely you are to see him as a reflection of your own limits, fears, and lack of integrity. Of this, however, you may not be aware. When you become aware of what you are, and your vision clears, the other person radiates his identity for what he really is.

Arthurs is a man easy to know because he inspires in us no fear, no need to become conscious of position, no desire to exploit him for a practical purpose. He helps us to know him because there is no sign of fear, class, or ulterior design in his attitude towards us, and we feel creative stirrings in his humour and kindness. Once you know him, you do not forget him. His interest in us stimulates us to be well disposed towards him. The interplay of this good will tends to compose us, as we relax and become ourselves in our relations with him. As we respond to him, he, too, enjoys a better sense of ease, and we all communicate without strain. Mutual self-respect thrives. In this way, both personal acquaintance, and the harmony of personal composure felt in one another, are achieved in one and the same act of mutual empathy. Truth and beauty are two facets of one action. The third facet is goodness. But it is not the goodness of a code of morals or a system of ethics. It is that basic goodness from which *any* code or system of values may arise.

By goodness we mean integrity. First there was identity, then harmony and form in the unique pattern of any person. Now we have integrity in knowing and respecting personal identity and harmony in oneself and others, and behaving in a way to show that we place personal integrity higher than any human goal.

The dynamic vital feeling which makes possible our personal identity, harmony, and integrity is simply good will.

Our personal identity each of us gets from the other in the way we are disposed towards one another. Our composure, or harmony of feeling and action within each and in one another, also depends upon our disposition. We cannot remain composed if we are hostile. And our integrity cannot be well known to us except in the way we feel about one another. Thus the feeling common to the three main qualities of being a person is good will, not an emotion, but a feeling of love and respect for the other as for oneself. Love, in the common ground I share with you; respect, in the distance required between us to insure to each his identity, harmony and integrity, and the freedom that each of us, in this relation, can achieve.

Good will is an ideal beyond human desires and hates. It is the ground of empathy, though it is reached only with much practice and deliberate effort, from the discipline and control of desire and hate—identification and resistance. Good will is the source of your freedom.

We have to get beyond desire, for desire urges us to possess or dominate rather than to know, and beyond hate because hate blocks knowledge and beauty, blinding us to the perception of integrity. Where there is hate, it conceals the person to be known, felt and appreciated. We cannot "see" a person if hate stands in the way, nor can we know him if we control or possess him, for to control or possess him is to rob him of his right to be a person, free to act as he likes. We have to reach a state of *wonder*, where we are raised above the tangle of human desire and hate, to feel the good will requisite to the act of empathy. Desire and hate are human emotions, movements towards and away from a human being, in the interests of self centred power, prestige or sex. Because all persons are human before they become personal, there will be much ado about money, power and sex in the life of any person, and there will be much devotion to science and the uses we make of it, because science is the effort to control nature for human purposes and needs. But beyond human desire, and science, and in harmony with them, there is the personal sense of wonder, in which we neither think nor feel nor act in the interests of any special human need, but of them all and more when we want to share and create new experiences with others, not control them, and to grow more free in our behaviour as persons.

Our sense of wonder is basic to the experience of mystery and adventure. It yields beauty because it is free of the dangers of addiction which threaten and obscure the truth about ourselves, and free of the lure of obsessions with money, power and sex, the great goals of human desire.

Control of the other is the aim of human desire. Kinship with the other is the experience of wonder. The tendency of the desire to control the other is to stifle and restrict him, and to keep him from growing in his own right. The tendency of the experience of wonder is to nourish good will and to foster personal growth both in the other and in oneself. The spirit of control over others is competition, domination, victory. The spirit of good will is sharing strength in common ground and achieving peace in mutual personal integrity. It is from good will that empathy arises. The only competition there is in good will is the effort to improve oneself, to beat one's own record, in the struggle to be a person. No one else gets hurt. But ceasing to compete with others does not mean that we become soft and grovelling. On the contrary, we do nothing but grow strong when we share experiences in team effort, respect one another in the process, and cease to waste energy in fighting to isolate ourselves as superior and apart.

Milton told Arthurs that the most rewarding experience of his life was that he did not feel obliged to compete any more. The fears of failure, and the desire for prestige, rather than genuine worthy practice, had formerly overshadowed any real merit there had been in his business life. "I realize now," he said, "that my best efforts come, not from trying to be better than the other fellow, not from trying to appear better than I am, but just by doing the best I can and trying to improve on that when I do it again. And I am astonished to find how much I can learn from people who have no pretensions at all, people willing to tell me what they know for what it is worth. The best way I can be myself is to share with others the things that matter most."

Arthurs marvelled at the wonderful feeling that was not like anything he ever felt before. Like Milton, he was astonished and impressed by this sense of wonder and the way it made him feel. It was not painful, and it was not pleasurable in any special physical way. It was not selfish, it was not unselfish. It was "nice", he said, but it was also "strange" and mysterious, because he had no words to describe it, except to imagine that it was what Sully called "peaceful".

Now Arthurs felt this peace through empathy, inspired to strive for it in the interests of his sobriety, and the sobriety of those he helped. But he was thrilled to learn that, besides the sobriety goal, there was deep lasting value in the way he reached that goal, a way of knowing people that was its own reward, not to be restricted to the sobriety goal, but a whole way of life, whether practised among alcoholics, or any other group of people. This way of knowing, empathy, is what enables Arthurs to be himself as a person.

Any tendency or attitude in our training that keeps us from being ourselves is an obstacle in the way of personal knowing. Every limit on our freedom, on our urge to create, on our capacity for love, makes us less able to appreciate similar needs for freedom, creation and love in others.

The practice of empathy for its own sake enables us to understand the meaning of human behaviour directly in personal knowing. And it is within empathy that actions speak for themselves. The meaning of life is thus in the practice of empathy, not a consequence or effect of it.

A person speaks for himself, if you are released from the urge to control him in a scientific technique, in business, or in any other human form of conquest. Hate, for example, a formidable block to personal knowing, can only arise within human desire—the need for money, power and sex. This danger is removed if you deliberately resolve to know him as *you* want to be known for what you are, by persons you respect. When you know him through goodwill, above the interests of control, use or amusement, you are in a state of wonder, not desire. And wonder is a personal feeling, not a human emotion.

In this state of wonder, in becoming acquainted with the other person, there is much you have to imagine him to be, because you go beyond ready-made controls and the habits of prejudice or custom. You are both on your own.

There is more to say about wonder than the limits of these talks can embrace. Here we content ourselves with its relation to the theme—adventure in empathy, in response to personal thirst.

There can be real pleasure in travel, but without the capacity for wonder we cannot imagine what it is to feel and think like our fellow man. Without wonder we will only be tourists, not adventurers. In genuine adventure, we do not move feverishly from place to place, betraying boredom in our anxiety to keep to a schedule, made out long in advance of the excursion.

The pleasure of travel, of any adventure, gets lost when we tend to regard leisure as we do business or science, looking for results and effects, and neglecting to savour the experience itself for its adventure value, for the zest of life that only wonder can yield. It would be wonderful if we could enjoy our work as genuine adventurers do their leisure, rather than to order our leisure in the tense cause-effect fashion of modern work.

Wonder is the ideal personal experience in which good will flourishes and makes empathy all that it can be. In an act of mutual empathy between you and me, each of us permits the other to speak for himself, to extend his freedom, to deepen his identity. Each of us becomes himself, speaks, feels and acts for himself—doing the same for the other, at the same time. In this relation, there is mutual good will, but there is also wonder and mystery—the sense of something more still to be felt and known, and of something more *never* to be felt and known as we now feel and know.

In wonder, then, we are urged to deepen our personal experiences and to relax in the peace which comes with our acceptance of limits, of the mystery beyond the area of human control.

To cultivate our sense of wonder will be to make us well disposed towards one another, and also well composed in the deepening of personal integrity. Within this interpersonal relation, the empathic act can flourish at its best. Besides the useful advantages that empathy brings, besides the enjoyment it radiates, there is the value it has in and for itself. In empathy, experienced for its own value, there is no fear of success or failure because we are not corrupted or stunted by exclusive concern for the control or use of others, we do not centre our attention on the worth of power or prestige, we are not overcome by the conceit of sexual mastery. Where there is excessive fear, there is anxiety, hate. And hate, we have seen, is a formidable threat to truth. But in empathy, for itself, where we are elevated above the human desire for power and control, we are released from the human tendency to hate and fear, from the impending threats of success and failure, of prestige and rejection. Thus released, we are well into the mature experience of personal life, the pursuit of fellowship for its own sake.

Empathy we now recognize as the central activity of mature personal life. It is grounded in the good will made possible by the sense of wonder and it proceeds to its goal, freedom in fellowship. That is the meaning of empathy for its own sake. It needs no other justification. It is useful in recovery from alcoholism, in creating sobriety, because it is primarily true, consistent and sound in its own right. Its universal scope as a way of life embraces the problem of alcoholism, or drug addiction, of the various obsessions, along with thousands of other personal problems, and offers the techniques of recovery to anyone suffering from a personal disorder.

It is natural that we first appreciate the practice of empathy as a useful technique in achieving freedom from alcoholism. But if we wish to move from the treatment of our problem to an enjoyment of our health, we shall not rest until we experience genuine adventure in life-long sobriety.

To do this will be at last to recognize that empathy is a personal way of life valuable in itself, beyond the sobriety goal.

The central aim of these talks has been to show that sobriety can be a thrilling adventure, positive and creative, rather than just a state of abstinence from alcohol. This adventure, within oneself, and among others, brings three gifts—grace, peace and fellowship. Grace is loss of the desire to drink, and a deepening desire for sobriety. Peace is an enduring and lively acceptance of life, whatever life may offer—beautiful, ugly, joyful, tragic, and a constant search for the truth, whatever it may be. To be at peace is to know that it is better to be free than happy. Peace is felt when we are released from addictions and obsessions, from the pull of human desires, and become free for the experience of wonder and mystery in which good will may flourish. And empathy for itself becomes daily practice when we seek fellowship and the personal freedom it fosters as a way of life. For empathy, grounded in good will, is a personal relation in which we find genuine love for others in the identification of common needs, and in the feeling of respect for others when we differ from them. Such love and mutual respect make up the meaning of fellowship, and within it we give personal freedom to one another. This is what it is to be a person, and this is the whole aim and purpose of human life in its best and highest form.

INDEX

Abstinence: inadequate as treatment, 37, 107-108; total, necessity of, 65, 78.

Acceptance, of self: in recovery, 98-99; necessity for, 116; as second step, 117.

Action: in sobriety, 217-219; from insight to, 240-282; allied to theory in sobriety, 316-320.

Addict, drug: treatment of, 24-25; genesis of, 26-32; social attitude toward, 34-35; purposes of, 36; and "devotion" to drug, 50; and search for personal freedom, 50-53; personal treatment of, 53-58.

Addiction: three classes of, 3; to morphine and heroin, 6-7; initial narratives of, 7-12; the "experimental" stage of, 18; genesis of, 26-27; scientific approach to, 35-37; mystery of, 36-53; as personal disorder, 44-46; three facts about, 49; negative estimate of, 50; as "devotion", 50; failure of negative approach to, 51; treatment of, 53-58; as magic, 321-322.

Adjustment: in personal growth, 143-144.

Adler, Alfred: and A.A., 137, 139.

Adventure: recovery as, 186-190, 220; gifts of, 340-359.

Aggression: as inducement to addiction, 25-29; in alcoholic, 83-84; to others and self, 85-86.

Agnosticism: and A.A., 135-136.

Alcohol: as means of finding self, 3; as addicting depressant, 6; drinking of, 60-66; as outlet, 61. (See Alcoholism and Drinking.)

"Alcohol Explored": by E. M. Jellinek and H. W. Haggard, 79.

Alcoholics: genesis of, 63; as minority group, 63; chronic, 65; drinking pattern of, 67-79; personality disturbances of, 67-68; fantasies of, 68; infantility of, 68; eight types of, 73-77; personal qualities of, 80-93; as dependent persons, 81; loneliness of, 82; as loving persons, 84; idealism of, 84-87; impulsiveness of, 87-88; intolerance of, 88; wishful thinking of, 89; "little dictator" in, 90-93; insight of, 100-108; mother-image and, 101-102; marriage and, 101-102; emotional immaturity of, 136-137; opposite to real selves, 153-154; six general tendencies in, 160-167, 252-253; women as, 253-272.

Alcoholics Anonymous: 34, 39, 42, 48, 52, 88, 110-111, 121-142, 143-147, 255-256, 269, 292, 305; success of, 121; twelve steps of, 122-129; four main ideas of, 122; and religion, 125-129; as personal fellowship, 126; spiritual reward of, 129-130; twelve traditions of, 131-133; anonymity of, 132, 335; religion, science, and, 133-142; clinical view of, 316-339; miracle of, 320-339.

Alcoholism: need for understanding of, 64; conditions engendering, 64-65; drinking pattern in, 67-79; eight types of, 73-77; as path to suicide, 77; physical explanation of, 77-78; sociological explanation of, 78, negative approach to, 112; and pleasure drinking, 152-153; five phases of, 154; six general tendencies in, 160-167, 252; as thirst, 170-187, 190-193; as symptom of disorder, 187; hopelessness of curing, 226-227; in women, 253-272; as slow death, 284.

Alexander the Great: as alcoholic, 104.

Amphetamine: see Dexedrine, Benzedrine.

Anxiety: free-floating, in alcoholic, 159; in dependent alcoholic, 161.

Aristotle: and formal cause, 45; and A.A., 140.
Arrogance: in alcoholic, 94-96.
Ataraxia: and tranquillizers, 2.
Atascadero State Hospital, Calif.: v.
Atheism: and A.A., 135-136.
Attention-absorbing: in recovery, 103.
Attention - getting: in alcoholic, 102 - 103.
Augustine, Saint: and time, 45; and A.A., 141.

Barbiturates: in initial addiction, 9-10; addiction to, 19-24.
Beatniks: and marihuana, 5-6.
Behaviour, human: dynamic nature of, 38-42.
Bell Clinic: v.
Bell, R. G.: v.
Benzedrine: 3-4.
Bergson, Henri: and time, 45.
Bingham, John: v.
Blame: alcoholic's shifting of, 294-297; as self-defence, 295.
British Journal of Addiction, 35, 59.
Bromides: addiction to, 19-20.
Brookside Clinic: v.
Buddhism, Zen: doctrine of, 1-2.
Byron, George Gordon Lord: as alcoholic, 104.

Cabot, John: and discovery, 217.
Calvin, John: and A.A., 141.
Carbromal: as addicting substance, 330.
Cause-effect: breakdown of, in alcoholics, 171.
Chloral hydrate: in withdrawal, 11; addiction to, 19-20.
Chlorpromazine: as addicting tranquillizer, 21.
Christ: and temptation, 184-185, 236.
Christianity: and A.A., 140-141.
Clinician: attitude and techniques of, 37-42, 46-48.
Cocaine: 3-4; in initial addiction, 9-11.
Codeine: as addicting depressant, 6-7.

Competitiveness: in women alcoholics, 257, 260, 263-265.
Compulsion: in alcoholism, 65, 69-70, 165-166; through physical discomfort, 70.
Conflict, basic: in alcoholic, 158-159.
Cook, R. H.: v.
"Cool" set: aims of, 1-2.
Crane, Stephen: "George's Mother", 179-180.
Craving, personal: in drug addict, 26, 30-31.
Creativeness: in sobriety, 200-209, 214-215, 240, 244-250.
Crichton Royal Hospital: v.
Cure for alcoholism: hopelessness of, 226-227.

Defectiveness: of alcoholic's thinking, 167, 299.
Defensiveness: in alcoholic, 94-96, 101.
Demerol: as addicting depressive, 6-7.
Dependence: of alcoholics, 81-84, 161, 295; shift of, from people to alcohol, 157, 296.
Depressants: varieties and effects of, 5-7.
DeRopp, Robert S.: "Drugs and the Mind," 35, 58n.
Devotion, compulsive, of addict, 50; free, of religionist, 50.
Dewey, John: in spiritual experience, 133.
Dexedrine: 3-4.
Dilaudid: as addicting depressant, 6-7.
Diorin: as addicting depressant, 6-7.
Discipline: in society, 62.
Dislocation: social, of alcoholic, 154.
Dodgers, Brooklyn: 334.
Doing: positive, in recovery, 119.
Drinking: reasons for, 60-66; sensible and social, 62-63; as a problem, 63; alcoholic's pattern of, 67-79; from physical discomfort, 70; alone, 71; three sets of facts about, 151-152; and loss of freedom, 153-154; pleasure, 154-155; problem, 155-

157; resistant, 158; resigned, 158; helpless, 160; six general tendencies in, 160-167, 252-253; as thirst, 170-187, 190-193, early, 178-181; as slow death, 284.
"Drinking And Intoxication," by R.G. McCarthy (ed.): 59n.
"Drug Addict As A Patient, The," by Marie Nyswander: 24-26, 58n.
"Drugs And The Mind," by Robert S. DeRopp: 35, 58n.
Dynamicism: in sobriety, 215-217.

Education: in prevention of addiction, 52.
Einstein, Albert: as artist, 308.
Elation: in idealistic alcoholic, 164-165.
Emotions: alcoholics' immaturity of, 77, 82-84.
Empathy: techniques of, 31-34; and recovery of addict, 45-48; 213-214, 303-306; danger inherent in, 45; in promoting freedom, 56-58; and non-addictive problems, 58; index of, 291-292; in adventure, 351-359.
Epicureans: and ataraxia, 2; and A.A., 140.

Fantasy: in alcoholic, 103-104, 167.
Father-image: in women alcoholics, 257-258, 264.
Fear: addiction as pattern of, 51, 95, 100-106.
Fleming, Sir Alexander: and discovery: 217.
Follow-up: of withdrawal, 37-42; results during, 42; surrender and the, 109-120; four phases of, 112-113.
Foreign: fear of the, 298-299.
Francis, Saint: and A.A., 144.
Freedom: addiction as loss of, 50-52, 158-159, 293; main goal of recovery, 51-53, 231-233; in sobriety, 240, 243-244, 284; practice of, 283-315.
Freud, Sigmund: 269; and A.A., 137-138.

"George's Mother," by Stephen Crane: 179-180.
Goals: human, of alcoholic, 201-209, 241, 307-308, 342; personal, of alcoholic, 201-209, 241, 307-311.
Government: Federal, of Canada, and restriction on tranquillizers, 23.
Grace: gift of, 341-343; as loss of desire to drink, 341.
Grandiosity: in idealistic alcoholic, 163.
"Grapevine, The": A.A. journal, 142.
Great Britain: and drug addiction, 35-36.
Greece: ancient, drinking in, 184.
Gregg, Milton F.: v.
Griffin, J. D. M.: v; 116.
Growth, personal: nature of, 47-48; sobriety as, 97-99, 102-103; and "becoming well," 115-116; the basic issue, 143-147; in women alcoholics, 270-272.
Guilt: alcoholic's feeling of, 67-69, 71, 95; in women alcoholics, 257-258.

Haggard, H. W., and Jellinek, E. M.: "Alcohol Explored," 79n.
Harbour Light Clinic: v.
Harris, Sara, and Murtagh, John M.: "Who Live In Shadow," 35, 59.
Health, physical: of addict, 53-55; breakdown of, 70.
Herodotus: on drinking.
Heroin: as addicting depressant, 6-7; in initial addiction, 7-12.
Hillil, Rabbi: teaching of, 135.
Honesty: drastic, in recovery, 170.
Horace (Quintus Horatius Flaccus): philosophy of, 117.
Huxley, Aldous Leonard: "Doors of Perception," 4.
Hypnotics: addiction to, 19-24.

Idealism: in alcoholics, 84-87, 162-163.
Ideals: of sobriety, 210-225.
Identification: in sobriety, 211-214.
Imagination: and sobriety, 198-209, 221-223, 309-311.

Imitation: free, and empathy, 32-33; imposed, and addiction, 32-33; imposed, in alcoholism, 181-183, 243; imposed, as aid to recovery, 192-196; free, in recovery, 241-243; transitional, 290, 292; conscious, 293.

Immaturity: emotional, of alcoholics, 136-137; in dependent alcoholic, 161.

Impulse: and action in sobriety, 218-219.

Impulsiveness: in alcoholics, 87-88, 165-166, 285-289.

Indians: and mescaline, 4; and alcohol, 61.

Insecurity: alcoholic's feeling of, 83-84.

Insight: of alcoholics, 97-108; in surrender, 109-120, 146-147; from, to action, 240-282.

Intolerance: in alcoholics, 88, 103-104, 219-220.

Intoxication: as early-stage addiction, 44, 229.

Isbell, Harris: v; 25, 28.

Islam: and A.A., 135.

James, William: v; and fallacy of wishful thinking, 104; "Varieties of Religious Experience," 136.

Jellinek, E. M.: v; on drinking away symptoms of drinking, 69, 79n; "Alcohol Addiction And Chronic Alcoholism," 79n; and H. W. Haggard, "Alcohol Explored," 79n; "doodle" of, 155n.

Johnson, Samuel: on drinking, 65.

Jonson, Ben: "To Celia," 185.

Judaism: and A.A., 135.

Jung, Carl Gustav: 269; and A.A., 137-138.

Kefauver Report: on tranquillizers, 21.

Knox, John: and A.A., 141.

Lamb, Charles: as alcoholic, 104.

Lindesmith, A. R.: "Opiate Addiction," 26.

Line, William: v.

"Little dictator": in alcoholics, 90-93, 109.

Lolli, Giorgio: v; on women alcoholics, 256-257, 260, 263.

Loneliness: of alcoholic, 71, 82, 159-160.

"Lost Weekend": movie, 94.

Love: in sobriety, 240, 248-250, 262-267, 333.

"Love's Philosophy," by Percy Bysshe Shelley: 185-186.

LSD: 3-4.

Luther, Martin: and A.A., 141.

Macmurray, John: v.

Man: nature of, 1.

Marihuana: derivation and effects of, 5-6.

Marriage: and alcoholic, 101-102.

Maurer, David, and Vogel, Victor H.: "Narcotics And Narcotic Addiction," 35, 58n.

McCarthy, R. G. (ed.): "Drinking And Intoxication," 59n.

Mead, George: and time, 45.

Medicine: inadequate to cure addiction, 49; in treatment, 55, 223; in early treatment, 327-328.

Meprobramate: addiction to, 23.

Mercer Clinic: v.

Mescaline: 3-4.

Metapon: as addicting depressant, 6-7.

Methadone: as addicting depressant, 6-7; in withdrawal, 13.

Mimico Clinic: v.

Miracle: of A.A., 320-339.

Moderation: impossible to alcoholic, 65.

Money: and the alcoholic, 242-244, 250.

Morphine: as addicting depressant, 6-7; in initial addiction, 10-12.

Mother-image: in alcoholic, 101-102.

Murtagh, John M., and Harris, Sara: "Who Live In Shadow" 35, 59n.

"Narcotics And Narcotic Addiction," by David W. Maurer and Victor H. Vogel: 35, 58n.

Narcotics Anonymous: 34-35.

Nembutal: in initial addiction, 9-10, 21.

Newton, Isaac: and science, 45.

Nyswander, Marie: v; "The Drug Addict As A Patient," 24-26, 58n.

Obsession: in alcoholics, 166-167, 176.

Omar Khayyam: philosophy of, 117.

"Opiate Addiction," by A. R. Lindesmith, 26, 58n.

Opium: and derivatives, as addicting depressants, 6-7; in initial addiction, 10-11.

Over-idealization: in alcoholics, 297-298; and resentment, 298.

Pain: as inducement to addiction, 25-29.

Pantopon: as addicting depressant, 6-7.

Paraldehyde: in withdrawal, 11; addiction to, 19-20.

Paranoia: and stimulants, 3-4; in alcoholic, 69-71; and sensitiveness, 84; in resigned drinking, 159; in sensitive alcoholic, 161-162.

Paregoric: addiction to, 6; in initial addiction, 11.

Paul, Saint: and A.A., 141.

Peace: in sobriety, 344-351; as acceptance, 347.

Personableness: in sobriety, 211-214.

"Pill people," the: 19-24.

Pity: alcoholic's search for, 85-87.

Plato: and sophrosyne, 1; and principle of action, 45; and A.A., 140.

Poe, Edgar Allen: as alcoholic, 104.

Positiveness: in recovery, 221-223.

Pratt, David: v.

Pride: false, in alcoholic, 94-96, 100-101, 157.

Promazine: as addicting tranquillizer, 21.

Provincial Hospital, Campbellton, N.B.: v.

Psychology: inadequate to cure addiction, 49; in treatment, 55-56.

Quarterly Journal Of Studies On Alcohol: 35, 59n.

Reason: and impulse, 286-289.

Recovery: true meaning of, 48; as personal freedom, 50-53; personal, under A.A., 123-124.

Rehabilitation, shift to, 37-42; decision for, 72.

Relapse: into narcotic addiction, 14-17; and mental attitude, 37; treatment of, 39-40; through fear, 41.

Religion: and sobriety, 48, 284; in recovery, 52-54, 328-332; and A.A., 125-129; science, and A.A., 133-142.

Resentment: in alcoholic, 95.

Reserpine: as addicting tranquillizer, 21.

Resistance: in sobriety, 211-214; making use of, 289-294; to recovery, 289; index of, 290-291; genuine, 300-306.

Respect: for self and others, 98-99.

Sartre, Jean Paul: philosophy of, 117.

Schopenhauer, Arthur: philosophy of, 117.

Science: religion, and A.A., 133-142; inadequacy of, for alcoholic, 171; natural, overreaching by, 286; limitations of, 306-315; and action, 316-320.

Seconal: in initial addiction, 9, 21.

Sedatives: and ataraxia, 2; addiction to, 19-24.

Self-denial: inimical to recovery, 114.

Sensitiveness: of alcoholic, 84, 161-162, 295; physical, in alcoholic, 153.

Service: to others, in recovery, 145-146.

Sex: as inducement to addiction, 25-29.

Shelley, Percy Bysshe: "Love's Philosophy," 185-186.

Single - mindedness: in sobriety, 219-221.

Sobriety: preference for, 28-29, 38; and empathy, 31-32; fear of, 41; as personal freedom, 50-51; desire for, 51-53, 56; and helping others, 145-146; reasons for, 151-168; search for creative, 169-196; as adventure, 186 - 190; and imagination, 198-209; ideals of, 210-223; across 12 years, 226-239; as life, 226-227; as paramount objective, 237; programme of, 272-286, 283; initial, 273, 275 - 276; learning, 273 - 274, 276-279; accepting, 274, 279-280; creative, 274-275, 280-281; pleasurable, 275, 281-282; and fear of the foreign, 299; as a lifetime job, 300; as adventure, 340-359.

Sociology: inadequate to cure addiction, 49.

Socrates: and self-knowledge, 80; and A.A., 140.

Sodium amytal: in initial addiction, 9-11.

Sophrosyne: and "cool", 1; three sources of, 2.

Spinoza, Benedictus de: and A.A., 141.

Steps: twelve, of A.A., 122-129.

Stimulants: varieties and effects of, 3-5.

Stoics: and ataraxia, 2; and A.A., 140.

Suicide: alcoholism as path to, 71-72, 77.

Surrender: and the follow-up, 109-120; to life, not to abstinence, 114; as personal act, 116-117; and A.A., 325.

Suttie, Ian: v; and "disorder of social disposition," 296.

Taboo: of tenderness, 290, 292, 295.

Theory: allied to action in sobriety, 316.

Thirst, personal: in alcoholic, 26; as means to recovery, 51-53, 250-251, 331-334; in alcoholism, 170-183; as imitation, 192; struggle to satisfy, 340.

Thomas Aquinas, Saint: and A.A., 141.

Tiebout, Harry: v; and the "positive phase," 111-112, 117; and surrender, 123.

Time: addict's indifference to, 45, 295-296.

"To Celia," by Ben Jonson: 185.

Traditions: twelve, of A.A., 131-132.

Tranquillizers: and ataraxia, 2; addiction to, 19-24.

Treatment: personal, of addicts, 53-58.

Tuinal: in initial addiction, 9.

Vogel, Victor H., and Maurer, David W.: "Narcotics and Narcotic Addiction," 35, 58n.

"Who Live In Shadow," by John M. Murtagh and Sara Harris: 35, 59n.

Wikler, A.: v; on opium addiction, 25.

Will power: in alcoholic, 69, 157-158, 318-320; as "little dictator," 90-93; failure of, 96, 221, 234; myth of, 106-108.

Winchell, Walter: on A.A., 334.

Wishful thinking: in alcoholics, 89, 167, 221, 255; tragic lesson of, 104-105; destruction of, 115-116.

Withdrawal: of stimulants, 5; first symptoms in stages of, 12; acute and chronic, 12-13; symptoms after addiction established, 14; the acute stage of, 18-19; the chronic stage, 19; from barbiturates and tranquillizers, 20-24; as "cold turkey," 23-24; long-term, 25.

Wolfe, Thomas: "You Can't Go Home Again," 199.

Women: as alcoholics, 253-272.

Wonder: in sobriety, 254-259.

Wordsworth, William: and recollection, 199.

Yale Center of Alcohol Studies: v; 59n.

"You Can't Go Home Again," by Thomas Wolfe: 199.